IMMUNOLOGY

HERMAN N. EISEN, M.D.

Professor of Immunology, Massachusetts Institute of Technology, Cambridge, Massachusetts; formerly Professor and Head, Department of Microbiology, Washington University School of Medicine, St. Louis, Missouri

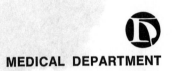

MEDICAL DEPARTMENT

*Harper & Row, Publishers
Hagerstown, Maryland
New York, Evanston, San Francisco, London*

immunology

AN INTRODUCTION TO MOLECULAR AND CELLULAR PRINCIPLES OF THE IMMUNE RESPONSES

IMMUNOLOGY   An Introduction to Molecular and Cellular Principles of the Immune Responses. Reprinted from Davis, Dulbecco, Eisen, Ginsberg, and Wood's MICRO-BIOLOGY, Second Edition, copyright © 1974 by Harper & Row, Publishers, Inc.

Standard Book Number: 06-140782-8

Library of Congress Catalog Card Number: 72-12233

CONTENTS

PREFACE

The immunology section of MICROBIOLOGY by Davis, Dulbecco, Eisen, Ginsberg, and Wood is reprinted here to make it available to those interested in just this part of the book. The numbering of pages and chapters has been left intact, but a new separate index has been prepared.

The special need for such a volume is suggested by the peculiar nature of immunology at this time. When this science took root, almost a century ago, it attracted wide attention among both the general public and the biomedical community because of the promise it offered for relief from epidemic infectious diseases. This promise was fulfilled beyond almost all expectation, and interest in the subject then lagged, although over the ensuing decades a small coterie continued to work in the field, fascinated by the fundamental biological problems raised by the exquisite specificity and diversity of immune responses. In the past 10–15 years, immunology has undergone another flowering, this time based on both its appeal as a fundamental biological science and its changing importance in clinical medicine, where it is contributing a rapidly growing number of diagnostic procedures and reagents, providing tools and concepts for probing mechanisms of diverse diseases, and raising the possibility that its contributions to the control of cancer may approach its earlier successes in controlling diseases of bacterial and viral origin.

These multiple sources of appeal have led to separate courses in immunology in many undergraduate, graduate, and medical school curricula, and I hope that this introductory text may be useful to them. Moreover, for established biologists and medical practitioners this volume may help satisfy a need for the kind of self-instruction that could be helpful in approaching the current flood in immunologic literature—estimated at about 7000 papers in 800 journals this year.

Much of this explosive growth derives from a change in the balance of scientific trade. Until recently, immunology imported more technics and concepts from related disciplines than it exported. This negative balance is being rapidly redressed: there is now hardly a field of biology or medicine in which antibodies are not useful as analytical or diagnostic reagents, and concepts stemming from clonal selection, the immense polymorphism of histocompatibility antigens at cell surfaces, the one cell–one antibody rule, the two genes–one chain hypothesis, and cell–cell cooperation in regulating the activities of antibody secreting cells are just beginning to have broad impact on the study of differentiation and many other areas.

For the satisfactions of writing about a rapidly expanding field one has to be prepared for early obsolescence and for more than the usual frequency of errors. Help in postponing the former and minimizing the latter has been generously provided by several colleagues to whom I am much indebted for careful review of various chapters: Fred Karush (Ch. 15), Lisa A. Steiner (Ch. 16), Joseph M. Davie (Ch. 17), Manfred M. Mayer and Steven Kinsky (Ch. 18), K. Frank Austen (Ch. 19), Barry R. Bloom (Ch. 20), Elvin A. Kabat and Ralph J. Graff (Ch. 21). Laura K. Bailey provided an unusually critical and valuable reading of the entire manuscript in proof. Finally, I am deeply grateful to Bernard D. Davis for many editorial contributions. In the end, of course, responsibility for all errors of fact or judgment are mine alone.

HNE

IMMUNOLOGY

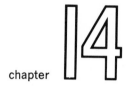

chapter 14

INTRODUCTION TO IMMUNE RESPONSES

Immune responses are remarkably versatile adaptive processes in which animals form specifically reactive proteins and cells in response to an immense variety of organic molecules and macromolecules. This ability seems to have been acquired relatively late in evolution since these responses are encountered only in vertebrates, for whose survival they are of vast importance: they constitute the principal means of defense not only against infection by pathogenic microorganisms and viruses but probably also against host cells that undergo transformation into cancer cells.

THE ORIGINS OF IMMUNOLOGY

From almost the earliest written observations of mankind it seems to have been suspected that persons who recover from certain diseases become incapable of suffering the same disease again: they become immune. Thucydides, for example, pointed out 2500 years ago, in a remarkable description of an epidemic in Athens (of what might have been typhus fever or plague), that fear of contagion led to neglect of the sick and dying, but whatever attention they received was "tended by the pitying care of those who had recovered, because they . . . were themselves free of apprehension. For no one was ever attacked a second time, or with a fatal result." This awareness led to deliberate attempts, beginning in the Middle Ages, to induce immunity by inoculating well persons with material scraped from skin lesions of persons suffering from smallpox. The procedure was hazardous, but in the late eighteenth century a safe, related procedure was established by the English physician Jenner.

Jenner shared the widely held impression that those individuals who had had cowpox (a benign disease acquired from cows infected with what seemed to be a mild form of smallpox) were spared in subsequent smallpox epidemics. To test this belief he inoculated a boy with pus from a lesion of a dairymaid who had cowpox; some weeks later reinoculation with infectious pus, from a patient in the active stage of smallpox, failed to cause illness. Repetition of the experiment many times led to Jenner's classic report, followed by widespread adoption of this procedure and confirmation of his conclusion that **vaccination** (L. *vacca* = cow) leads to immunity against smallpox.

It is remarkable that Jenner's work was not extended until nearly 100 years later, when a fortuitous observation led Pasteur to recognize and exploit the general principles underlying vaccination. While studying chicken cholera Pasteur happened to use an old culture of the causative agent (*Pasteurella aviseptica*) to inoculate some chickens, who failed to become ill. When the same animals were reinoculated with a fresh culture, which was known to be virulent, they again failed to become ill. The finding that aged cultures lose virulence but retain the capacity to induce immunity against cholera may have prompted Pasteur's epigram that "chance favors only the prepared mind." His observations were soon applied to many other infectious diseases.

A variety of procedures have been used to destroy the viability or attenuate the virulence of pathogenic organisms for purposes of vaccination; examples are aging of cultures or passing the microorganisms through "unnatural hosts" (e.g., the agent of rabies through the rabbit). The latter effect provides a plausible explanation for Jenner's earlier success: passage of smallpox virus through cows had probably selected for a variant virus that multiplied unusually well in cows but poorly in humans, while retaining ability to induce immunity against the virus that is virulent in man.

Induction of immunity to infectious diseases does not always require inoculation of the causative microorganism. Following the demonstration of a powerful toxin in culture filtrates of diphtheria bacilli in 1888, von Behring showed that nonlethal doses of the bacteria-free filtrates could induce immunity to diphtheria. These results were then generalized when Ehrlich and Calmette similarly established immunity to toxins of nonmicrobial origin, e.g., snake venoms and ricin from castor beans.

The basis for these immune responses was revealed in 1890, when von Behring and Kitasato demonstrated that induced immunity to tetanus was due to the appearance in the serum of a capacity to neutralize the toxin; this activity was so stable it could be transferred to normal animals by infusions of blood or serum. Moreover, Ehrlich showed that protection against the toxic effects of ricin on red cells in vitro involved the combination of specifically reactive components of the sera with the toxin; a similar combination presumably accounted for the effects of immune sera on infectious agents. These observations opened the way to analyses of substances responsible for immunity and to the practical treatment of many infectious diseases by infusions of serum from immune animals.

Within the ensuing 10 years most of the now known serological* reactions were discovered. For example:

1) **Bacteriolysis:** Cholera vibrio disintegrated when incubated with serum from animals that had previously been inoculated with this organism (Pfeiffer and Issaeff, 1894).

2) **Precipitation:** Cell-free culture filtrates of plague bacilli formed a precipitate on being added to serum from animals previously inoculated with cultures of plague bacilli (Kraus, 1897).

3) **Agglutination:** Bacterial cells suspended in serum from an animal previously injected with these bacteria underwent clumping (Gruber and Durham, 1898).

These reactions were all specific: the immune serum reacted only with the substance inoculated for induction of the immune response, or, as we shall see later, with substances of similar chemical structure. By about 1900 it

was realized that immune responses can also be elicited by nontoxic agents, such as proteins of milk or egg white injected into rabbits.

DEFINITIONS

The inoculated agents, and the substances whose appearance in serum they evoked, were called antigens (Ags) and antibodies (Abs), respectively.

An **antigen** has two properties: **immunogenicity,**† i.e., the capacity to stimulate the formation of the corresponding Abs; and the **ability to react** specifically with these Abs. The distinction is important, because substances known as **haptens** (described more fully below) are not immunogenic but react specifically with the appropriate Abs. "Specific" means here that the Ag will react in a highly selective fashion with the corresponding Ab and not with a multitude of other Abs evoked by other Ags.

The term **antibody** refers to the proteins that are formed in response to an Ag and react specifically with that Ag. All Abs belong to a special group of serum proteins, the **immunoglobulins,** whose properties will be considered in Chapter 16.

Though the definition states that Abs are formed in response to Ag, sera may contain immunoglobulins that react specifically with certain Ags to which the individuals concerned have had no **known** exposure. These immunoglobulins are called **natural antibodies.** When present in serum they are usually in low titer, but they may exercise a significant role in conferring resistance to certain infections. It is not clear whether natural Abs are formed without an immunogenic stimulus or in response to unknown exposure to naturally occurring Ags, e.g., in inapparent infections or in food.

In contrast to the restricted group of proteins that possess Ab activity, an enormous variety of macromolecules can behave as Ags —virtually all proteins, many polysaccharides, nucleoproteins, lipoproteins, numerous synthetic polypeptides, and many small mole-

---

* The specific reactions of immune sera are generally referred to as serological reactions.

† The term immunogen is often used for the substance that stimulates the formation of the corresponding Abs.

cules if they are suitably linked to proteins or to synthetic polypeptides.

It is important to recognize the operational nature of the definition of Ag. For example, when rabbit serum albumin (RSA) is isolated from a rabbit and then injected back into the same animal, Abs specific for RSA are **not** formed. Yet the same preparation of RSA injected into virtually any other species of vertebrate may evoke copious amounts of anti-RSA Abs. Moreover, the formation of these Abs depends not only on the injection of RSA into an appropriate species, but also on the other conditions employed: viz., the quantity of RSA injected and the route and frequency of injection. It is clear, therefore, that **immunogenicity is not an inherent property of a macromolecule,** as is, for example, its molecular weight or absorption spectrum; immunogenicity is operationally dependent on the biological system and conditions employed. One cardinal condition is that the putative immunogen be somehow recognized as alien (i.e., not self) by the responding organism.

ANTIGENIC DETERMINANTS

The reaction between an Ag and the corresponding Ab in an immune serum involves an actual combination of the two. We shall consider in Chapter 15 the nature of this combination, which is the fundamental reaction common to most immunological phenomena. For the present, however, it is useful to distinguish between the Ag molecule as a whole and its **antigenic determinants,** i.e., those restricted portions of the Ag molecule that determine the specificity of Ab-Ag reactions.

Attempts to evaluate the size and conformation of an antigenic determinant involve indirect approximations (Ch. 16, Size of active sites of antibodies) which indicate that these determinants are much smaller than a typical macromolecule, being equivalent in volume to, perhaps, five or six amino acid residues.

The great diversity of antigenic substances was first emphasized by Obermayer and Pick (1903), who attached NO_2 groups to rabbit serum proteins, injected these proteins into rabbits, and found that the serum obtained reacted with the nitrated proteins of rabbit, horse, or chicken sera, but not with the corresponding unmodified proteins. They inferred, therefore, that the Abs formed were capable of specifically recognizing the nitro groups or other uniquely altered structures in the nitrated proteins.

Such responses to chemically defined substituents of modified proteins were vigorously developed by Landsteiner to explore the chemical basis of antigenic specificity. Diazonium salts were used to couple a wide variety of aromatic amines to proteins, as indicated by the representative reactions in Figure 14-1.

Rabbits injected with p-azobenzenearsonate globulin form Abs that react with this protein and with other proteins containing p-azobenzenearsonate substitutuents, but not with the latter proteins in unsubstituted form. Landsteiner and Lampl showed in 1920 that p-aminobenzenearsonate alone can competitively inhibit the reaction with p-azobenzenearsonate proteins, whereas other aromatic amines (with a few important exceptions) do not.

Though benzenearsonate combines in a highly selective manner with the Abs formed

Fig. 14-1. Attachment of an aromatic amine to a protein via azo linkage (-N=N-) formed by reaction with diazonium ions.

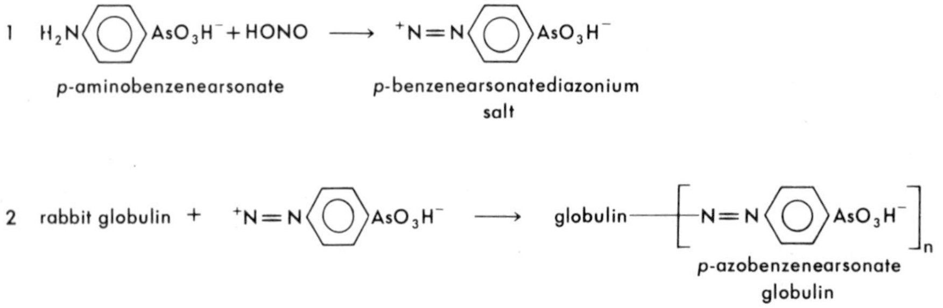

1 H_2N〈◯〉AsO_3H^- + HONO ⟶ $^+N=N$〈◯〉AsO_3H^-

   p-aminobenzenearsonate   p-benzenearsonatediazonium
                                            salt

2 rabbit globulin + $^+N=N$〈◯〉AsO_3H^- ⟶ globulin—$\left[N=N 〈◯〉 AsO_3H^- \right]_n$

                                            p-azobenzenearsonate
                                            globulin

in response to injection of the corresponding azoprotein (as further described in Ch. 15), injections of benzenearsonate itself do not evoke the formation of Abs. Substances of this type are defined as **haptens: they are not immunogenic but they react selectively with Abs of the appropriate specificity.** In the example cited the hapten is a small molecule; it should be noted that the definition does not say anything about molecular weight; even some macromolecules can function as haptens.

While the formal difference between Ag and hapten is clear, in practice it may be difficult to decide whether a substance is weakly immunogenic or completely non-immunogenic. Generally, however, small molecules (MW <1000) are not immunogenic, unless covalently linked to proteins in vitro or in vivo (Fig. 14-2; for other examples see Ch. 17, Contact skin sensitivity). Certain macromolecules also become immunogenic only when bound by proteins: however, covalent bonds are unnecessary here, probably because the cumulative effect of many weak noncovalent ones between large interacting molecules (e.g., between DNA and protein) can establish stable (nondissociating) complexes.

The diazo reaction introduces azo groups as substituents in tyrosine, tryptophan, histidine, and lysine residues (Fig. 14-2). Other methods for coupling haptens to proteins will be referred to in subsequent chapters; some are even more useful because they provide a more stable linkage and substitute fewer kinds of amino acid residues.

Proteins with substituents covalently linked to their side chains are referred to as **conjugated proteins;** and the substituents, sometimes including the amino acid residues to which they are linked (when these are known), are called **haptenic groups.** These distinctions are shown in Figure 14-3. While a haptenic group is thus part of an antigenic determinant, it is not yet clear just how much of the complete antigenic determinant it represents.

CELLULAR IMMUNITY

Coincident with early studies on the role of serum Abs, Metchnikoff's observation of phagocytosis suggested that ingestion and destruction of microbes by polymorphonuclear leukocytes and macrophages are responsible for resistance to most infectious agents. The resulting controversy between advocates of Abs and of cells was reconciled by the finding, in 1903, that coating of particles with Abs (opsonins; Gr., "to prepare food") increased their susceptibility to phagocytosis.

Fig. 14-2. Some azo substituents on tyrosine, lysine, and histidine residues of a representative azoprotein.

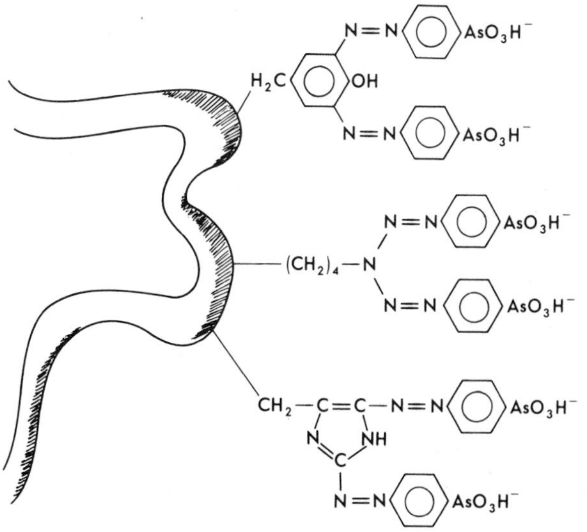

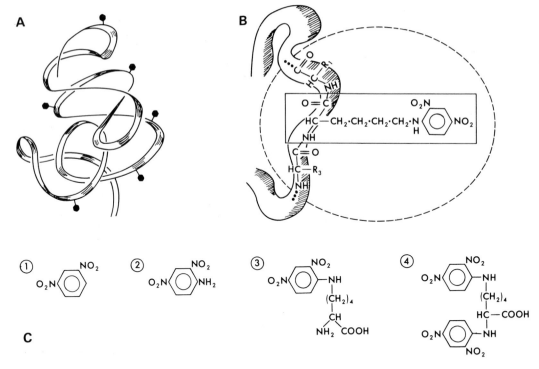

Fig. 14-3. Distinctions between conjugated proteins, antigenic determinants, haptenic groups, and haptens.

A. Conjugated protein with substituents represented as solid hexagons.

B. A representative **haptenic group:** a 2,4-dinitrophenyl (Dnp) group substituted in the ε-NH₂ group of a lysine residue. The haptenic group is outlined by solid line, whereas the **antigenic determinant** might be visualized as the area outlined by the broken line. Amino acid residues contributing to the antigenic determinant need not be the nearest covalently linked neighbors of the ε-Dnp-lysine residue, as shown; they could be parts of distant segments of the polypeptide chain looped back to come into contiguity with the Dnp-lysyl residue.

C. Some **haptens** that correspond to the haptenic group in **B.** 1) m-dinitrobenzene; 2) 2,4-dinitroaniline; 3) ε-Dnp-lysine; 4) α,ε-bis-Dnp-lysine. With respect to antibodies specific for the Dnp group, haptens 1, 2, and 3 are univalent haptens (one combining group per molecule), and hapten 4 is bivalent.

However, the Ab-cell controversy reappeared in different form in the 1920s as a result of studies of allergy (hypersensitivity)—a state induced by an Ag, in which a subsequent response to the Ag causes inflammation or even acute shock and death. Though many allergic states can be transferred by the Abs in serum, Landsteiner and Chase showed (1942) that transfer of others can be accomplished only with living leukocytes (later shown to be lymphocytes).

Various other immune responses were subsequently also found to be mediated by living lymphocytes rather than by Ab molecules, e.g., immunity to tubercle bacilli and many other infectious agents, the capacity for accelerated rejection of allografts (i.e., grafted cells from genetically different individuals of the same species), and resistance to many experimental cancers. In all these **cell-mediated immune reactions** the Ag apparently combines specifically with particular lymphocytes. Thus mediators of immune responses can be either freely diffusible Ab molecules **(humoral immunity)** or specifically reactive lymphocytes **(cell-mediated immunity):** whether the Ag-binding receptors on these cells are surface immunoglobulins (cell-bound Abs) or a different type of molecule is still uncertain.

IMMUNOLOGY AND IMMUNITY

Though immune responses were originally of interest because of their role in **immunity** to infection, it has long been evident that these responses can be induced against an almost limitless variety of substances, of which microbial Ags are a small minority: hence immunity represents only a limited facet of a more general adaptive response. Coincident with this expanded view of immunology, diverse pathological effects have been traced to immune responses to noninfectious and nontoxic Ags (e.g., allografts, red blood cells, pollens, drugs), and even to an individual's own constitutents (autoimmunity); hence immunological considerations have now come to pervade almost all segments of modern medicine. In addition, interest has grown in 1) the Ab-Ag reaction as a model for specific noncovalent interactions in general (e.g., those between viruses and their host cell membranes, or those causing cell aggregation in such phenomena as fertilization and morpho-

genesis); 2) Ab formation as a model for cellular differentiation; and 3) the use of Ab molecules as highly specific and sensitive analytical reagents for exploring the structure of complex macromolecules (e.g., enzymes, blood group glycopeptides, cell surface macromolecules) and for measuring trace amounts of many physiologically important substances (e.g., hormones, vasoactive peptides, cyclic AMP, prostaglandins).

While there is thus much more to immunology than immunity in the literal sense, the historical role of infectious diseases has left an indelible imprint on nomenclature, which is not always appropriate: for example, induction of Ab formation and of specific cellular responses is referred to as immunization even when infectious agents are not involved. **Vaccination** is the term reserved for immunization in which a suspension of infec-

TABLE 14-1. Comparison of Enzymes and Antibodies

Property	Enzymes	Antibodies
Phylogenetic distribution	Ubiquitous; made by all cells	A late evolutionary acquisition; made only in vertebrates (and in certain cells of the lymphatic system)
Structure	Proteins with variable chemical and physical properties; an enzyme of a given specificity and from any particular organism is homogeneous; many have been crystallized	A group of closely related proteins having a common multichain structure with the chains held together by —SS— bonds. Molecules of a given specificity are heterogeneous in structure and function
Constitutive	Yes	"Natural" antibodies?
Inducible	Often	Yes
Function	Specific reversible binding of ligands* with breaking and forming covalent bonds	Specific reversible binding of ligands* without breaking or forming covalent bonds
Reaction with ligands*	Wide range of affinities; populations of enzyme molecules of a given specificity are uniform in affinity for their ligand	Wide range of affinities; but populations of antibody molecules of the same specificity are usually heterogeneous in affinity for their ligand
Affinity	Usually measured kinetically	Usually measured with reactants at equilibrium (because the reactions are so fast)
Number of specific ligand-binding sites per molecule	Different in different enzymes, depending on number of polypeptide chains per molecule; usually one site per chain	2 per molecule of the most prevalent type (MW ∼ 150,000); each site is formed by a pair of chains (a light plus a heavy chain)
Inducers	Primarily small molecules	Usually macromolecules, especially proteins and conjugated proteins

* Ligand = substrate or coenzyme in case of enzymes, and antigen or hapten in case of antibodies.

tious agents (or some part of them), called a **vaccine,** is given to establish resistance to an infectious disease.

In the chapters that follow we shall consider the molecular before the cellular aspects of immune responses: not only are structure and functions of Ab molecules better understood than those of the relevant cells, but the properties of Abs and their interactions with Ags provide the conceptual framework in which immune cellular reactions are viewed.

It would be logical to consider first the structure of Abs and then, perhaps, how these molecules are made and function. However, the present view of Ab structure is extensively based on the use of Ab molecules themselves as analytical reagents. We shall therefore begin with a consideration of specific Ab-Ag reactions. Some properties that will be emphasized are summarized in Table 14-1, where Abs are compared with enzymes.

SELECTED REFERENCES

Books and Review Articles

AMOS, B. (ed.). *Progress in Immunology.* Proceedings of the First International Congress of Immunology. Academic Press, New York, 1971.

ARRHENIUS, S. *Immunochemistry.* Macmillan, New York, 1907.

BURNET, F. M. *Cellular Immunology.* Cambridge Univ. Press, London, 1970.

EHRLICH, P. *Studies in Immunity.* Wiley, New York, 1910.

HEIDELBERGER, M. *Lectures in Immunochemistry.* Academic Press, New York, 1956.

HAUROWITZ, S. *Immunochemistry and the Biosynthesis of Antibodies.* Interscience Publishers, New York, 1968.

LANDSTEINER, K. *The Specificity of Serological Reactions,* rev. ed. Harvard Univ. Press, Cambridge, Mass., 1945; reprinted by Dover Publications, New York, 1962 (paperback).

TOPLEY, W. W. C., and WILSON, G. S. *The Principles of Bacteriology and Immunity,* 2nd ed. Williams & Wilkins, Baltimore, 1936.

ZINSSER, H., ENDERS, J. F., and FOTHERGILL, L. D. *Immunity: Principles and Applications in Medicine and Public Health,* 5th ed. Macmillan, New York, 1939.

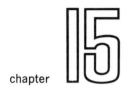

chapter 15

ANTIBODY-ANTIGEN REACTIONS

The combination of antibody (Ab) with antigen (Ag) underlies most immunological phenomena. However, most Ags in wide use are macromolecules, especially proteins, and even when their covalent structure is completely established we hardly ever know the identity and conformation of their functional groups or even the number and variety per molecule. We shall therefore first consider specific Ab reactions with simple haptens, on which most of our understanding of the Ab-Ag reaction is based. Subsequently the more complicated reactions with macromolecular Ags will be taken up. Since the distinction between haptens and Ags, based on immunogenicity, is largely irrelevant for the present discussion (Ch. 14, Definitions), we shall frequently use the generic term **ligand** to include both.

REACTIONS WITH SIMPLE HAPTENS

Abs specific for simple haptens are usually obtained with immunogens prepared by attaching the hapten covalently to a protein. In addition, Abs formed in response to high molecular weight polysaccharides may react with small oligosaccharides corresponding to short sequences in the immunogen, e.g., the cellobiuronic acid of type 3 pneumococcus (below, Fig. 15-18). Since the Abs that react with haptens are easily isolated (Appendix, this chapter), the formation of specific Ab-ligand complexes can be examined in detail with relatively simple systems.

VALENCE AND AFFINITY OF ANTIBODIES

In the simplest reaction a small **univalent ligand,** with one combining group per molecule, binds reversibly to a specific site on the Ab. At low concentrations of unbound ligand only a small proportion of the Ab's combining sites are occupied by ligand molecules; and as the ligand concentration increases the number of occupied Ab sites rises until all are filled. At saturation the number of univalent ligand molecules bound per Ab molecule is the **antibody valence** (or n, see below).

If we assume that the binding sites on Ab molecules are equivalent and act independently of each other the **intrinsic binding reaction** can be represented as

$$S + L \underset{k'}{\overset{k}{\rightleftharpoons}} SL \qquad (1)$$

where S is a representative binding site on Ab, L is ligand, and k and k' are the rate constants for association and dissociation, respectively. The ratio of these rates (k/k') is the **intrinsic association constant** $K,$ which measures the tendency of site and ligand to form a stable complex; i.e., **K represents the intrinsic affinity of the representative Ab binding site** for the ligand, or

$$K = \frac{k}{k'} = \frac{[SL]}{[S][L]} \qquad (2)$$

the terms in brackets referring to the concentrations, at equilibrium, of the occupied Ab sites (SL), vacant Ab sites (S), and free (unbound) ligand molecules (L). If the total concentration of binding sites $(S + SL)$ and of ligand molecules $(L + SL)$ are known, a measurement at equilibrium of any one term on the right side of equation (2) can lead to the association constant. It is usually most convenient to measure the free ligand concen-

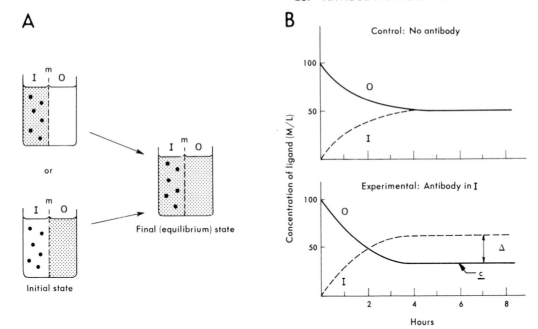

Fig. 15-1. Equilibrium dialysis. **A.** Small univalent haptens (small dots) can diffuse freely between the compartments (I, O), but Ab molecules (large dots) cannot. At equilibrium the greater concentration of hapten in I is due to binding by Ab. **B.** Change in hapten concentration with time. Equilibrium is reached in about 4 hours (the time varies with temperature, volumes of the compartments, nature and surface area of the membrane (m), etc.). In **B** the hapten was initially in compartment O; c is the concentration of free (unbound) hapten at equilbrium in I and O; Δ is the concentration of Ab-bound ligand in compartment I at equilibrium.

tration, and several methods are available to distinguish free (L) from bound (SL) ligand. The most generally applicable is equilibrium dialysis (below); it is also the most satisfactory method because it avoids perturbing the equilibrium, unlike some more rapid methods that physically separate free and Ab-bound ligands (e.g., precipitation of Ab with high salt concentration, below).*

EQUILIBRIUM DIALYSIS

The principles are shown in Figure 15-1. A solution containing Ab molecules specific for a simple haptenic group, such as 2,4-dinitrophenyl, is placed in a compartment (I, for

---

* Hapten inhibition of precipitation, described later in this chapter, is widely used to obtain relative values of association constants for a series of homologous haptens in relation to a reference hapten and a reference Ag. Other methods are also useful with special systems, e.g., ultracentrifugation, fluorescence quenching (see below).

"inside") which is separated by a membrane (m) from another compartment (O, for "outside") that contains a solution of an appropriate univalent ligand (e.g., 2,4-dinitroaniline; Ch. 14, Fig. 14-3). The membranes used are impermeable to Abs, but freely permeable to small molecules (MW <1000). If the concentration of ligand is measured periodically, it is observed to decline in O and to rise in I until equilibrium is reached; thereafter the concentrations in the two compartments remain unchanged. If compartment I had simply contained the solvent, or a protein that was incapable of binding, the ligand's concentration would ultimately become the same in both compartments. But if I contains Ab molecules that can bind dinitroaniline, the final (equilibrium) concentration of total ligand in I will exceed its concentration in O.† The difference represents

---

† Even without specific binding by Ab, charged ligands could be unevenly distributed across the membrane at equilibrium because of the net charge

ligand molecules bound to Ab molecules. Because the reaction is **readily reversible** the same final state is attained regardless of whether the Ab and ligand are placed initially in the same or in adjacent compartments (Fig. 15-1A).

By dividing the numerator [SL] and the denominator [S] by the Ab concentration, equation (2) may be expressed as:

$$K = \frac{r}{(n-r)c},$$ (3)

or, more conveniently, as:

$$\frac{r}{c} = Kn - Kr,$$ (4)

where, at equilibrium, r represents the number of ligand molecules bound per Ab molecule at c free concentration of ligand, and n is the maximum number of ligand molecules that can be bound per Ab molecule (i.e., the Ab valence). A set of values for r and c is obtained by examining a series of dialysis chambers at equilibrium, each with the same amount of Ab but a different amount of ligand. The derivation of equation (4) is outlined in the Appendix, this chapter.

Two features of equation (4) are notable. 1) A plot of r/c vs. r should give a straight line of slope $-K$, provided the original assumption was correct that all Ab sites are identical and independent. As we shall see, linearity or nonlinearity of this plot provides information on the uniformity of the ligand-binding sites in the sample of Ab molecules. 2) When the concentration of unbound ligand (c) becomes very large r/c approaches 0 and r approaches n; i.e., the number of ligand molecules bound per Ab molecule approaches the number of ligand-binding sites, or Ab valence.

Antibody Valence. Figure 15-2 shows representative data for the binding of univalent ligands by Abs of the most prevalent type (MW 150,000, IgG class; see Ch. 16). The limiting value for r is 2 as c approaches

infinity. That is, there are two binding sites per Ab molecule of this molecular weight. Bivalence of Abs has been repeatedly observed with many systems in which the ligands are small dialyzable molecules. Even in the more complex reactions with macromolecular Ags the same stoichiometry has been observed (Fig. 15-11).

Heterogeneity with Respect to Affinity. The relation between r/c and r is **not** linear for most Ab-ligand systems (Fig. 15-2, A–C). According to the assumptions made above, nonlinearity means that the Ab's binding sites are not uniform or not independent. However, bivalent Ab molecules can be cleaved by proteolytic enzymes into univalent fragments (Ch. 16), which exhibit similar nonlinearity in the reaction with their ligands. Hence the nonlinearity cannot be due to interactions between sites, e.g., to the modification of a vacant binding site by occupancy of the other site on the same molecule. Rather, as we shall see, several independent lines of evidence demonstrate that Ab molecules of any particular specificity are usually highly diversified with respect to affinity for the ligand.

However, occasional animals form Abs (particularly to certain Ags, such as polysaccharides of streptococcal cell walls and pneumococcal capsules) that have greatly restricted heterogeneity. In their uniform affinity for ligands these **homogeneous Abs** resemble enzymes and the immunoglobulins produced by plasma cell tumors (the neoplastic counterparts of the cells that normally synthesize Abs; see Ch. 16, Myeloma proteins; Fig. 15-2 D–F).

For an Ab-ligand pair with diverse binding constants (nonlinearity in r/c vs. r) it is useful to determine an average value, K_0, which is defined by the free ligand concentration required for occupancy of half the Ab-binding sites. Thus, substitution of $r = n/2$ in equation (4) leads to

$$K_0 = \frac{1}{c}.$$ (5)

K_0 is designated the **average intrinsic association constant;** it is a measure of **average affinity,** and is usually referred to simply as "the affinity." Its unit is the reciprocal of con-

---

on the protein. This inequality, or Donnan effect, is avoided by carrying out the dialysis in the presence of a sufficiently high salt concentration, e.g., 0.15 M NaCl. Donnan effects are irrelevant with uncharged ligands.

Fig. 15-2. Specific binding of ligands plotted according to equation (4). For all Ab-ligand systems **(A–E)** the extrapolation indicates two ligand-binding sites per Ab molecule (MW 150,000, IgG class; see Ch. 16). In **B** affinity is higher at 7.1° than at 25°. In **C** two purified anti-2,4-dinitrophenyl (anti-Dnp) Abs differ about 30-fold in affinity for dinitroaniline, and even larger variations occur (Ch. 17, Changes in affinity). In **E** the anti-Dnp protein was produced by a plasma cell tumor (Ch. 16, Multiple myeloma). Non-linearity, showing heterogeneity with respect to affinities of binding sites, is pronounced in **B** and **C**, but slight in **A**; linearity, showing uniformity of binding sites, is evident with the antipolysaccharide Abs **(D)**, the anti-Dnp myeloma protein **(E)**, and the enzyme muscle phosphorylase a, which has four binding sites per molecule (MW 495,000) for Amp **(F)**. [Data based on: **(A)** Eisen, H. N., and Karush, F., *J Am Chem Soc* 71:363 (1949); **(B)** Karush, F., *J Am Chem Soc* 79:3380 (1957); **(C)** Eisen, H. N., and Siskind, G., *Biochemistry* 3:996 (1964); **(D)** Pappenheimer, A. M., Redd, W. R., and Brown, R., *J Immunol* 100:1237 (1968); **(E)** Eisen, H. N., Little, J. R., Osterland, C. K., and Simms, E. S., *Cold Spring Harbor Symp Quant Biol* 32:75 (1967); **(F)** Madsen, N. B., and Cori, C. F., *J Biol Chem* 224:899 (1957).]

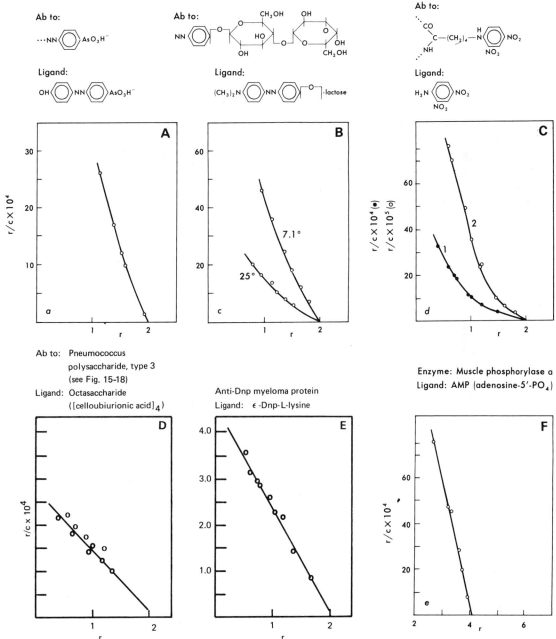

centration, i.e., liters mole^{-1} when c is in moles liter^{-1}. The higher the affinity of a given population of Ab molecules for ligand, the lower the concentration of free ligand need be for the binding sites to become occupied to any specified extent. (The analogy to the equilibrium constant for ionization reactions should be evident; by convention, however, the ionization constant is expressed as the dissociation constant [reciprocal of the association constant], which for the reaction $HA \rightleftharpoons H^+ + A^-$ is the H^+ concentration at which half of A binds a hydrogen ion.)

The heterogeneity of Abs with respect to affinity is often evaluated by the Sips distribution function,

which is similar to the normal distribution function commonly used in statistics. The Sips function leads to the explicit statement:

$$\log \frac{r}{n-r} = a \log K + a \log c \qquad (6)$$

where r, n, K, and c have the same meanings as before, and a is an index of the dispersion of equilibrium constants about the average constant, K_0. The term a is similar to the standard deviation in the more familiar normal distribution.

As is shown in Figure 15-3, a plot of $\log (r/n-r)$ vs. $\log c$ is indeed a straight line, and a, the index of heterogeneity with respect to affinity, is obtained as its slope. Values for a range from 1 to 0. When $a = 1.0$, all sites are identical with respect to K, and equation (6) is then equivalent to equations (3) and (4); the smaller the a value, the greater the degree of heterogeneity.

Some representative average association constants are shown in Table 15-1. With different conditions of immunization substantial differences are observed among Ab molecules of the same specificity (Ch. 16); for example, different populations of anti-Dnp antibodies differ as much as 100,000-fold in affinity for ε-Dnp-lysine.

Thus **the term antibody, which is used in the singular, is in most instances a collective noun referring to a population or set of molecules defined by the capacity to bind a given functional group.** With simple ligands it is relatively easy to specify the functional group and thereby the corresponding set of Ab molecules. For example, the set that binds lactose is the "antilactose antibody." With protein Ags, however, the functional groups (antigenic determinants) have only rarely been identified; but it is reasonable to assume that each of the groups on a protein also specifies a set of heterogeneous Ab molecules.

Fig. 15-3. Contrast between uniform binding of substrate by enzyme (AMP by phosphorylase) and heterogeneous binding of a ligand by Ab (dinitroaniline by anti-Dnp). Data are from Figure 15-2 and plotted according to equation (6). The slopes (a) are 1.0 for the enzyme-substrate pair and 0.5 for the Ab-ligand pair. (At $a = 0.5$ about 20% of the protein's binding sites fall outside the range $K_0/40$ to $40 K_0$.)

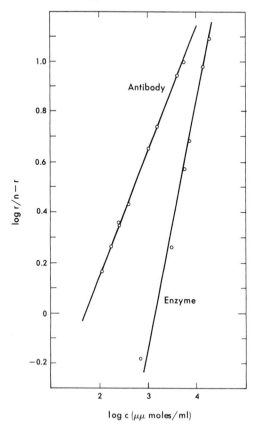

log c ($\mu\mu$ moles/ml)

EFFECTS OF TEMPERATURE, pH, IONIC STRENGTH; RATES OF REACTION

Because Abs are relatively stable proteins, their reactions can be studied over a wide range of conditions. The resulting changes in association constants provide some insight into the forces that stabilize the Ab-ligand complex. For example, the binding of ionic ligands, such as p-aminobenzoate by antibenzoate, decreases as pH is dropped from 7 to 4 and as salt concentration is raised from

TABLE 15-1. Average Intrinsic Association Constants for Representative Antibody-Ligand Interactions

Antibody specific for	Ligand	Average intrinsic association constants (K_0) in liters mole^{-1}
p-Azobenzenearsonate	OH⟨◯⟩NN⟨◯⟩AsO$_3$H$^-$	3.5×10^5
p-Azobenzoate	I⟨◯⟩COO$^-$	3.8×10^4
ε-2,4-Dinitrophenyl-lysyl	$^-$OOC(NH$_2$)CH—(CH$_2$)$_4$NH⟨◯⟩—NO$_2$ (NO$_2$)	1×10^7
p-Azophenyl-β-lactoside	(CH$_3$)$_2$N⟨◯⟩NN⟨◯⟩—O-lactose	1.6×10^5
Mono-Dnp-ribonuclease	Mono-Dnp-ribonuclease	1×10^6

Based on references given in Karush, F., *Adv Immunol* 2:1 (1962); Singer, S. J., in *The Proteins,* vol. 3, p. 269, Academic Press, N.Y., 1965; Eisen, H. N., and Pearce, J. H., *Annu Rev Microbiol* 16:101 (1962).

0.1 to 1.0 M NaCl. But similar changes do not affect the binding of nonionic ligands, such as 2,4-dinitroaniline by anti-Dnp Abs. This means that the COO$^-$ group of benzoate probably interacts with a positively charged group of the Ab combining site, but ionic interactions are not important for the binding of the neutral Dnp group.

Temperature variations have, broadly speaking, two kinds of effects. With some systems **increasing** temperature **decreases** the association constant; i.e., binding is exothermal. In others, association constants are unaltered between 4 and 40°. But no Ab–simple ligand systems have increasing affinity with increasing temperature. Nevertheless, the general practice of incubating mixtures of antisera and Ags at 37° is often helpful in speeding up some of the secondary reactions of Ab-Ag complexes, e.g., precipitation, agglutination, and complement fixation (see below and Ch. 18).

Thermodynamics. The formation of the Ab-ligand complex results in a change in free energy, ΔF, which is exponentially related to the average association constant by

$$\Delta F = RT \ln K_0, \tag{7}$$

where R is the gas constant (1.987 cal/mole-deg.), T the absolute temperature, and $\ln K_0$ the natural logarithm of the average intrinsic association constant. $\Delta F°$, the standard free energy change, is the gain or loss of free energy in calories, as 1 mole of Ab sites and 1 mole of free ligand combine to form 1 mole of bound ligand; when the units of K_0 are

liters per mole (i.e., reactant concentrations are in moles per liter) ΔF in equation (7) is $\Delta F°$.

$\Delta F°$ values for various Ab-hapten pairs range from about −6000 to −11,000 calories (per mole hapten bound), corresponding to association constants of 10^5 to 10^9 liters mole^{-1} at 30° (Table 15-1).

It is sometimes useful to determine whether the free energy change comes about from a change in heat content (enthalpy) or in the entropy of the system. This determination is based on

$$\Delta F° = \Delta H° - T\Delta S° \tag{8}$$

where $\Delta H°$ is the change in enthalpy (measured in calories), T is absolute temperature, and $\Delta S°$ is the entropy change. $\Delta H°$ is determined experimentally in sensitive calorimeters or by measuring the average intrinsic association constant (K_0) at two or more temperatures:

$$\Delta H° = \frac{R \ln \dfrac{K_2}{K_1}}{\dfrac{1}{T_1} - \dfrac{1}{T_2}}, \tag{9}$$

where K_1 and K_2 are average association constants (K_0) at temperatures T_1 and T_2. $\Delta H°$ values range from 0 (no change in affinity with temperature), in which case the driving force for complex formation is the $T\Delta S$ term of equation (8), to −30,000 cal/mole ligand bound, in which case the decrease in heat content drives the reaction. The formation of apolar or hydrophobic bonds is essentially athermal ($\Delta H° \cong 0$), whereas the formation of hydrogen bonds is exothermal ($\Delta H° \cong -1000$ cal/hydrogen bond).

Rates of Reaction. Abs combine with ligands so rapidly that rates can be measured only with special technics. In one approach ligand is added at extremely low concentration (e.g., 10^{-10} M). This slows the rate to where changes can be measured at ca. 5-min intervals, but unusually sensitive methods are then required for determining the changing, low ligand concentrations. One effective procedure exploits the finding that haptens, such as Dnp, can be coupled to bacteriophage, which remain infectious and can be counted by plaque technics at concentrations as low as 10^{-17} M (a virion is taken as equivalent to a single macromolecule). The rate of decreasing infectivity following addition of Abs to the haptenic group measures the forward (association) rate, and reappearance of infectivity after adding an excess of the simple hapten measures the backward (dissociation) rate. In a second approach Ab and hapten are present initially at concentrations that present no unusual analytical problems (10^{-4} to 10^{-5} M), but the resulting extremely rapid reaction can be followed only in special instruments for measuring changes at microsecond (10^{-6}) intervals.

The forward (association) reaction for binding small haptens is one of the fastest biochemical reactions known: the rate constant (k in equations 1 and 2) is only about 10 times less than the theoretical limit of 10^9 liters/mole/second for diffusion-limited reactions. This implies that a high proportion of collisions between ligand and Ab are fruitful (i.e., they lead to specific binding), perhaps because of a "cage effect" of the water solvent, which holds collided ligand and Ab molecules together until the ligand slips into the protein's binding site. Forward rate constants for binding protein Ags are about 10 to 100 times lower than for small haptens.

Forward rate constants differ only slightly for Ab-hapten pairs that differ enormously in intrinsic affinity (Table 15-1); hence the differences in affinity are due almost entirely to wide variations in reverse (dissociation) rate constants. The activation energy of the forward reaction (measured by effects of temperature on association rate constants) is low, suggesting that the Ab's combining site is rigid. In contrast to enzymatic reactions, where binding of substrate is usually complicated by sequential conformational modifications of the enzyme, the combination of Ab and hapten appears to be a straightforward and uncomplicated bimolecular reaction.

Phage Neutralization as Assay for Antibody. The rate of neutralization of phage has been developed into perhaps the most sensitive general assay method for measuring Abs because, as is noted above, the infectivity of phage with covalently attached ligands can be blocked ("neutralized") by Abs to the attached ligand. The initial rate of neutralization is proportional to Ab concentration: it measures the forward (association) reaction which, as we have just emphasized, is essentially independent of the

Ab's affinity for the ligand. Because phage with a wide variety of attached ligands, including proteins, can remain infectious for bacteria, and can be measured at exceedingly low concentrations (ca. 10^{-17} M, above), the assays based on neutralization are widely applicable and extremely sensitive: for example, they have been used to measure Ab production by single cells (Ch. 17) and trace levels in serum of the Abs that cause human hypersensitivity to penicillin (Ch. 19; see Table 15-5, below). Unbound ligand competes with the ligand attached to phage and can inhibit the neutralization of phage infectivity caused by a standard amount of a standard antiserum to the attached ligand. From the extent of inhibition it is possible to measure trace amounts of unbound ligand in diverse biological fluids (serum, lymph, urine) following the same principle and with about the same sensitivity as in radioimmunoassays (e.g., see Fig. 15-33, below).

SPECIFICITY

Immune reactions are highly specific: a given population of Ab molecules will usually have different affinities for ligands whose structures differ only in the most minute detail. The basis for this discrimination lies in the forces responsible for the stability of the Ab-ligand complex. Insight into the nature of these forces has been acquired by comparing the binding of structurally related ligands.

The early classic studies by Landsteiner were elegant and illuminating. They were based on ability of antisera to a conjugated protein, such as sulfanilate-azoglobulin, to form specific insoluble complexes (precipitates) with other proteins conjugated with the same azo substituent, e.g., sulfanilate azoalbumin, but not with the albumin itself. Thus the reaction was specific for the sulfanilate azo group. The Abs' reactivity with diverse groups could be evaluated by comparing the precipitating effectiveness of various conjugates, each substituted with a different azo group. Some representative results are shown in Figures 15-4 and 15-5.

Some more recent examples of the dependence of affinity on the structure of ligands are given in Figures 15-6 and 15-7. From these and many other examples the generalizations discussed below have been drawn.

1) The ligands bound most strongly by a given set of Ab molecules are those that most closely simulate the structure of the deter-

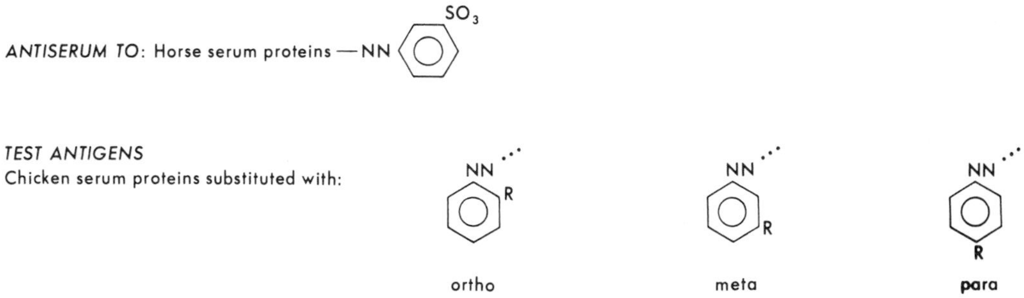

ANTISERUM TO: Horse serum proteins — NN ⟨○⟩ SO₃

TEST ANTIGENS
Chicken serum proteins substituted with:

	ortho	meta	para
R = SO₃⁻	+±	**++**	±
R = AsO₃H⁻	0	+	0
R = COO⁻	0	±	0

Fig. 15-4. Prominent effect of position and nature of acidic substituents of haptenic groups on the reaction between Abs to *m*-azobenzenesulfonate and various test Ags. R in the test Ag refers to the acidic substituents SO_3^-, AsO_3H^-, and COO^-. The homologous reaction is most intense (largest amount of precipitation) and is shown in heavy type. [From Landsteiner, K., and van der Scheer, J. *J Exp Med 63*:325 (1936).]

minant groups of the immunogen. This generalization is part of the broader rule that Abs react more effectively with the Ag that stimulated their formation than with other Ags; within this context the former is generally designated **homologous antigen** and the latter **heterologous antigens.** Similarly, haptens that resemble most closely the haptenic groups of the immunogen are the **homologous haptens** (Ch. 14, Fig. 14-3).

2) Those structural elements of the determinant group that project distally from the central mass of the immunizing Ag are **immunodominant,** i.e., they are especially influential in determining the Ab's specificity. Thus, Abs to *p*-azophenyl-*β*-lactoside and to 2,4-dinitrophenyl bind the **terminal residues** almost as well as the larger haptenic structures of which these residues constitute the end groups: for example, compare lactose with a phenyl-*β*-lactoside (Fig. 15-6), and dinitroaniline with *ε*-Dnp-lysine (Fig. 15-7). A particularly striking example is provided by Abs to the human blood group substances: anti-A is specific for terminal N-acetyl galactosamine residues, and anti-B is specific for

Fig. 15-5. Effect of nature and position of uncharged substituents of haptenic groups on the reactions between Abs to the *p*-azotoluidine group and various test Ags. The homologous reaction is shown in heavy type. [From Landsteiner, K., and van der Scheer, J. *J Exp Med 45*:1045 (1927).]

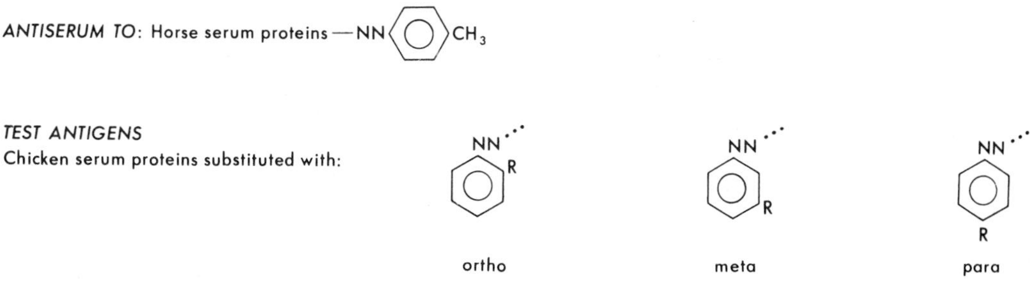

ANTISERUM TO: Horse serum proteins — NN ⟨○⟩ CH₃

TEST ANTIGENS
Chicken serum proteins substituted with:

	ortho	meta	para
R = CH₃	+±	+±	**++**
R = Cl	+	+±	++
R = NO₂	±	+	+±

Antibody Prepared Against	Test Hapten	Average Affinity K_0, liters mole^{-1} $\times 10^4$
L-phenyl (*p-azo benzoylamino*) acetate		
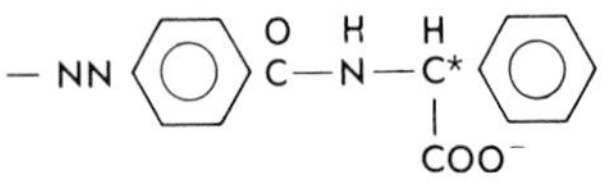	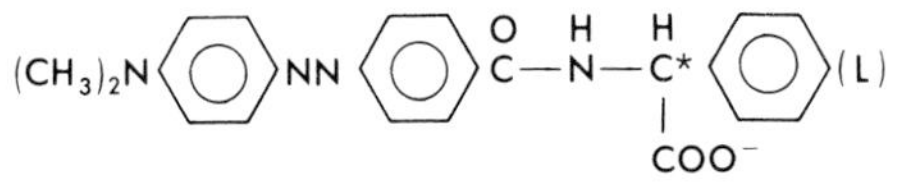	50
		1
	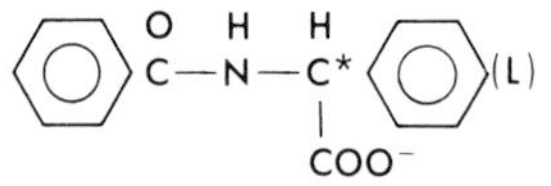	10
	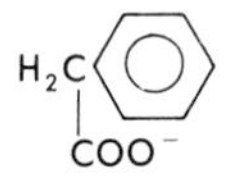	0.15
	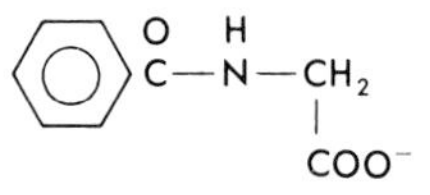	0.01
p-azophenyl-β-lactoside		13
	CH_3—O—β-lactose	2
	lactose (1, 4-β-galactosyl glucose)	1
	cellobiose (1, 4-β-glucosyl glucose)	0.03
	β—CH_3—O—galactose	0.007
	α—CH_3—O—galactose	0.001

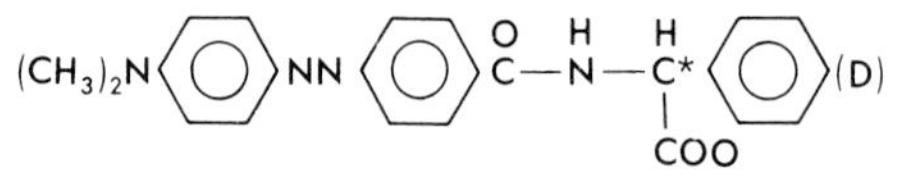

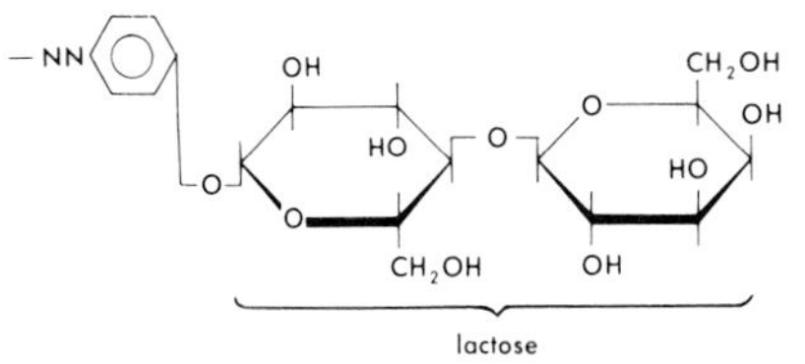

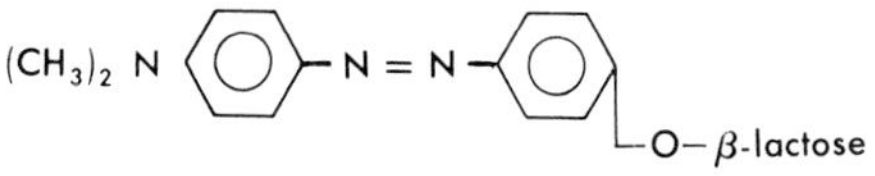

Fig. 15-6. Specificity of Ab-hapten reactions: Dependence of affinity on structure of the hapten. [From Karush, F. *J Am Chem Soc 78*:5519 (1956); *79*:3380 (1957).]

terminal galactose residues (Ch. 21, ABO system).

However, nonterminal residues also contribute to specific binding, sometimes decisively. For example, in the cell wall lipopolysaccharide that determines the serological specificity of various groups of *Salmonella* the sugars that react specifically with Abs to group E organisms are nonterminal mannosyl galactose residues (Fig. 15-20).

3) The **resolving powers** of Abs are, in general, comparable to those of enzymes. Some Abs readily distinguish between two molecules that differ only in the configuration about one carbon (e.g., glucose and galac-

tose, or D- and L-tartrate; see also Fig. 15-6).

4) The specific binding of a ligand by an Ab molecule may be regarded as a competitive **partition** of ligand between water and Ab-binding sites, which are relatively hydrophobic. Hence **ligands that are sparingly soluble in water,** such as dinitrophenyl haptens, tend to form particularly **stable complexes** with Ab, whereas ligands that are highly soluble in water, such as sugars and organic ions (e.g., benzonate), tend to form more dissociable complexes.

Many observations on the interactions between Abs and their ligands have made clear that the strength of the over-all bond between

Antibody Prepared Against	Test Hapten	Average Affinity K_0, liters mole^{-1} $\times 10^5$
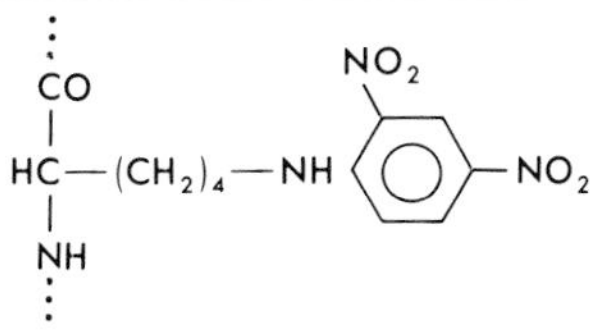 2,4-dinitrophenyl-L-lysyl group of Dnp protein	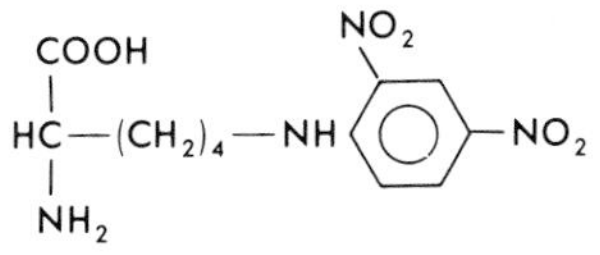 ε-Dnp-L-lysine	200
	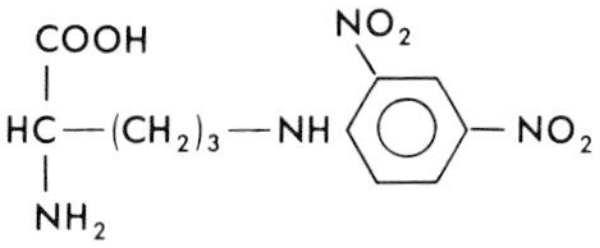 δ-Dnp-L-ornithine	80
	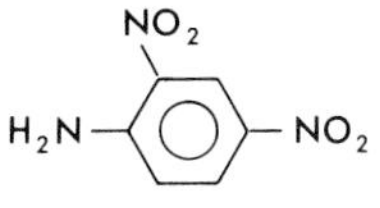 2,4-dinitroaniline	20
	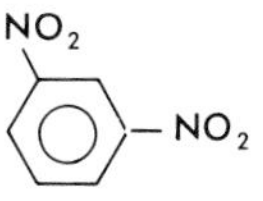 m-dinitrobenzene	8
	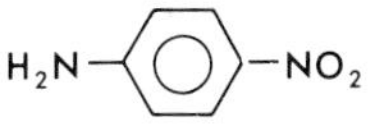 p-mononitroaniline	0.5

Fig. 15-7. Specificity of Ab-hapten reactions: Dependence of affinity on structure of the hapten. The haptens that approximate the haptenic group of the immunogen are bound more strongly. [From Eisen, H. N., and Siskind, G. W. *Biochemistry* 3:996 (1964).]

an Ab and a ligand reflects the sum of many constituent noncovalent interactions among atomic groups of the ligand and side chains of amino acid residues in the binding site of Ab. The greater the number and strength of the constituent interactions the more stable (i.e., the less dissociable) is the Ab-ligand complex. It is apparent intuitively that the number of bonds formed is greater the more closely the three-dimensional surface of the ligand matches, in a complementary sense, the three-dimensional contour of the Ab site. However, binding strength depends not only on geometrical complementarity but on chemical features of the paired groups: for example, it is greater when the groups attract, as when an anionic group of the ligand is contiguous to a cationic group of the Ab, or a hydrogen-bond acceptor of the ligand is adjacent to a hydrogen-bond donor of the Ab.

Virtually all the known noncovalent bonds appear to participate in various Ab-ligand interactions: ionic bonds, hydrogen bonds, apolar (hydrophobic) bonds, charge-transfer bonds. The strength of these bonds depends on distance between the interacting groups; for some bonds their strength is inversely proportional to distance to the sixth or seventh power. Hence the stability of immune complexes is critically dependent on the closeness of approach of ligand groups to Ab groups. Bulky substituents on ligands can hinder close approach and thereby diminish the strength of binding (**steric hindrance;** for example, see Fig. 15-16).

The binding sites of Ab molecules probably exist on the surface as shallow depressions, rather than as deep clefts, since they are accessible to determinant groups on macromolecules, including those on cell surfaces.

SPECIFICITY AND AFFINITY

As noted above, the specificity of an Ab population refers to its capacity to discriminate between ligands of similar structure by combining with them to detectably different extents: **the greater the difference in affinity for two closely related structures, the more specific the antibody.** Long before affinity was measurable this viewpoint was recognized by Landsteiner, who defined specificity as "the disproportional action of a number of related agents on a variety of related substrates"; by "related agents" he meant Abs, and by "related substrates" he meant haptens and Ags.

Sera differ greatly in specificity: for example, antiserum to *m*-azobenzenesulfonate is highly specific (it distinguishes sharply among *p*-, *o*-, and *m*-azobenzenesulfonates), whereas antiserum to *p*-azotoluidine is poorly specific (it does not differentiate methyl, chloro, or nitro in the para positions; Figs. 15-4 and 15-5). This difference in specificity probably arises because of the following considerations: 1) uncharged toluidine is more apolar than charged benzenesulfonate; 2) Abs to apolar groups tend to have higher affinity than Abs to polar groups for their respective ligands (see item 4 under Specificity, above); 3) high-affinity Abs usually appear to be less specific than low-affinity Abs, probably because Abs with high affinity for the homologous ligand often give easily detectable reactions with related ligands (for which their affinity may be very much lower), but Abs whose affinity for the homologous ligand is so low as just to permit a detectable reaction are not likely to react perceptibly with any other ligand. The high specificity (resolving power) of low-affinity Abs and the low affinity of Abs for carbohydrates could account for the exquisite specificity of some anticarbohydrate antisera and their resulting practical value in diagnostic typing of blood groups (Ch. 21), salmonellae (Chs. 6, 29), etc.

CARRIER SPECIFICITY

Some of the Abs made against a hapten-protein conjugate seem to react exclusively with the haptenic group, for they combine no better with the immunogen than with conjugates of the same hapten with unrelated proteins. However, many other Abs exhibit "carrier specificity": for maximal reactivity (highest affinity) they require not only the haptenic group and the amino acid residue to which it is attached but also (in varying degree) neighboring, unsubstituted residues of the immunogen. Other carrier-specific Abs react only with the protein moiety of the conjugate. Carrier specificity is particularly significant in some of the reactions of Ags with specific receptors on cell surfaces, as we shall see in connection with Ab formation (Ch. 17) and cell-mediated immunity (Ch. 20).

REACTIONS WITH SOLUBLE MACROMOLECULES

All complexes formed by Abs and small univalent ligands, considered in previous sections, are soluble. With macromolecular Ags, however, the complexes frequently become insoluble and precipitate from solution. Though the Abs responsible for this **precipitin reaction** used to be regarded as members of a unique class, called "precipitins," it is now clear that most Abs are capable of precipitating with their Ags (for exceptions see Blocking Abs and the Unitarian hypothesis, below).

PRECIPITIN REACTION IN LIQUID MEDIA

Since its discovery in 1897 the precipitin reaction has been used extensively as a qualitative or semiquantitative assay for estimating Ab titers in sera. Attempts to measure precipitates quantitatively were of limited value until Heidelberger and Avery discovered, in 1923, that an important Ag of the pneumococcus, the capsule, was a polysaccharide. This discovery had several important consequences: 1) it established that some macromolecules besides proteins could be immunogenic; 2) the structural basis for the specificity of natural Ags could be explored because the antigenic determinants of polysaccharides, unlike those of proteins, are not markedly influenced by the macromolecule's conformation; hence small oligosaccharides, derived from polysaccharides, could be used as simple haptens; 3) the Ab precipitated from serum could be identified as proteins; and 4) quantitative procedures for measuring proteins in general could be applied to the analysis of precipitated Abs since the included Ag did not interfere.

THE QUANTITATIVE PRECIPITIN REACTION

For purposes of illustration consider an antiserum prepared by immunizing a rabbit with type 3 pneumococci. When the purified capsular polysaccharide is added to the antiserum a precipitate appears. The reaction is specific: it does not occur with serum obtained before immunization or from rabbits immunized with other Ags. Analysis of the precipitate after thorough washing reveals only protein and the type 3 polysaccharide. Moreover, when the precipitated protein is separated from the polysaccharide (Appendix, this chapter) it can be precipitated completely and specifically by the type 3 polysaccharide. Thus, all the precipitated protein is evidently Ab, which can be measured with precision by a variety of quantitative procedures, e.g., by Kjeldahl analysis for nitrogen. (Trace amounts of some other proteins, called complement, are also precipitated; these are considered in Ch. 18.)

As is shown in Figure 15-8 and in Table 15-2, the amount of protein precipitated in a series of tubes, each with the same volume of antiserum, increases with the amount of polysaccharide added up to a maximum, beyond which larger amounts of the Ag lead to progressively less precipitation. The precipitation of a **maximum** amount of Ab by an **optimal** amount of Ag may appear inconsistent with the binding reaction discussed earlier, in which the number of Ab sites occupied by ligand increased monotonically without going through a maximum. This apparent discrepancy is due to special features of precipitation, which are discussed below (Lattice theory).

When the Ag is a protein instead of a polysaccharide the precipitated Ag protein must be deducted from the total precipitated protein. One must therefore know the Ag content of the precipitate. Fortunately, in certain regions of the precipitin curve (Ab-excess and equivalence zones in Fig. 15-8) the precipitated Ag is essentially equivalent to the total amount of Ag added, as had been inferred many years ago from the absence of Ag (in qualitative precipitin tests) in the corresponding supernatants. Subsequently a direct demonstration was provided by the use of Ags labeled with radioactive iodine or with intensely colored substituents.

Fig. 15-8. Precipitin curve for a monospecific system: One Ag and the corresponding Abs.

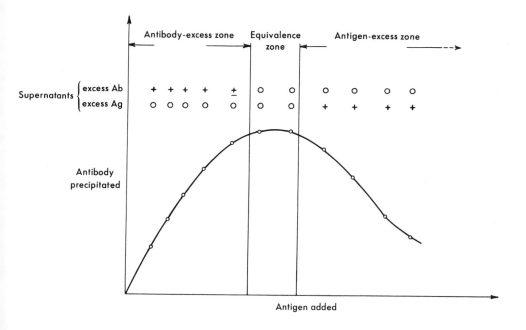

Zones of the Precipitin Curve. Useful information can be obtained from an examination of the supernatants by qualitative tests to detect unreacted Ab and unreacted Ag. For this purpose each supernatant is divided into aliquots, to one of which is added a small amount of fresh Ag (to detect excess Ab), and to the second a small amount of fresh antiserum (to detect excess Ag). If the Ag is homogeneous (i.e., consists of a single uniform group of molecules), or if the Ag preparation is heterogeneous but the antiserum is capable of reacting with only one of the components, then **none** of the supernatants contains **both** unreacted Abs and unreacted Ag in detectable amounts. Instead, the residual soluble reactants are distributed as shown in the precipitin curve of Figure 15-8: on the ascending limb, or **Ab-excess zone,** the supernatants contain free Ab; on the descending limb, or **Ag-excess zone,** the supernatants contain free Ag. In the region of maximum precipitation, the **equivalence zone** or **equivalence point,** the supernatants are usually devoid of both detectable Ab and detectable Ag, and the amount of Ab in the corresponding precipitate is taken to represent the weight of Ab in the volume of serum tested. Sometimes, as in Tables 15-2 and 15-3, the maximum amount of Ab is precipitated when there is a slight excess of free Ag in the supernatant; this is commented on below (see Nonprecipitating antibodies).

Up to this point we have been considering a **monospecific** system, i.e., one in which only one Ag and the corresponding Abs form the precipitates. However, most Ags, including those that satisfy the usual physical and chemical criteria of purity, are actually contaminated by small amounts of unrelated Ags, which may provoke independent immune responses. The precipitin reaction between such a contaminated Ag and its antiserum is thus usually the sum of two or more independent precipitin reactions, each monospecific.

This complex (but commonplace) situation is shown schematically in Figure 15-9. Contrary to what was observed with a monospecific system, some supernatants contain **both** unreacted Abs and unreacted Ag, because the Ag-excess zone of one system overlaps the Ab-excess zone of another. Qualitative testing of supernatants in the precipitin reaction thus provides a simple means for detecting the existence of multiple systems. However, as we shall see later the precipitin reaction in agar gel provides a more sensitive way to detect multispecificity, and can also indicate how many monospecific systems are present in a given pair of reactants.

Antibody/Antigen Ratios in the Precipitin Reaction. With most monospecific systems the Ab/Ag ratio in precipitates varies nearly linearly over the Ab-excess zone with the

TABLE 15-2.   Precipitin Reaction with a Polysaccharide as Antigen

Tube No.	S3 added (mg)	Total protein (or antibody) precipitated (mg)	Supernatant test
1	0.02	1.82	Excess Ab
2	0.06	4.79	Excess Ab
3	0.08	5.41	Excess Ab
4	0.10	5.79	Excess Ab
5	0.15	6.13	No Ab, no S3
6	**0.20**	**6.23**	**Slight excess S3**
7	0.50	5.87	Excess S3
8	1.00	3.76	Excess S3
9	2.00	2.10	Excess S3

The antigen (S3) is purified capsular polysaccharide of type 3 pneumococcus. Each tube contained 0.7 ml of antiserum obtained by injecting rabbits repeatedly with formalin-killed, encapsulated type 3 pneumococci. The supernatant of tube 6, which had the maximum amount of precipitated Ab, contained a slight excess of Ag; this is often observed and reflects the presence of some nonprecipitable or poorly precipitable Ab (see text).

Based on Heidelberger, M., and Kendall, F. E. *J Exp Med* 65:647 (1937).

TABLE 15-3. Precipitin Reaction with a Protein as Antigen

Tube No.	EAc added (mg)	Total protein precipitated (mg)	Antibody precipitated, by difference (mg)	Supernatant test	Ab/Ag in precipitates	
					Weight ratio	Mole ratio
1	0.057	0.975	0.918	Excess Ab	16.1	4.0
2	0.250	3.29	3.04	Excess Ab	12.1	3.0
3	0.312	3.95	3.64	Excess Ab	11.7	2.9
4	0.463	4.96	4.50	No Ab, no EAc	9.7	2.4
5	**0.513**	**5.19**	**4.68**	**No Ab, trace EAc**	**9.1**	**2.3**
6	0.562	5.16	(4.60)	Excess EAc	(8.2)	(2.1)
7	0.775	4.56	(3.79)	Excess EAc	(4.9)	(1.2)
8	1.22	2.58	—	Excess EAc	—	—
9	3.06	0.262	—	Excess EAc	—	—

Each tube contained 1.0 ml of antiserum obtained by injecting rabbits repeatedly with alum-precipitated crystallized chicken ovalbumin (EAc).

Ab content of precipitates in tubes 6–9 could not be determined by difference because too much EAc remained in the supernatants. The latter was measured independently in the supernatants of tubes 6 and 7, allowing an estimate to be made of EAc and Ab in the corresponding precipitates (values in parentheses).

Mole ratio Ab/Ag was estimated by assuming molecular weights for EAc and Ab of 40,000 and 160,000, respectively.

Based on Heidelberger, M., and Kendall, F. E. *J Exp Med* 62:697 (1935).

amount of Ag added (Fig. 15-10). With Ab in large excess the mole ratio greatly exceeds 1.0, showing that many Ab molecules can combine simultaneously with one molecule of Ag; i.e., **Ag is multivalent.** In the Ag-excess zone the role ratio of Ab/Ag tends to plateau with a limiting value of slightly over 1.0 (Table 15-3, Fig. 15-10). These variations are explicable in terms of the lattice theory (below).

LATTICE THEORY

Multivalency of Ags suggested to Marrack, and to Heidelberger and Kendall, that precipitation could be a consequence of the growth

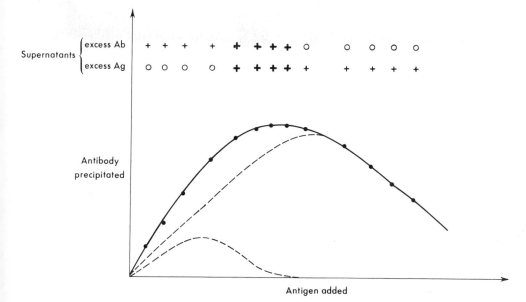

Fig. 15-9. Precipitin curve for a multispecific system. The precipitation observed (—•—) is the sum of two or more precipitin reactions (– – –). The significant difference from the monospecific system shown in Figure 15-8 is that some supernatants have **both** excess Ag and excess Abs (indicated by pluses in heavy type).

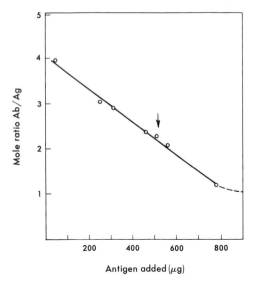

Fig. 15-10. Continuous decline in Ab/Ag ratio of precipitates with increasing amount of Ag added to a fixed volume of antiserum. Chicken ovalbumin (EAc) is the Ag and the serum is rabbit anti-EAc. The limiting mole ratio and slope vary about 30% in different sera. The arrow marks the equivalence zone. (Data are those of Table 15-3.)

to more than one Ab molecule and, in turn, each Ab molecule is linked to more than one Ag molecule. When the aggregates exceed some critical volume they settle out of solution spontaneously (because sedimentation rate is proportional to $V(\rho - \rho_0)g$, where V is the volume of a particle, ρ and ρ_0 are the densities of the particle and solvent, respectively, and g is the gravitational field). The assumption that Abs are multivalent was subsequently validated by equilibrium dialysis with univalent haptens (Fig. 15-2).

As is shown in Figure 15-11, the suggested **alternation** of multivalent Ag and Ab molecules (i.e., the **lattice theory**) accounts for the wide and continuous variations in Ab/Ag ratios of specific precipitates (Fig. 15-10), which for some time previously had defied rational explanation and seemed to be in conflict with the law of fixed proportions in formation of chemical compounds. With systems in which the Ag is distinctively labeled, and thus can be measured directly, it can be shown that precipitates formed in the presence of excess Ag have Ab/Ag ratios that approach 1.0 as a limiting value. This suggests that the least complicated precipitating complex is a large linear aggregate with alter-

of Ab-Ag aggregates in such a way that, broadly speaking, each Ag molecule is linked

Fig. 15-11. Hypothetical structure of immune precipitates and soluble complexes according to the lattice theory. Numbers refer to mole ratios of Ab to Ag. Dotted lines with precipitates are intended to indicate that the complexes continue to extend as shown. The precipitates may be visualized as those found in the Ab-excess zone **(A)**, the equivalence zone **(B)**, and the Ag-excess zone **(C)**. The soluble complexes correspond to those in supernatants in moderate **(D)**, far **(E)**, or extreme **(F)** Ag excess. Black circles, Ag molecules; open ellipses, Ab molecules.

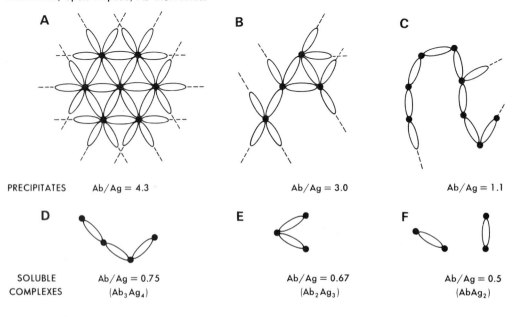

nating Ab and Ag molecules (. . . Ab·Ag·Ab· Ag·Ab·Ag . . .). Moreover, in the region of Ag-excess complexes of even lower Ab/Ag ratios are found, but they remain in the supernatant because they are small (Fig. 15-11D–F); they account for the "descending limb" of the precipitin curve. The soluble complexes have been demonstrated by ultracentrifugation and electrophoresis, and their mole ratios vary considerably; e.g., 0.75 (Ab$_3$Ag$_4$) in slight Ag excess and 0.67 (Ab$_2$Ag$_3$) in substantial Ag excess. In extreme excess the ratio approaches 0.5 (AbAg$_2$), as expected from the bivalence of Ab molecules.

VALENCE AND COMPLEXITY OF PROTEIN ANTIGENS

The limiting mole ratio of Ab/Ag in extreme Ab excess is often taken as a measure of the Ag molecule's valence (e.g., 4 in Fig. 15-10). Since Ab molecules are bivalent, however, the actual number of binding sites on the Ag can approach twice the limiting mole ratio. And the limiting ratio provides only a **minimal** estimate of the Ag valence: a larger number of reactive sites could exist but fail to be expressed, either because the spatial limitations at the surface preclude the packing of more Ab molecules about one Ag molecule, or else because the particular antiserum used lacks Abs for some potentially functional groups.

An Ag molecule of high molecular weight should be able to bind more Ab molecules simultaneously than an Ag of low molecular weight; as Table 15-4 shows, this relation is, in general, found. It should be especially noticed that all Ags capable of giving a precipitin reaction have a valence of at least two. Even some small bivalent haptens form specific precipitates; for example, some Abs to the 2,4-dinitrophenyl (Dnp) group are specifically precipitated by α,ε-bis-Dnp-lysine (Ch. 14, Fig. 14-3; Fig. 15-13).

The multivalency of many **polysaccharides** is readily understandable, since they are made up of repeating residues (e.g., Fig. 15-18). With **proteins,** however, the chemical basis for their multivalency is less obvious. The covalent structures of many proteins (e.g., ribonuclease, myoglobin) make clear that groups of amino acid residues almost never recur as repetitive sequences in a given polypeptide chain. Hence each antigenic determinant should occur once per chain, and two or more times only in those molecules with multiple copies of a particular chain. Nevertheless, protein molecules made up of a single chain behave as though multivalent. This is because there are a variety of determinants per chain and a particular determinant need occur only once per molecule of immunogen in order to stimulate the formation of the corresponding Abs.

The consequences can be illustrated with bovine pancreatic ribonuclease, with one

TABLE 15-4. Correlation Between Molecular Weight and Valence of Antigens

Antigen	Molecular weight	Approximate mole ratio Ab/Ag of precipitates in extreme antibody excess*
Bovine pancreatic ribonuclease	13,600	3
Chicken ovalbumin	42,000	5
Horse serum albumin	69,000	6
Human γ-globulin	160,000	7
Horse apoferritin	465,000	26
Thyroglobulin	700,000	40
Tomato bushy stunt virus	8,000,000	90
Tobacco mosaic virus	40,000,000	650

* The mole ratios are representative, and tend to be higher with antisera obtained late in the course of immunization. Since the Ab molecules involved are at least bivalent (cf. IgG and IgM Abs in Ch. 16), the Ag valences must be somewhat higher than the ratios listed.

Based on Kabat, E. A. In *Kabat and Mayer's Experimental Immunochemistry,* 2nd ed. Thomas, Springfield, Ill., 1961.

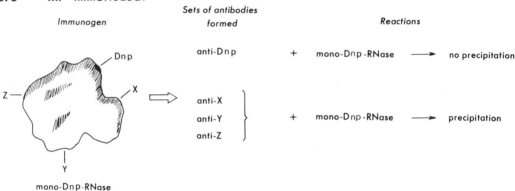

Fig. 15-12. Antigen valence illustrated with mono-Dnp-RNase, which induces the formation of anti-Dnp and other Abs, arbitrarily called anti-X, anti-Y, and anti-Z. The immunogen is **univalent** with respect to the anti-Dnp Abs, with which it forms soluble complexes. The same immunogen, however, is **multivalent** with respect to the mixture of diverse sets of Abs (anti-X, anti-Y, etc.) that are formed against its various nonhaptenic determinants (X, Y, Z). [Based on Eisen, H. N., Simms, E. S., Little, J. R., and Steiner, L. A. *Fed Proc 23*:559 (1964).]

chain per molecule, carrying one Dnp group (mono-Dnp-RNase). In the antiserum made against this immunogen some Abs are anti-Dnp and others are specific for different determinant groups (X, Y, Z in Fig. 15-12). Mono-Dnp-RNase behaves as a multivalent molecule with this antiserum, giving a classic precipitin reaction. But if the anti-Dnp molecules are isolated from the antiserum and then mixed with mono-Dnp-RNase only soluble complexes are formed, because the same Ag is univalent with respect to this particular set of Ab molecules. These observations emphasize the operational nature of the definition of valence: **a given molecule of antigen can be univalent with respect to some antibody molecules and multivalent with respect to others.**

These observations also reinforce the view that a typical globular protein is a mosaic within one molecule of many determinants, and that an antiserum to a protein consists of many sets of Ab molecules, each with the capacity to react with a single kind of functional group. Thus, proteolytic cleavage of bovine serum albumin (BSA, MW 70,000) yields several large fragments, each of which gives a precipitin reaction with different sets of Abs in antiserum prepared against the whole BSA molecule.

The minimum number of sets of Abs in an antiserum to a globular protein is indicated by the limiting mole ratio of Ab/Ag in the far Ab-excess region of its precipitin curve.

Since each set is probably made up of Ab molecules of different affinities and even of somewhat different structures (see Ch. 16), terms such as "the anti-BSA Ab" or "tetanus antitoxin" are deceptively simple.

From the argument that a protein Ag is a constellation of determinants, it follows that **the precipitin reaction usually involves cooperation between different Abs.** This conclusion is supported by the observations in Figure 15-13: the small ligand R-X, in which the functional groups R and X each occurs once per molecule, does not precipitate with an anti-R serum or with an anti-X serum, but does precipitate with a mixture of the two. These considerations lead to the schematic view of the precipitin reaction shown in Figure 15-14.

Homospecificity of Antibodies. Since there are diverse functional groups in most Ags it may be asked whether a bivalent Ab molecule can have binding sites that are specific for two different ligand groups. All existing evidence indicates that this does not occur: **bivalent Abs are homospecific.** For example, in antisera prepared against dinitrophenylated bovine γ-globulin (Dnp-BγG) one could imagine Ab molecules with one binding site specific for Dnp and one specific for a nonhaptenic group of BγG. However, removal of all the Abs that can react with BγG does not reduce the capacity of the antiserum to bind Dnp ligands. This finding is in accord with

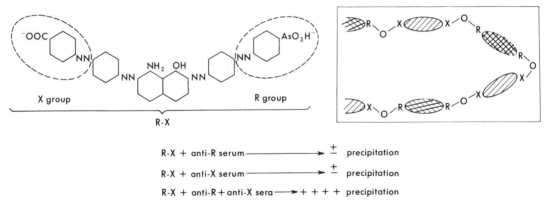

Fig. 15-13. Cooperation between Abs of different specificities (anti-R and anti-X) in the precipitin reaction with a synthetic ligand, R-X. (The small amount of precipitate (±) formed by R-X with anti-R alone or with anti-X alone is probably due to some aggregation of R-X.) The inset shows a hypothetical segment of the precipitate with alternation of anti-R and anti-X molecules in a linear aggregate. [Based on Pauling, L., Pressman, D., and Campbell, D. H. *J Am Chem Soc 66*:330 (1944).]

and explained by the symmetrical structure of Ab molecules (Ch. 16).

NONSPECIFIC FACTORS IN THE PRECIPITIN REACTION

The precipitin reaction involves two distinct stages: rapid formation of soluble Ab-Ag complexes and **slow** aggregation of these complexes to form visible precipitates. Thus, by measuring free Ag concentrations it has been found that the specific interactions are completed within a few minutes, but precipitate formation usually requires several days to reach completion.

While the lattice theory is clearly relevant for the first stage, an older view, that of Bordet, contains elements of interest for the second. This view suggests that the close packing of Ab molecules when bound to an Ag molecule provides opportunities for neighboring Ab molecules to react with each other, mostly by way of ionic bonds between oppositely charged groups (Fig. 15-11). As a consequence the complexes, which are usually predominantly made up of Ab molecules, become relatively hydrophobic and so tend progressively to associate with each other and to become increasingly insoluble. This view is supported by the effects of ionic strength on precipitation (less precipitation at low salt concentrations) and by observations on chemically modified Abs. For instance, when the negative charge on Ab molecules is increased by acetylation of free amino groups the ability to pre-

cipitate can be lost without impairing the Ab's ability to form a specific, soluble complex with Ag.

NONPRECIPITATING ANTIBODIES

Nonprecipitating Abs were first recognized because of discrepancies between the amounts of Ab precipitated after the addition of Ag by two different procedures. In **procedure A** each of a series of tubes, containing the same amount of antiserum, receives a different amount of Ag systematically increasing as in Table 15-2. By analysis of the precipitates the quantity of Ag necessary to precipitate the maximal amount of Ab is established. In **procedure B** about 1/10 the equivalent amount of Ag is added repeatedly to a single volume of antiserum, from which the precipitate formed after each addition is removed before the next addition. The sum of all the Ab precipitated is usually considerably less than that precipitated at the equivalence point in procedure A. The difference represents **nonprecipitating antibodies,** i.e., molecules that cannot alone precipitate with Ag but can become incorporated into Ab-Ag precipitates of the same specificity.

Under the influence of the lattice theory, **nonprecipitating Ab molecules** were assumed to have a single combining site. However, careful studies have never demonstrated intact Ab molecules to be truly univalent, and the inability of some Abs to precipitate with Ags arises from other mechanisms. For example, some Abs have too low an affinity for Ag. Hence the Ag must be added at relatively high concentrations in order to occupy a significant proportion of Ab combining sites; because

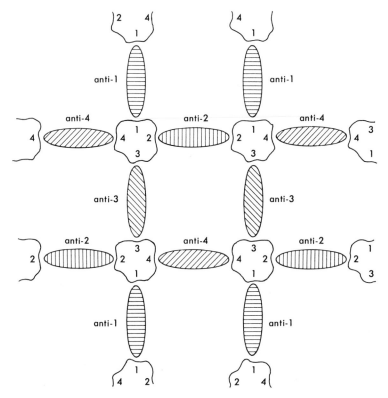

Fig. 15-14. Schematic illustration of the diversity of Abs formed against a pure Ag and their cooperation in the precipitin reaction with that Ag. Further complexities arise because each set of Abs (anti-1, anti-2, etc.) is probably heterogeneous with respect to affinity for the corresponding antigenic determinant; in addition Abs of the same specificity may differ considerably in structure (Ch. 16). Antigenic determinants are labeled 1,2,3,4.

this level of Ag is likely to be in excess, relative to Ab, only small soluble Ab-Ag complexes are formed. Another mechanism arises from monogamous bivalency (below).

Monogamous Bivalency. Some bivalent Ab molecules with high affinity for Ag do not form specific precipitates because they preferentially combine with two determinant groups of a **single** Ag particle, forming cyclic complexes (Ab:Ag) rather than cross-linked ones (Ag·Ab·Ag; Fig. 15-15). This type of binding, called "monogamous bivalency" by Karush, requires that a given antigenic group occur repetitively on the Ag surface. Besides hapten-protein conjugates, polysaccharides, and multichain proteins, this commonly occurs with surface determinants of bacteria, red cells, and viruses. The commonplace and important "blocking Abs" (which do not agglutinate bacteria, red cells, etc., but combine specifically with them) could also owe their behavior to monogamous bivalency (see below, Incomplete Abs).

Abs in general would be expected to engage preferentially in monogamous bivalent binding (because it is energetically advantageous to form binary Ab:Ag rather than ternary Ag·Ab·Ag complexes). However, most seem unable to do so, and act instead to cross-link Ags, perhaps because insufficient flexibility prevents the two combining sites in most Ab molecules from being adjusted to fit neighboring antigenic sites on a given Ag particle (Fig. 15-15; see Ch. 16, Overall structure of Abs).

For Ab-ligand pairs that can form monogamous complexes the equilibrium constant with multivalent ligands can be many orders of magnitude higher than the same Ab's intrinsic affinity for the corresponding univalent hapten. For instance, the reaction between anti-Dnp Abs and Dnp bacteriophage, with many Dnp groups per phage particle, has an association constant about 100,000-fold greater than the reaction between the same Abs and univalent Dnp-lysine (e.g., 10^{12} vs. 10^7 liters/mole): evidently the two bonds involved in the monogamous complex greatly decrease the probability that the Ab:Ag pair will dissociate. Because similar cyclic complexes are probably formed with unmodified

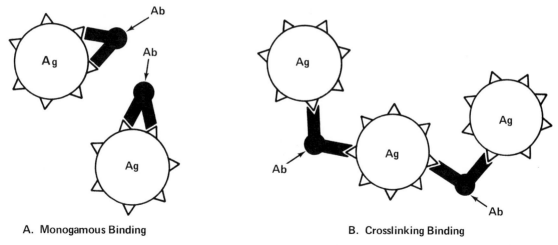

A. Monogamous Binding   B. Crosslinking Binding

Fig. 15-15. Monogamous bivalent binding, leading to cyclic Ab:Ag complexes, is contrasted with conventional binding, which leads to cross-linking of Ag particles (. . . Ag · Ab · Ag . . .).

viruses and bacteria, whose surfaces often have identical, repeating antigenic groups (e.g., various structural subunits of wall or envelope), some Abs can probably combine with and neutralize pathogenic microbes under in vivo conditions where the free Ab concentration is exceedingly low (e.g., 10^{-12} M).

REVERSIBILITY OF PRECIPITATION

After a precipitate has formed, its complexes can dissociate and reequilibrate with a fresh charge of Ag. When the latter is in sufficient excess small soluble complexes are formed and the precipitate dissolves. This reversibility provides the basis for many of the procedures used to isolate purified Abs (see Appendix, this chapter). In practice, however, it may be difficult to observe dissociation: hence the formation of Ab-Ag aggregates was formerly held to be irreversible, as in a particularly striking example described by Danysz.

The **Danysz phenomenon** is well illustrated with the diphtheria toxin-antitoxin system. When an equivalent amount of toxin is added to an antitoxin serum the residual toxicity depends upon how the reagents are mixed. If the toxin is added to the antiserum all at once the mixture is nontoxic; but if the same quantity of toxin is divided into two or more portions and added at intervals of about 30 minutes the mixture is toxic. This phenomenon was interpreted to mean that the first addition of toxin led to the formation of irreversible complexes with a

high Ab/Ag ratio, leaving insufficient free Ab to neutralize all the toxin subsequently added.

However, all Ab-Ag reactions are reversible in principle; those that appear irreversible probably have unusually slow dissociation rates, requiring days or even months, rather than minutes, to reestablish equilibrium when the system is perturbed. **Apparent irreversibility** is especially striking with many Ab-virus complexes: some are so stable that they do not perceptibly dissociate even when a mixture of virus and antiserum is diluted many thousandfold, with a corresponding reduction in the concentrations of free virus and free Ab (Ch. 50). The extraordinary stability of such complexes, reflecting unusually high equilibrium constants, probably derives from monogamous multivalent binding (above). Even ordinary single-bonded complexes of Ab with small univalent haptens can appear to be irreversible if the intrinsic association constant is sufficiently high ($> 10^8$ liters/mole); e.g., the hapten cannot be separated from the Ab by dialysis. Nevertheless, reversibility can always be demonstrated by "exchange": addition of more ligand, in great excess, will replace the molecules that appeared to be irreversibly bound.

APPLICATIONS OF THE PRECIPITIN REACTION

Measurement of Antibody Concentration. The quantitative precipitin reaction is performed as described above: various amounts of Ag are added to a constant volume of antiserum, and the resulting specific precipitates are washed and analyzed for total protein: the results, plotted as shown in Figure 15-8, measure the amount of precipitable Ab.

The precipitin assay is highly reproducible and precise. However, it requires the analysis of multiple precipitates, and its accuracy (i.e., its relation to "true" values) is limited because a proportion of the Abs, varying from serum to serum, may not bind to the Ag or precipitate under the conditions of the assay (see Nonprecipitating antibodies, above). Despite these reservations the quantitative precipitin reaction remains the most reliable general method for measuring Ab concentrations.

Measurement of Antigen Concentration. Once a precipitin curve has been constructed for a given antiserum and its Ag, the serum can be used to measure the concentration of that Ag in unknown solutions. The assay is carried out in the Ab-excess region; and it is only necessary to establish that the antiserum is free of extraneous Abs that could precipitate other Ags in the test solution. Antisera are stable on prolonged storage, and the precipitin reaction can measure small quantities (microgram range) of Ags in complex solutions; e.g., rabbit antisera have been used to measure immunoglobulins in human spinal fluid. However, more sensitive assays are often preferred (e.g., Radioimmunoassays, see below and Table 15-5).

HAPTEN INHIBITION OF PRECIPITATION

Qualitative Hapten Inhibition. Long before its quantitative features were characterized by Heidelberger and his associates the precipitin reaction was widely used as a visual, qualitative test to detect Ab-Ag reactions. It was, in fact, in just this simple fashion that Landsteiner had exploited it, by means of hapten inhibition, in his classic investigations of immunological specificity. In general terms, in the precipitin system he used the antiserum was prepared against one conjugated protein, which may be designated X-azoprotein A, and the precipitating agent was another conjugate with the same azo substituent attached to a different protein, X-azoprotein B. A and B were chosen so that they did not react with other's antisera (e.g., horse and chicken serum

proteins, Figs. 15-4 and 15-5), and X-azoprotein B was prepared with many X-azo groups per molecule, so that it formed precipitating complexes with anti-X Abs. In contrast, simple haptens with one X group per molecule formed soluble complexes with anti-X and could competitively inhibit the precipitin reaction (Fig. 15-16). The greater the Ab's affinity for the hapten, relative to its affinity for the precipitating azoprotein, the more effectively was its precipitation inhibited.

Quantitative Hapten Inhibition. By combining hapten inhibition with quantitative measurements of precipitates, Pauling and Pressman were able to obtain more insight into the specificity of Ab reactions than had been possible with the qualitative method. In their assay analyses are carried out by adding equal volumes of an anti-X serum to a series of tubes with varying amounts of univalent X haptens. After a few minutes a multivalent precipitating agent (e.g., an X-azoprotein) is added in that amount which, in the absence of hapten, would give roughly maximal precipitation of anti-X Abs. The amount of Ab precipitated decreases as the concentration of added hapten increases (Fig. 15-17). The binding sites in a heterogeneous population of anti-X molecules differ in capacity to discriminate between the univalent and the multivalent ligand, and the relative effectiveness of univalent ligands is characterized by specifying the concentration required to inhibit precipitation by 50%. The concentration required of the reference hapten for 50% inhibition, divided by the concentration required of a second hapten, provides an index of the Ab's affinity for the second hapten, relative to the reference hapten. Some representative results are shown in Figure 15-17.

Hapten inhibition of precipitation has been used effectively to identify determinant groups of complex Ags, such as proteins and blood group substances (Ch. 21). The reactions of globular protein Ags are usually inhibitable by some of the large fragments (MW $\gg$ 1000) derived from the Ag by proteolytic enzymes, but not by small peptides or by the denatured protein. Such results suggest that **most determinant groups of proteins are "conformational,"** representing a particular three-dimensional spatial arrangement of a cluster of amino acids, rather than simply their sequence. However, a few protein-antiprotein reactions are inhibited specifically to some extent by small dialyzable peptides (derived from the Ag); these determinants appear to be **"sequential,"** their reactivity being manifested whether the sequence is part of the intact protein or a small oligopeptide. Such determinants are conspicuous in fibrous proteins (e.g., silk fibroin, synthetic polypeptides), but are evident only in exceptional globular proteins (e.g., coat protein of tobacco mosaic virus).

Fig. 15-16. Competitive inhibition of the precipitin reaction by a univalent ligand. Ag, multivalent ligand; Ab, antibody; H, univalent ligand.

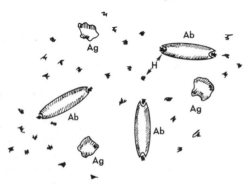

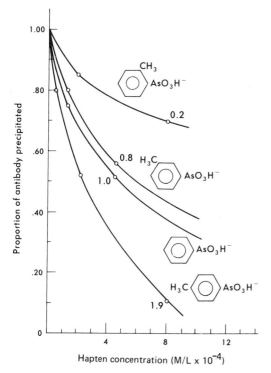

Fig. 15-17. Hapten inhibition of the precipitin reaction, illustrated with various univalent benzenearsonates. The number on each curve gives the affinity for the corresponding hapten **relative** to benzenearsonate (= 1.0). The antiserum was prepared against *p*-azobenzenearsonate; hence the hapten with -CH$_3$ in the para position is bound best, i.e., it is most inhibitory (K' = 1.9). With the methyl group in the meta or ortho position steric hindrance reduces affinity for Ab. [From Pressman, D. *Adv Biol Med Phys 3*:99 (1953).]

CROSS-REACTIONS

Besides reacting with its immunogen, an antiserum usually reacts with certain other Ags (heterologous Ags) that are sufficiently similar to the immunogen; some cross-reactions are illustrated in Figures 15-18 and 15-19.

Cross-Reactions Due to Impurities in Antigens. Most immunogens are complex mixtures of many different kinds of antigenic molecules. This is obviously true when the immunogen is a cell. It is also usually true, though less obvious, with purified proteins, since these are nearly always contaminated with other immunogenic proteins. Even at trace levels (e.g., 1%) the contaminants can often

provoke the formation of detectable amounts of Ab. Hence, antisera prepared against these mixtures consist of several Ab populations, each reactive with one Ag.

If, for example, crystallized chicken ovalbumin (EAc) contaminated with trace amounts of chicken serum proteins were used as immunogen, the anti-EAc serum would probably contain low levels of Abs to the contaminants and would probably form precipitates (i.e., cross-react) with some chicken serum proteins. Supernatant tests would probably reveal that the precipitin reaction was not monospecific; and this would be even easier to establish by reactions in agar gel (see below, Fig. 15-27).

Cross-Reactions Due to Common or Similar Functional Groups in Different Antigens. We have already discussed some of the evidence that a single protein contains many different antigenic determinants, each of which can potentially evoke the formation of a corresponding set of Ab molecules. If two different molecules happen to have one or more groups in common they usually cross-react.

This type of cross-reaction is frequently observed with polysaccharides and provides the basis for classifying many groups of closely related bacteria. The 500 or more varieties of salmonellae, for example, have been arranged into several serological groups, each identified by mutual cross-reactions: an antiserum to any strain of a particular group reacts with the other strains of that group. The common antigenic determinants responsible for the group-specific cross-reactions have been shown to be short sequences of particular sugar residues. For example, the determinant that defines group O *Salmonella* has as its principle residue colitose (3,6-dideoxy-L-galactose), attached as a terminal sugar on a branch of the cell wall lipopolysaccharide. Other terminally attached dideoxyhexoses are responsible for the cross-reactions that characterize other groups of salmonellae. The determinants responsible for cross-reactions need not, however, be terminal residues. The strains of group E *Salmonella,* for example, cross-react because their cell wall lipopolysaccharides all possess nonterminal mannosyl-rhamnose residues as repeating units (Fig. 15-20).

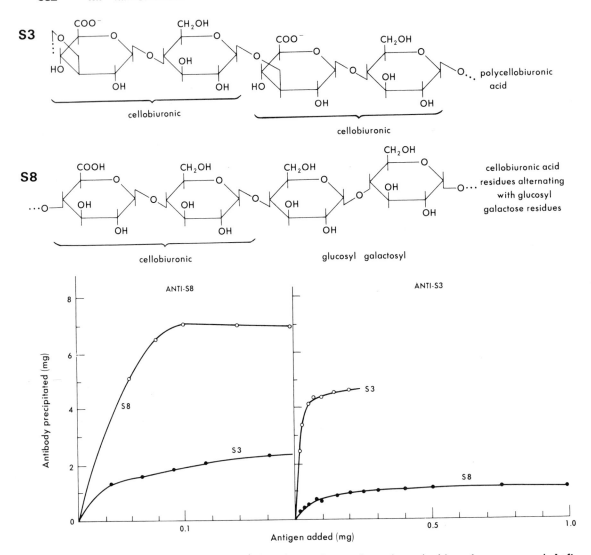

Fig. 15-18. Cross-reactions between type 3 and type 8 capsular polysaccharides of pneumococci. **Left:** Horse antiserum to type 8 pneumococcus, reacted with purified S8 and S3 polysaccharide. **Right:** Horse antiserum to type 3 pneumococcus, reacted with S3 and S8 polysaccharide. [Based on Heidelberger, M., Kabat, E. A., and Shrivastava, D. L., *J Exp Med* 65:487 (1937); and Heidelberger, M., Kabat, E. A., and Mayer, M., *J Exp Med* 75:35 (1942).]

Another example is provided by the pneumococcus. The capsular polysaccharide of type 3 is a linear polymer of repeating cellobiuronic acid residues (β-1,4-glucuronidoglucose), while in that of type 8 these residues alternate with glucosyl-galactose residues. Hence antisera to either Ag cross-react extensively with the other (Fig. 15-18).

A similar principle accounts for the cross-reactions that are commonplace with conjugated proteins; for example, antisera to 2,4-dinitrophenyl (Dnp)-bovine γ-globulin react with Dnp-human serum albumin because Dnp groups are present in both conjugates.

Cross-reactivity does not require that a functional group of the heterologous ligand be **identical** with the corresponding group of the immunogen; it need only be sufficiently **similar.** For example, Abs to *m*-azobenzenesulfonate cross-react with *m*-azobenzenearsonate (Fig. 15-4), and Abs to the 2,4-dinitrophenyl-lysyl group cross-react with

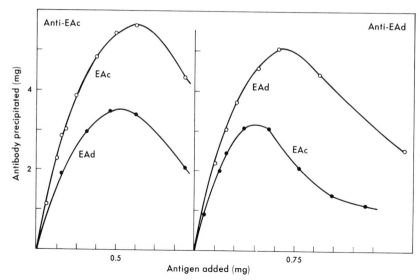

Fig. 15-19. Cross-reactions between chicken and duck ovalbumin, EAc and EAd, respectively. **Left:** Rabbit antiserum to EAc, reacted with EAc and EAd. **Right:** Rabbit antiserum to EAd, reacted with EAd and EAc. [Based on Osler, A. G., and Heidelberger, M. *J Immunol* 60:327 (1948).]

Fig. 15-20. Portion of the cell wall lipopolysaccharide of three strains of salmonellae. The strains are assigned to the same group (O) because of their serological cross-reaction, due to their common mannosyl rhamnose residues (boxed in). They are also distinguishable serologically because each has some unique structural feature, e.g., the terminal glucose (G) residue in *S. minneapolis,* and the α or β glycosidic bond linking galactose (Gal) to mannose (M). [Based on Robbins, P. W., and Uchida, T. *Fed Proc* 21:702 (1962).]

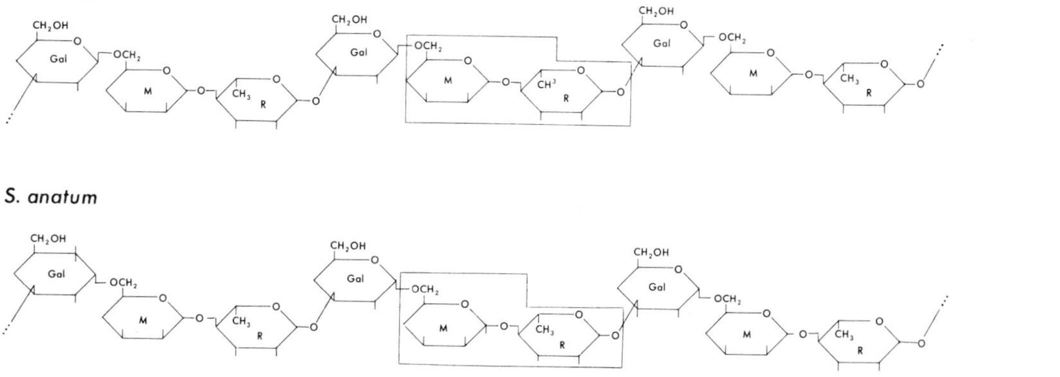

S. minneapolis

S. newington

S. anatum

2,4,6-trinitrobenzene. All Abs exhibit some cross-reactions: i.e., they bind some Ags with determinant groups that are not identical with those in the immunogen.

General Characteristics of Cross-Reactions. The following generalizations are drawn from the study of many cross-reactions.

1) An antiserum precipitates **more copiously** with its immunogen than with cross-reacting Ags (Figs. 15-18 and 15-19), because a heterologous ligand usually reacts only with some proportion of the total Ab to the immunogen. In addition, purified Abs of a given specificity will almost always have **greater affinity** for the homologous ligand than for cross-reacting ligands (Figs. 15-6 and 15-7).

2) The mutual cross-reactions between a pair of Ags are usually not quantitatively equivalent; Abs to the first Ag may react more extensively with the second Ag than Abs to the second react with the first (Fig. 15-18).

3) Different antisera to a given immunogen are likely to vary in the extent of their cross-reactions with diverse heterologous Ags, even when the antisera are obtained from the same animal (at different times after immunization, Ch. 17).

4) Cross-reacting ligands tend to be bound more strongly by Abs with high affinity than by those with low affinity for the homologous ligand. Thus, fewer cross-reactions are exhibited by low- than by high-affinity Abs (see Specificity and affinity, above). Since polysaccharide-antipolysaccharide systems are, in general, characterized by low affinities (see above), this rule may account for the extraordinary specificity of the sera used in typing bacteria and red blood cells according to the saccharides on their surfaces (Ch. 21).

Comparison of Various Types of Cross-Reactions. The cross-reactions discussed above may be contrasted as follows. 1) The presence of antigenic impurities is trivial conceptually but of considerable importance technically in practical applications of serological reactions. 2) The presence of **identical** functional groups in different Ags is particularly relevant for those groups that are relatively insensitive to the fine structure of macromolecules, such as lactose, 2,4-dinitrophenyl, etc. Groups of this type are usually found in polysaccharides, nucleic acids, and conjugated proteins. 3) Cross-reactions based on **similarity** rather than identity of determinants are probably of particular importance among proteins, whose determinant groups are mainly conformational (see Hapten inhibition, above) and not likely to be precisely duplicated in different proteins. While the second and third types of cross-reactions may be distinguished formally, it is not usually possible to differentiate between them experimentally.

Removal of Cross-Reacting Antibodies (Adsorption and Absorption). It is usually necessary to remove certain cross-reacting Abs before an antiserum is sufficiently **monospecific** for use as an analytical reagent, e.g., in typing bacteria, measuring enzyme levels in bacterial extracts, etc. Removal is accomplished simply by allowing the antiserum to react with the appropriate cross-reacting Ags. Large complexes (e.g., precipitates or Abs bound to cells) are easily removed along with the cross-reacting Abs. When, however, the complexes are soluble and difficult to remove, cross-reacting ligand may be added in large excess to saturate the cross-reacting Abs, eliminating them functionally without excluding them physically. An effective alternative is to pass the serum over a column of agarose beads to which the cross-reacting Ags are covalently attached, removing the corresponding Abs. We shall use the terms **adsorption** and adsorbed serum when Abs are removed by specific binding on the surface of **particulate** Ags (e.g., red cells, bacteria, agarose beads coated with Ag), and **absorption** and absorbed serum when Abs are neutralized by reaction with **soluble** Ags.

AVIDITY

Early in this chapter we saw that an Ab's affinity for univalent ligands is measured by the intrinsic association constant, K, which is the property of a representative **single** site (see also Appendix, below). However, Ab molecules and most Ag particles are multivalent, and their tendency to pair depends not only on intrinsic affinities (per site), but also upon the **number** of sites involved per reactant. For instance, the equilibrium constant in the formation of multivalent monogamous Ab:Ag complexes (above) can exceed by perhaps 100,000-fold the intrinsic equilibrium constant of the Ab for the homologous univalent ligand. In most reactions the number of functional groups on Ag particles is usually obscure and different ones are likely to be engaged by different sets of Abs (see Fig. 15-12); in addition, the pairing of Ab and Ag can also be influenced by nonspecific factors involved in aggregation or close-packing of macromolecules.

Because of these complexities the term **avidity** is used to denote the over-all tendency of Abs to combine with Ag particles, reserving the term **affinity** for the intrinsic association constant that characterizes the binding of a univalent ligand (see Appendix, below).

Differences in the avidity of different antisera for the same Ag can sometimes be demonstrated simply by diluting antiserum-Ag mixtures. The concentrations of free Ab and free Ag are reduced, causing dissociation of the immune complexes: **dissociation is less evident with more avid antisera.** This procedure is particularly useful when the unbound Ag can be measured with high sensitivity (as toxin or infectious virus). Variations in the shape of precipitin curves also reveal differences in avidity. For example, in Figure 15-21 antiserum A is more avid than B, which is more avid than C, etc.

Antisera can differ in avidity because their

Abs differ in intrinsic affinity for a given determinant (Fig. 15-21); or they might differ in the number of sets of Abs for diverse determinants of the Ag, or in the proportion of Ab molecules that can engage in monogamous binding. Abs with more available combining sites also have a greater tendency to bind ligands than Abs with fewer available sites, even when both Abs have the same intrinsic association constant (see Appendix, especially equation 16); hence sera can differ in avidity if they have different proportions of Abs with 2 or 10 combining sites per molecule (see Ch. 16, IgG and IgM). Avidity differences among antisera are commonplace and easily recognized, but the basis for the differences is usually obscure.

THE FLOCCULATION REACTION

The precipitin reactions of certain antisera differ from the classic precipitin reaction in that insoluble aggregates are not observed until the amount of Ag added exceeds some relatively large value (cf. Figs. 15-18, 15-19, and 15-22). In these anomalous **flocculation** reactions precipitation is inhibited by extreme Ab excess as well as by Ag excess: precipitation is observed only over a narrow range of Ab/Ag ratios.

Flocculation reactions are regularly given by certain horse antisera, particularly those prepared against diphtheria toxin and some streptococcal toxins; but horse antisera to most other proteins and to polysaccharides give the usual precipitin re-

Fig. 15-21. Precipitin curves showing differences in avidity of four antisera for the same Ag. The sera were prepared against 2,4-dinitrophenyl (Dnp)-bovine γ-globulin and tested with human serum albumin substituted with about 30 Dnp groups per molecule (Dnp-HSA). The order of avidity of the sera is A>B>C>D. A similar order in affinity for ε-Dnp-lysine was found for anti-Dnp molecules isolated from each of the sera: K_o in liters mole^{-1} were: (A) $> 10^8$, (B) 1×10^7, (C) 5×10^6, and (D) 1×10^6. (From Steiner, L. A,. and Eisen, H. N. In *Immunological Diseases*. M. Samter, ed. Little, Brown, Boston, 1965.)

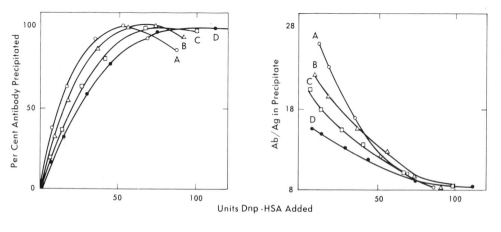

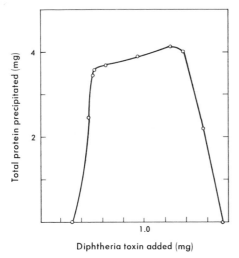

Fig. 15-22. Precipitin reaction of the flocculation type. The indicated amount of toxin was added to one ml of horse antiserum to diphtheria toxin. [Based on Pappenheimer, A. M., Jr., and Robinson, E. S. *J Immunol* 32:291 (1937).]

actions. The explanation for the special features of the flocculation reaction must lie in the properties of the Abs involved, rather than the Ags, because the same Ags (and all others tested) give only typical precipitin reactions with rabbit antisera. Some human antisera to thyroglobulin give flocculation reactions.

The basis for the flocculation reaction has not been clarified. Possibly the involved Abs are unusually soluble or the special antisera that give this reaction contain some high-affinity, nonprecipitating Abs (see Monogamous binding, above), and it is only after

they are saturated that the remaining conventional Abs can react and precipitate with additional Ag.

PRECIPITIN REACTION IN GELS

When Abs and Ag are introduced into different regions of an agar gel they diffuse freely toward each other and form readily visible opaque bands of precipitate at the junction of their diffusion fronts. Simple and ingenious applications of this principle provide powerful methods for analyzing the multiplicity of Ab-Ag reactions within a system. The most widely used methods are illustrated in Figure 15-23 and are described below.

Single Diffusion in One Dimension. This procedure, developed by Oudin in France, is generally performed by placing a solution of Ag over an antiserum that has been incorporated in a column of agar gel. By diffusion, a concentration gradient of Ag advances down the agar column (provided the concentration of Ag in the upper reservoir is high relative to the concentration of Ab in the agar phase), and a precipitate forms in the agar at the advancing diffusion front. This precipitate extends upward to that level in the gradient at which Ag excess is sufficient to prevent precipitation. With continuing diffusion of Ag from the reservoir, the leading edge of the precipitate advances downward. The trailing edge of the precipitate likewise advances, since the additional Ag migrating into the

Fig. 15-23. Some arrangements for gel diffusion precipitin reactions. **A.** Single diffusion in one dimension. **B.** Double diffusion in one dimension (Preer method). **C.** Double diffusion in two dimensions. Arrows show direction of diffusion. Stippled areas are opaque precipitation bands.

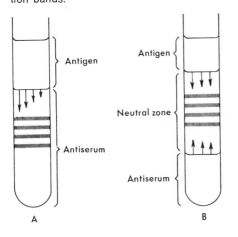

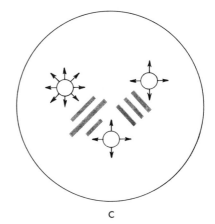

region of the specific precipitate dissolves it by forming soluble complexes, as expected from the precipitin reaction in liquid. Thus, a **band** of precipitate migrates down the column of agar. The distance traveled is proportional to the square root of time, in accord with the laws of diffusion.

The rate of migration depends on the diffusion coefficient of the Ag (which varies with molecular weight and shape) and on its **concentration** in the upper reservoir (Fig. 15-23A). Accordingly, when several Ags diffuse into an antiserum that can react with each of them, several bands of precipitation are observed, and each migrates at a distinctive rate. It is possible, though, that different Ab-Ag systems will form overlapping bands that migrate at indistinguishable rates; hence the number of bands observed represents the **minimum** number of Ab-Ag systems in the substances being analyzed.

The rate of band migration varies with the concentration of Ag introduced, and the optical density of a precipitate (which can be measured by suitable photometers) depends on the concentration of Ab in the antiserum. Hence it is possible, with the use of appropriate standards (solutions of known Ag concentration and antisera of known Ab concentration), to measure the concentration of Ag in unknown solutions and the concentration of precipitating Abs in antisera.

The arrangement shown in Figure 15-23A can be reversed by incorporating Ag in the agar column below and overlaying it with antiserum. If the concentration of Abs greatly exceeds the concentration of relevant Ags, precipitation takes place at the interface and migrates into the lower gel phase. This arrangement can distinguish between precipitin and flocculation reactions (Fig. 15-24).

Double Diffusion in One Dimension. In this procedure the antiserum in agar is overlaid by a column of clear agar which in turn is overlaid by Ag, added either as liquid or incorporated into agar. Ag and Ab molecules diffuse across the respective interfaces into the clear neutral zone and advance toward each other. At that junction of their diffusion fronts where Ab and Ag are in equivalent proportions a precipitation band forms, and it increases in density with time as more Ab and Ag molecules continue to enter this zone in optimal (i.e., equivalent) proportions (Fig. 15-23B). If the Ag and Ab are added to their respective reservoirs in proportions that correspond to the equivalence zone in solution, the precipitation band has maximal sharpness and is

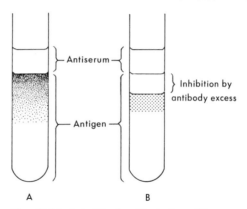

Fig. 15-24. Gel diffusion illustrating differences between the usual type of precipitin reaction **(A)** and the flocculation reaction **(B)**. Precipitation is inhibited by excess Ab in the flocculation reaction but not in the precipitin reaction. Compare Ab-excess zones of Figures 15-17, 15-18, and 15-21.

stationary. If, however, either is added in relative excess, the band migrates slowly away from the excess.

This method can detect as little as 10 μg Ab per milliliter. It is particularly valuable for determining the number of Ab-Ag systems in complex reagents. For example, with highly purified diphtheria toxin and a human antiserum to diphtheria toxin as many as six bands of precipitation have been observed. These same reactants in liquid solution would very likely have displayed a precipitin curve with a single zone of maximum precipitation; with careful supernatant analysis it might have been possible to recognize that more than one Ab-Ag system was involved, but not how many.

Double Diffusion in Two Dimensions. Additional insight can be obtained by the simple but elegant procedure, developed mainly by Ouchterlony in Sweden, of placing Ag and Ab solutions in separate wells cut in an agar plate (Fig. 15-23C). A large number of geometric arrangements are possible; some of the simpler ones are shown in Figures 15-25 to 15-27. The reactants diffuse from the wells, and precipitation bands form where they meet at equivalent proportions. If the concentration of Ab introduced is in relative excess over Ag, the band forms closer to the Ag well; and the converse occurs if the Ag is introduced in relative excess.

The arrangements shown in Figures 15-25 to 15-27 are particularly useful for comparing Ags for the presence of identical or cross-reacting components. If a solution of Ag is

Identity

Nonidentity

Partial identity

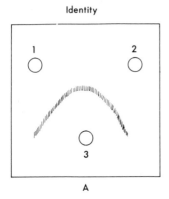

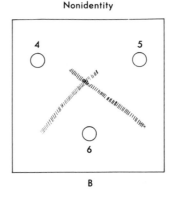

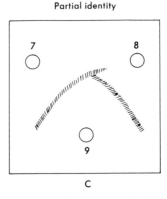

A

B

C

Fig. 15-25. Double diffusion precipitin reactions in agar gel illustrating reactions of identity, nonidentity, and partial identity. In **A** the same Ag was placed in wells 1 and 2, and the antiserum was in well 3. In **B** different Ags were placed in wells 4 and 5, and antisera to both were placed in well 6. In **C** an Ag and its antiserum were placed in wells 7 and 9, respectively, and a cross-reacting Ag was placed in well 8.

placed in two adjacent wells and the corresponding Ab is placed in the center well, the two precipitin bands eventually join at their contiguous ends and fuse (Fig. 15-25A). This pattern, known as the **reaction of identity,** is seen whenever indistinguishable Ab-Ag systems react in adjacent fields. If, on the other hand, unrelated Ags are placed in adjacent wells and diffuse toward a central well that contains Abs for each, the two precipitin bands form independently of each other and cross (**reaction of nonidentity,** Fig. 15-25B). If, however, the Ag in one of the wells and the antiserum in the central well constitute a homologous pair, and the Ag in an adjoining well is a cross-reacting Ag, the precipitation bands fuse, but in addition form a spur-like projection that extends toward the cross-reacting Ag (**reaction of partial identity** or **cross-reaction,** Fig. 15-25C). From what is known of precipitin reactions in liquid the spur can be readily interpreted: it represents the reaction between homologous Ag and those Ab molecules that do **not** combine with the cross-reacting Ag and hence diffuse past its precipitation band. Since these non-cross-reacting Abs represent only a fraction of the total Ab involved in the homologous precipitin reaction (see Figs. 15-18 and 15-19, for example), the spur is usually less dense than the band from which it projects and tends to have increased curvature toward the antiserum well (Fig. 15-25C).

In the event that neither of the Ags is homologous with respect to the antiserum (i.e., neither is the immunogen) a pattern of partial identity might be observed, with the spur projecting toward the less reactive Ag; or there might be partial fusion with two crossing spurs, indicating that some Abs react only with one of the cross-reacting Ags and

Fig. 15-26. The use of purified Ags to identify components of a complex series of precipitin bands. The center well (AS) contains rabbit antiserum prepared against unfractionated human serum. Wells a and c contain human serum; well b has purified human serum albumin (HSA); and well d has a purified human immunoglobulin (HIg). Thus, bands 4 and 6 correspond to HIg and HSA, respectively.

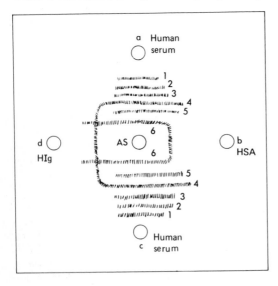

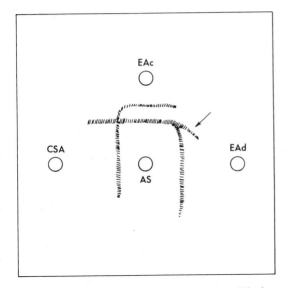

Fig. 15-27. An example of the use of gel diffusion to discriminate between two types of cross-reactions. In liquid medium an antiserum (AS) prepared against crystallized chicken ovalbumin (EAc) precipitates copiously with EAc and less well with crystallized duck ovalbumin (EAd; see Fig. 15-19); it also precipitates slightly with crystallized chicken serum albumin (CSA). From the gel precipitin pattern shown it is concluded that 1) EAc is contaminated with CSA, hence the antiserum contains some antibodies to CSA; 2) CSA and the main component of EAc are unrelated antigenically (reaction of nonidentity); and 3) some antigenic determinants of EAd are similar to or identical with some determinants of EAc (reaction of partial identity). The Abs that cause the spur (arrow) are those that in the quantitative precipitin reaction of Figure 15-19 precipitate with EAc but not with EAd.

some only with the other. Unless inspected carefully for attenuation and curvature of the spurs, double spur formation can be mistakenly interpreted to mean that the adjacent systems are unrelated.

As in diffusion in one dimension, if one well contains a mixture of different Ags and the facing well contains Abs to several of them, the number of bands formed between the wells represents the minimum number of Ab-Ag systems involved. These bands may be identified if the appropriate pure Ags are placed in adjacent wells, as illustrated in Figure 15-26.

Double diffusion in two dimensions provides a simple means for evaluating, to a limited extent, the basis for cross-reactions observed in liquid media. Thus, of the several

classes of cross-reactions discussed earlier, that which arises from a common impurity can usually be recognized unambiguously, as is shown in Figure 15-27. On the other hand, when two purified Ags, such as chicken and duck ovalbumins (Fig. 15-19), give rise to a cross-reaction it is not possible by gel diffusion analysis to decide whether their common determinant groups are identical or only similar; in both cases partial fusion would be observed, with projection of the spur toward the cross-reacting Ag (Fig. 15-27).

Because rates of diffusion vary inversely with molecular weight, the curvature of the precipitin band also provides a clue to the molecular weight of the Ag (provided Ag and Ab are present in roughly equivalent amounts). If the Ag and Ab have about the same molecular weight the precipitation band appears as a straight line; if the Ag has a higher molecular weight the band is concave toward the Ag source; and if the Ag is of lower molecular weight the band is concave toward the Ab reservoir.

Radial Immunodiffusion. This procedure is carried out in a layer of agar (e.g., on a glass slide) containing a uniformly dispersed monospecific antiserum. Diffusion of Ag from a well cut in the agar leads to the formation of a ring of precipitation, whose diameter is proportional to the initial concentration of the Ag (Fig. 15-28). From the results obtained with known concentrations a calibration curve is constructed, permitting quantitation of the concentration of the Ag. This simple procedure has been widely adopted for measurement of many Ags (e.g., immunoglobulins in diverse biological fluids).

IMMUNOELECTROPHORESIS

By combining electrophoresis with precipitation in agar, Grabar and Williams developed a simple but exceedingly powerful method for identifying Ags in complex mixtures (Fig. 15-29). The mixture of Ags is introduced into a small well in agar that has been cast on a plate, say an ordinary microscope slide. By applying an electric field across the plate for 1 to 2 hours the proteins are made to migrate, each according to its own electrophoretic mobility. The electric gradient is then discontinued, and antiserum is introduced into a trough whose long axis

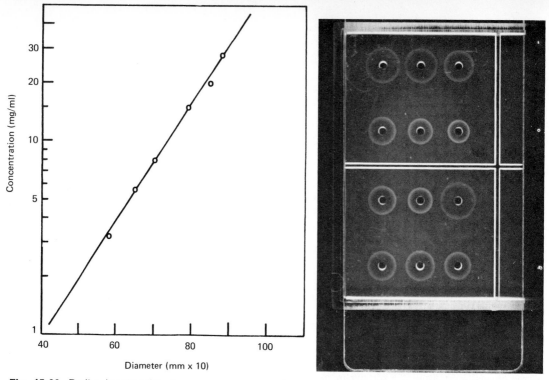

Fig. 15-28. Radial immunodiffusion measurement of Ag concentrations. A standard preparation of Ag, human immunoglobulin G (HIgG), was added at six different concentrations to wells in agar containing goat antiserum to HIgG (upper panel). The diameters of the resulting circular precipitates are plotted on the left. The lower panel (rignt) shows six human sera with different concentrations of HIgG. (Courtesy of Dr. C. Kirk Osterland.)

Fig. 15-29. Immunoelectrophoresis. **A.** A thin layer of agar gel (ca. 1 to 2 mm) covers a glass slide, and a small well near the center (marked origin) receives a solution containing various Ags. After electrophoresis of the Ags the current is discontinued and antiserum is added to the trough. Precipitation bands form as in double diffusion in two dimensions. The apex of each precipitin band corresponds to the center of the corresponding Ag. **B.** Human serum, placed at the origin, was analyzed with an antiserum prepared against unfractionated human serum. (Courtesy of Dr. Curtis Williams.)

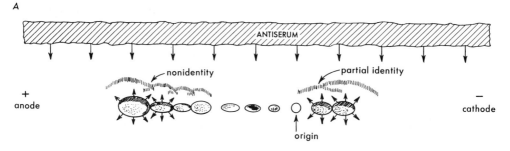

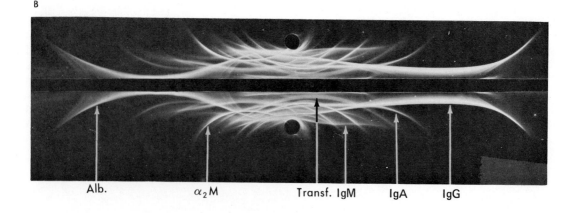

parallels the axis of electrophoretic migration. The Abs and Ags now diffuse toward each other, and precipitin bands form at the intersection of their diffusion fronts. The principles involved in the precipitation stage are those described above: the familiar reactions of identity, nonidentity, and partial identity may be seen.

Immunoelectrophoresis has revealed as many as 30 different Ags in human serum. Many applications of this method appear in subsequent chapters.

REACTIONS WITH PARTICULATE ANTIGENS

THE AGGLUTINATION REACTION

Bacterial and other cells in suspension are usually clumped (agglutinated) when mixed with antisera prepared against them. The principles involved are fundamentally the same as those described above for reactions with soluble Ags. Nevertheless, agglutination requires special consideration, for it is widely used as a simple and rapid method for identifying various bacteria, fungi, and types of erythrocytes; and, conversely, with the use of known cells it provides a simple test to detect and roughly quantitate Abs in sera.

Mechanisms of Agglutination. Agglutination is carried out in physiological salt solution (0.15 M NaCl). The ionic strength is important, for at neutral pH bacteria ordinarily bear a net negative surface charge which must be adequately damped by counter-ions before cells can approach each other closely enough for Ab molecules to form specific bridges between them. Hence even with Abs bound specifically to bacterial cell surfaces agglutination may not occur if the salt concentration is too low (e.g., $< 10^{-3}$ M NaCl). Conversely, the addition of sufficient salt can lead to agglutination even in the absence of Abs.

When a mixture of readily distinguishable particles, such as nucleated avian erythrocytes and nonnucleated mammalian erythrocytes, is added to a mixture of their respective antisera, each clump that forms consists of cells of one or the other type (Ch. 16, Fig. 16-10). Thus, as expected from the lattice theory (above), **each cell-Ab system agglutinates independently of the others in the same mixture.** The basic similarity between agglutination and precipitation is also brought out by the quantitative agglutination reaction, which measures the amount of Ab adsorbed by bacteria; e.g., the maximum amount taken up by encapsulated pneumococci is identical with the maximum amount precipitated from the same volume of serum by the cells' isolated, soluble capsular polysaccharide (see Unitarian hypothesis, below).

Titration of Sera. The agglutination reaction is widely used as a semiquantitative assay. A given volume of a cell suspension is added to a series of tubes, each with the same volume of antiserum at a different dilution, usually increasing in twofold steps. The reaction is speeded up by shaking and warming to 37° (sometimes to 56°); then, after the cells have been allowed to settle, or have been centrifuged lightly, the clumping is detected by direct inspection. The relative strength of an antiserum is expressed as the reciprocal of the highest dilution that causes agglutination. If, for example, a 1:512 dilution gives perceptible agglutination but a 1:1024 dilution does not, the titer is 512.

Agglutination titers are not precise ($\pm 100\%$), but they are easily obtained and provide valid indications of the **relative** Ab concentrations of various sera with respect to a particular strain of bacteria. Hence agglutination titrations are of immense practical value in following changes in Ab titer during the course of acute bacterial infections (see below, Diagnostic application of serological tests).

Agglutination titers obtained with **different** sera and their respective Ags are, however, not necessarily comparable: for example, an antiserum to type 1 pneumococcus with 1.5 mg of Ab per milliliter agglutinated these organisms at a dilution of 1:800, while an antiserum to type 1R pneumococcus with 9.6 mg of Ab per milliliter agglutinated the latter organisms to a titer of only 1:80. Apparently the number and distribution of determinant groups on the bacterial cell surface can markedly influence titer.

Agglutination reactions are, in principle, neither more nor less specific than other serological reactions. However, they present difficulties in actual practice because a cell surface possesses a great diversity of antigenic determinants, of which some will usually cross-react with different but related cells. Hence in order to achieve a high level of specificity it is nearly always necessary to adsorb antisera with sufficient amounts of appropriate cross-reacting cells.

Surface vs. Internal Antigens of Cells. When a bacterial, fungal, or alien animal cell is introduced as an "immunogen" it is broken up in the host animal and many of its surface and internal components (of cytoplasm and nucleus) are immunogenic. However, the Abs that cause agglutination are those specific for surface determinants, which are often called **agglutinogens** (i.e., they induce formation of **agglutinins,** the agglutinating Abs). Surface Ags are much more potent immunogenically when administered as part of a morphologically intact cell that when given in purified form, possibly because in the former condition they are more likely to facilitate interactions among precursors of Ab-forming cells (Ch. 17, Immunogenicity).

Prozone. By analogy with the precipitin reaction it would be expected that agglutinating activity would decrease progressively with dilution of an antiserum. Curiously, however, some sera give effective agglutination reactions only when diluted several hundred- or thousandfold: when undiluted or slightly diluted they do not visibly react with the Ag. The latter region of the titration is called the **prozone,** as in tubes 1 to 3 below.

Tube No.	1	2	3	4	5	6	7	8	9
Serum dilution	1:8	1:16	1:32	1:64	1:128	1:256	1:512	1:1024	1:2048
Clumping	0	0	0	+	+	+	+	+	0

By means of labeled Abs, or the antiglobulin test described below, it can be shown that unagglutinated cells in the prozone actually have Abs adsorbed on their surface. Indeed, it might be expected, on statistical grounds, that when Ab molecules are in great excess relative to the number of functional groups on the cells, the simultaneous attachment of both sites of individual bivalent Ab molecules to different cells would be improbable. Nevertheless, the prozone phenomenon is not due simply to Ab excess, but often involves special blocking or incomplete Abs.

BLOCKING OR INCOMPLETE ANTIBODIES

In certain sera with a pronounced prozone a portion of the total Ab appears to react with Ag particles in an anomalous manner: the bound Ab not only fails to elicit agglutination but actively inhibits it, as shown by subsequently mixing the particles with antiserum at a dilution that would otherwise evoke a brisk clumping reaction. These inhibitory Ab molecules are referred to as **blocking** or **incomplete** Abs, and they are particularly evident in certain human antierythrocyte sera (anti-Rh; see Ch. 21). Some sera, in fact, contain only blocking Abs; their presence is revealed by the ability to inhibit specifically a standard agglutinating mixture.

Blocking Abs were once thought to be univalent. However, they must be bivalent, because they can agglutinate the cells to which they are adsorbed if the reaction is carried out under special conditions, e.g., in the presence of serum albumin at high concentration (instead of in conventional salt solutions) or if the red cells are first treated with a proteolytic enzyme (trypsin or ficin). It is possible that blocking Abs can engage in monogamous binding (to repeating antigenic groups of the cell surface), like some nonprecipitating Abs in the precipitin reaction. (Some entirely different Abs are also called "blocking Abs" for a different reason: they seem to protect the cells on which they are adsorbed against destructive attack by specifically reactive lymphocytes; see Chs. 20, 21, Enhancement in tumor immunity and in allograft reaction.)

The Antiglobulin Test. An ingenious method for detecting incomplete or blocking Abs,

Fig. 15-30. The antiglobulin (Coombs) test for incomplete Abs. Cells coated with specifically bound, incomplete (nonagglutinating) Abs are clumped by other Ab molecules (from another species), which react specifically with antigenic determinants of the incomplete Abs.

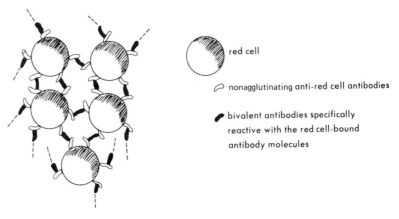

○ red cell

⌒ nonagglutinating anti-red cell antibodies

▰ bivalent antibodies specifically reactive with the red cell-bound antibody molecules

called the Coombs or antiglobulin test, is of considerable importance in the recognition of certain hemolytic diseases. The test exploits the ability of Ab molecules to participate simultaneously in binding to an Ag on the red cell surface and in complexing with Ab to itself (Fig. 15-30). As we shall see subsequently (Ch. 16), Abs are highly immunogenic in a foreign species.

For example, rabbits injected with human immunoglobulins (HIg) form anti-HIg that reacts with most HIg molecules, regardless of their specificities as Abs (Ch. 16). Hence erythrocytes with incomplete human Abs bound specifically to their surface can be agglutinated by rabbit anti-HIg serum. Since an Ab molecule can function both as an Ab and as a ligand in two independent and simultaneous reactions, the ligand-binding sites of Abs must be different from, or represent only a fraction of, their numerous and diverse antigenic determinant groups (Ch. 16).

PASSIVE AGGLUTINATION

In the agglutination reactions described above the functional ligand groups are components of cell wall or cell surface membrane. It has also been possible to extend the agglutination reaction to a wide variety of soluble Ags by attaching them to the surface of particles. In such **passive agglutination** reactions the particles most widely used are erythrocytes **(passive hemagglutination),** a synthetic polymer such as polystyrene, or a mineral colloid such as bentonite. Adsorption ordinarily depends on noncovalent bonds and is generally achieved by simply mixing the particles with

the Ags. Thus erythrocytes readily adsorb many polysaccharides. For the attachment of proteins, however, it is usually necessary first to treat the cells with **tannic acid** or chromic chloride (whose mechanisms of action are not established). Covalent linkage of proteins to the red cell surface has also been achieved by the use of bifunctional cross-linking reagents (Fig. 15-31).

As in conventional agglutination tests, passive agglutination is highly sensitive (see below), but its precision is low (at best ± 100%); and Ab levels are measured only in relative terms, not in weight units.

Inhibition of passive agglutination provides a sensitive assay for Ags, and it has been widely used for this purpose to measure certain hormones in plasma and urine (e.g., urinary chorionic gonadotropin in a rapid test for pregnancy). For example, polystyrene particles or tanned red cells with an adsorbed purified protein or polypeptide hormone can be agglutinated by the corresponding antiserum; and added free ligand specifically inhibits agglutination by competing for Ab. Thus, by comparison with standard Ag solutions, the concentration of Ag in biological fluids, e.g., blood or urine, can be evaluated (see Radioimmunoassays, below).

DIFFERENCES IN SENSITIVITY OF PRECIPITATION, AGGLUTINATION, AND OTHER REACTIONS

The methods used for measuring Ab levels differ considerably in the minimal amounts of Ab that can be detected and measured. Of the two considered so far in this chapter, aggluti-

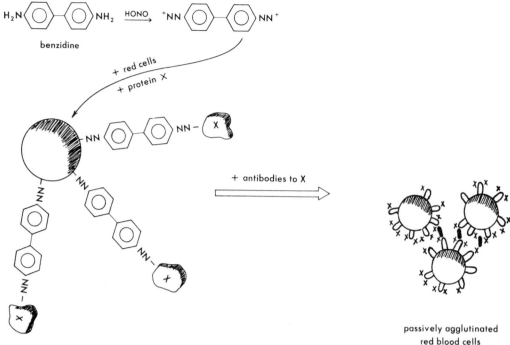

Fig. 15-31. Passive hemagglutination. Bis-diazotized benzidine is used to attach protein X to the red cell surface. Red cells coated with X are specifically clumped by anti-X Abs. The antiglobulin test shown in Figure 15-30 may be regarded as another form of passive hemagglutination, the Ag attached to the red cell surface being an adsorbed, noncovalently bound, incomplete Ab molecule. Besides benzidine, a variety of other bifunctional reagents have been used, e.g., toluene-2,4-diisocyanate (Fig. 15-37).

nation is considerably more sensitive than precipitation: the relatively voluminous particle, coated with a thin layer of Ag, serves to **amplify** the reaction.

Thus, precipitin reactions in liquid media or gels are usually not observed when antisera are diluted more than ten- to fiftyfold, while many antisera to bacteria or red blood cells retain agglutinating activity after being diluted many thousandfold. Passive agglutination, especially passive hemagglutination, is particularly sensitive: some mouse antisera to hemocyanin have titers of almost 10^5.

The difference in sensitivity is clearly illustrated when agglutination and precipitation involve the same Ag. In one instance, for example, an antiserum to hen ovalbumin (EA) lost ability to precipitate EA when diluted 1:5, but at 1:10,000 dilution it could still agglutinate collodion particles coated with EA. These large differences are probably related to the difference in the number of particles needed for a visible reaction; e.g., about 10^7 bacterial cells (corresponding to perhaps 10^9 surface Ag mole-cules), but about 6×10^{12} molecules of soluble Ag (1 μg of a protein of MW 100,000). The sensitivities of some routine assay methods for Abs are compared in Table 15-5.

TABLE 15-5. Minimal Concentrations of Antibody Detectable by Various Quantitative and Semi-Quantitative Methods
(Approximate Values)

Method	μg antibody/ml
Precipitin reactions in liquid media	20
Precipitin reactions in agar gel	60
Bacterial agglutination	0.1
Passive hemagglutination	0.01
Complement fixation*	1
Passive cutaneous anaphylaxis†	0.02
Phage neutralization‡	0.001–0.0001

* See Chapter 18.
† See Chapter 19.
‡ See Rates of reaction, above, this chapter.

RADIOIMMUNOASSAYS

The most versatile and sensitive of the various assays that use Ags or haptens with radioactive labels was introduced by Berson and Yalow for measurement of serum insulin concentrations. The method, which can measure trace concentrations of any substance that can serve as Ag or hapten (Table 15-6), is based on competition for Ab between a standard radioactive indicator ligand (*L) and its unlabeled counterpart (L) at unknown concentration in the test sample: the higher the concentration of unlabeled competitor the lower the ratio of bound (B) to unbound or free (F) indicator (B/F). Specific precipitates do not form even if the ligand is multivalent, because Ags and ligands are used at exceedingly low concentrations. Nevertheless, bound and free ligands are readily separated (and counted) by using either special technics for particular ligands (e.g., chromatography, electrophesis, adsorption of certain free ligands on talc) or the general method in which soluble Ab-*L complexes are specifically precipitated with antisera to the Ab moiety of the immune complex (Fig. 15-32).

The double Ab approach is feasible because, as noted before, the Abs of one species (donor) are usually immunogenic in other species: the resulting antisera (anti-antibodies) react with essentially all Abs of the donor species, regardless of their ligand-binding specificities (e.g., rabbit antihuman immunoglobulins in the antiglobulin test,

above; see also Ch. 16). The concentration of unlabeled ligand in the test sample is determined by comparison with the inhibitory effect of known standards (Fig. 15-33).

In the double Ab reaction the first Ab (antiligand) is added at a level that enhances competition between labeled and unlabeled ligand, i.e., the Ab/L ratio corresponds to the Ag-excess side of the equivalence zone in a liquid precipitin reaction (see Fig. 15-8). The second Ab (anti-Ab) is introduced in excess to ensure complete precipitation of the first Ab and its complexes with ligand (i.e., Ab-excess side of the equivalence zone in Fig. 15-8). The method is exceedingly discriminating because it is possible to choose antisera with great specificity for the test ligand. Its sensitivity is limited only by the amount of radioactivity that can be introduced into the indicator ligand: with carrier-free radioactive iodine as extrinsic label it is possible to detect ligands at almost the picogram level (e.g., at ca. 10^{-10} gm). However, the method is sometimes limited by difficulty in determining whether the inhibitor in the unknown is identical with the radioactive indicator or only similar enough to cross-react.

Ammonium Sulfate Precipitation. Abs and soluble Ag-ligand complexes are precipitated by ammonium sulfate at high concentration (40% of saturation), but many unbound ligands are soluble at this ionic strength. Hence addition of the salt at this concentration to a mixture of Ab and radioactive ligand can provide a measure of bound ligand if the specific

TABLE 15-6. Substances Measured by Radioimmunoassays: A Partial List

Insulin	Testosterone
Growth hormone	Estradiol
Parathyroid hormone	Aldosterone
Adrenocorticotropic hormone	Intrinsic factor (see Ch. 20)
Glucagon	Digitalis
Secretin	Cyclic AMP (cAMP), cGMP, cIMP, cUMP
Vasopressin	Prostaglandins
Bradykinin (see Ch. 19)	Australia antigen (see Ch. 16)
Thyroglobulin	Carcinoembryonic antigen (see Ch. 21)
Gastrin	Human IgE (see Ch. 19)
Calcitonin	Morphine

Each substance corresponds to ligand X in Figure 15-32. The same principle has been applied in nonimmune assays, in which Abs are replaced by particular proteins; for example, vitamin B_{12} is measured by its binding to intrinsic factor.

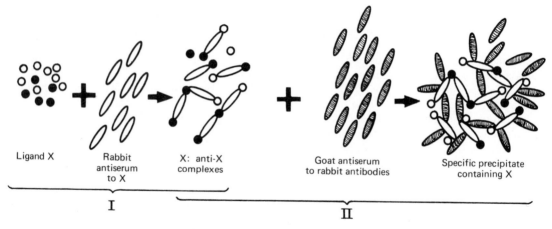

Ligand X   Rabbit   X: anti-X   Goat antiserum   Specific precipitate
            antiserum   complexes   to rabbit antibodies   containing X
            to X

I

II

Fig. 15-32. Radioimmunoassay. The Ab-ligand complexes formed in step I are separated from unbound ligand by specific precipitation in step II with goat antiserum prepared against rabbit Abs. The effect of competition between labeled (●) and unlabeled (O) ligand molecules is illustrated in Figure 15-33.

binding reaction does not depend on ionic interactions (i.e., is not affected by high ionic strength). This approach has been used in the **Farr technic** to measure Ab concentrations in serum: by titrating the serum sample with increasing amounts of labeled ligand (or testing the ligand with increasing dilutions of the antiserum) the **Ag-binding capacity** of the serum can be established: 1 nmole of bound ligand is equivalent to 75 μg of Ab (i.e., one occupied site in Ab corresponds to half the molecular weight of

150,000, see Fig. 15-2). This approach has also been used with radioactive univalent ligands to estimate intrinsic association constants. Even though the high salt concentration might modify the over-all Ab structure (e.g., cause the molecule to become highly insoluble) the ligand-binding site seems to be largely unperturbed: under these conditions the affinity for at least some ligands has been close to that measured in solution by equilibrium dialysis (see above).

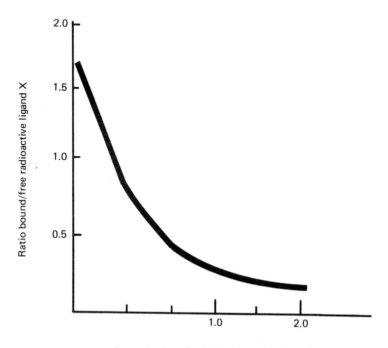

Fig. 15-33. Calibration curve for a radioimmunoassay. A fixed amount of radioiodine-labeled ligand X competes with various amounts of unlabeled ligand X for a limiting amount of anti-X Abs.

FLUORESCENCE AND IMMUNE REACTIONS

The fluorescent* properties of Ab molecules and of certain organic residues that can be attached to them provide the basis for a number of analytical methods. The most important of these is called **immunofluorescence.** Introduced by Coons, this method is widely used for rapid identification of bacteria in infected materials and for the identification

and localization of cellular Ags (and Abs, Ch. 17).

IMMUNOFLUORESCENCE

Of the several reagents that introduce fluorescent groups into proteins, the most widely used with Abs is fluorescein isothiocyanate (Fig. 15-34). Abs substituted with one or two fluorescein residues per molecule are intensely fluorescent but retain their specific reactivity; e.g., they can specifically bind to bacteria in smears and tissue sections. After a specimen on a slide has been covered for several minutes with a solution of fluorescein-labeled Abs (usually in the form of the globulin fraction of an antiserum), the slide is rinsed to remove

---

* When molecules absorb light they subsequently dispose of their increased energy by various means, one of which is the emission of light of longer wave length. When the emission is of short duration (10^{-8} to 10^{-9} seconds for return of the excited molecule to the ground state) the process is called **fluorescence.** (When the emission is of long duration the process is called phosphorescence.)

Fig. 15-34. Immunofluorescence. The fluorescent isothiocyanates **(1)** form thioureas, substituted with the fluorescent group and ε-NH$_2$ groups of lysine residues of Abs or other proteins **(2)**. In the **direct** staining reaction **(3)** the labeled Abs are specific for the Ag of interest. In the **indirect** reaction **(4)** the labeled Abs are specific for the Abs of another species (e.g., goat anti-rabbit immunoglobulin; see Ch. 16).

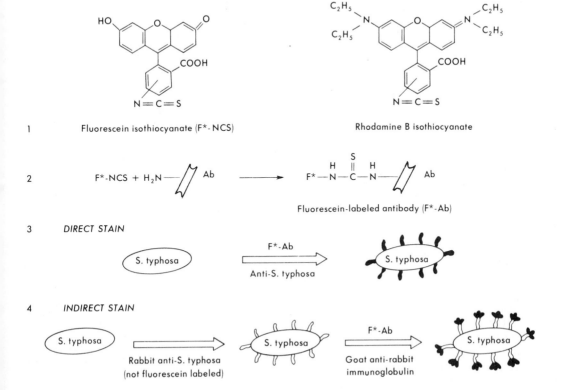

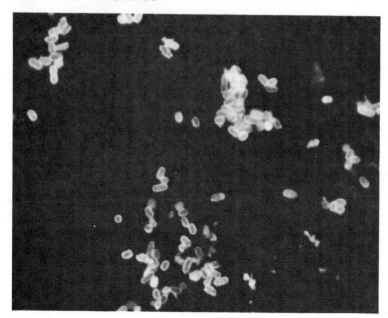

Fig. 15-35. Immunofluorescence staining. Stained with a fluorescein-labeled globulin fraction of a specific antiserum, *E. coli* 0127:B8 is clearly visible in a fecal smear from a patient with infantile diarrhea. Many other types of bacteria are abundant in the smear but are not stained. Ca. × 1000. (Photograph supplied by National Communicable Disease Center, Atlanta.)

unbound fluorescent protein and then is examined in the light microscope, with suitable light source and filters to provide the proper incident light. Since the emitted light (about 530 nm) is of longer wave length than the background incident light (about 490 nm), the Ab-coated cell stands out as a sharply visible yellow-green mass (Fig. 15-35).

As with all immunological reactions it is necessary to establish specificity with suitable controls. Thus staining should be blocked by preliminary treatment of the smear or tissue section with unlabeled Abs (to saturate antigenic sites) and by addition of excess soluble Ag (to saturate the labeled Abs).

Fluorescein-labeled Abs can be used in both direct and indirect reaction sequences, outlined in Figure 15-34, for the detection and localization of a wide variety of Ags. The indirect reaction both amplifies the response and permits one labeled preparation to be used as a stain for a wide variety of serologically specific reactions.

Different chromophores can be introduced into Abs with other reagents, e.g., orange-red fluorescence with rhodamine B isothiocyanate (Fig. 15-34). This modification provides opportunities for applying immunofluorescence to a number of special problems, e.g., to the possible coexistence of different Abs in the same cell (Ch. 17, Antibody formation).

In all these applications a recurrent problem arises from the nonspecific staining of tissues, especially by labeled proteins with more than two or three fluorescein residues per molecule. To minimize this difficulty ion-exchange chromatography and adsorption with acetone-dried tissue powders are used to remove the more highly substituted proteins. In addition, the use of high-titer antisera (e.g., > 2 mg of Ab per milliliter) reduces nonspecific staining by making it possible to use dilute solutions of labeled protein.

FLUORESCENCE QUENCHING

Like other proteins, unlabeled Ab molecules fluoresce in the upper ultraviolet region by virtue of their aromatic amino acid residues. Ab fluorescence is excited maximally at 290 nm and the emitted light has maximal intensity at about 345 nm (characteristic of the absorption and emission spectrum of tryptophan). When the binding sites in the Ab are specifically occupied by certain kinds of haptens (or Ags) the energy absorbed by the irradiated tryptophan residues is transferred to the bound ligand, which emits light at some still longer wave length or does not fluoresce at all. The net result is quenching or damping of the Ab's characteristic fluorescence. Thus the binding sites of a preparation of purified Abs can be titrated as shown in Figure 15-36; and the titrations can be used to calculate average intrinsic association constants, which agree with those determined by equilibrium dialysis. Quenching is particularly effective with those ligands whose absorption spectrum overlaps the protein's

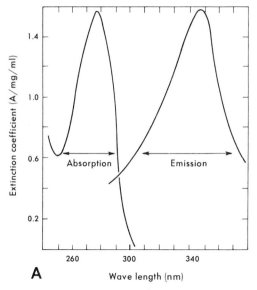

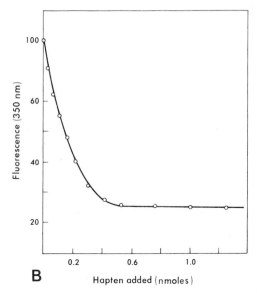

Fig. 15-36. Fluorescence quenching. **A.** Absorption and emission spectra of a purified Ab, specific for the 2,4-dinitrophenyl group. The height of the emission band maximum is set, by convention, equal to that of the absorption maximum, though only about 20% of the energy absorbed by Abs appears as fluorescence emission. **B.** Decline in fluorescence of the Ab as it binds ε-Dnp-lysine; about 75% of the fluorescence is quenched when the Ab's ligand-binding sites are saturated. [From Velick, S. F., Parker, C. W., and Eisen, H. N. *Proc Natl Acad Sci USA 46*:1470 (1960).]

emission spectrum; but the overlap need not be extensive.

The fluorescence quenching method is not as generally useful as equilibrium dialysis, since many haptens, such as simple sugars, do not quench. However, the method offers a number of advantages: it is rapid, requires only small amounts of Ab, and can be carried out with ligands that are too large to be dialyzable (for example, cytochrome c quenches Ab to cytochrome c).

FLUORESCENCE POLARIZATION

When fluorescent molecules are excited by a beam of polarized light the extent of polarization of the emitted light varies with the molecule's size: emission from small molecules, with much rotational motion, exhibits little polarization. If, however, the fluorescent molecule is bound to a relatively large particle, such as an Ab molecule, its rotational movement is restricted and the polarization of its fluorescence is increased. Hence the proportion of

ligand molecules bound by Abs can be determined from the polarization of fluorescent emission. This method is potentially useful with those small Ags and haptens whose fluorescence spectrum (natural or introduced by fluorescent substituents) is distinctly different from that of Abs (see Fluorescence quenching, above).

FLUORESCENCE ENHANCEMENT

Certain small organic molecules, such an anilinonaphthalenesulfonates, have strikingly different fluorescence spectra when they exist as free molecules in water and when bound in the active sites of Abs, which have a much lower dielectric constant than water. It is thus possible to measure the specific binding of such ligands to the corresponding Abs by following the appearance of fluorescence at the appropriate wave length. The method is exquisitely sensitive and can be used with Abs in complex media, such as serum.

DIAGNOSTIC APPLICATIONS OF SEROLOGICAL TESTS

The etiological diagnosis of infectious diseases is usually established both by isolating the putative causative microorganism and by demonstrating Abs to it. Several principles are involved in the diagnostic use of serological tests.

Changing Titer. The Ab formation initiated by an infectious agent may continue for months or even years after the clinically apparent infection has subsided. Hence the presence of an elevated titer of Abs to a given microbe indicates only that infection (or vaccination) has occurred at some time in the past. In order to establish that an acute illness is due to a particular agent it is desirable to show a **change** in titer to that agent during the illness, i.e., the absence (or low level) of detectable Abs during the first week, their appearance and progressive increase in titer during the second and subsequent weeks, and perhaps their eventual decline. For practical purposes a pair of serum samples is compared, one drawn in the acute phase of the illness, the other during convalescence. If only a single serum sample is available, from late in the illness, a high titer is sometimes accepted as provisional diagnostic evidence; the critical level depends on the disease and the assay, and it is necessary to be sure that the high titer is not the result of prior vaccination.

Identification of Etiological Agent. Even when no likely agent has been isolated, a provisional etiological diagnosis can be established by testing the serum with Ags from microbial strains under suspicion: the Ag that elicits the highest titer reaction is assumed to be from the etiological agent. This procedure can be misleading: thus other Ags, not tested, might have elicited a still higher titer. Moreover, some curious cross-reactions between very different microorganisms may also serve

to mislead: in a classic example persons with rickettsial infections form Abs that react in high titer with certain *Proteus* strains (Ch. 38, Weil-Felix reaction).

Time-Course of Immune Response in Infectious Disease. In the course of a given infectious disease the appearance and the persistence of Abs to the etiological agent follow a different time course when measured with different antigenic preparations and different assays. In brucellosis, for example, agglutination titers appear early in infection and persist at low levels for years afterward, whereas precipitin levels appear later and disappear much sooner; and in many rickettsial and viral diseases the Ab titers measured by complement fixation (Ch. 18) appear later and subside sooner than those measured by neutralization of infectivity (Ch. 50).

A number of possibilities can account for these variations. 1) The many Ags in a microbe differ in amount, immunogenicity, and stability in the animal host. 2) There are structural and functional differences in the Abs specific for a given antigenic determinant, and different types of Abs are formed at different stages of the immune response, e.g., IgM Abs (Ch. 16) are formed early in the response and are especially effective in the agglutination assay (Ch. 17, Antibody formation). 3) The various serological methods differ in their sensitivity (Table 15-5), and a method that requires less Ab will, other things being equal, detect Ab earlier and more persistently. Though the basis for the differences between different assays is not always clear, it is important for practical purposes to be aware that such differences exist.

THE UNITARIAN HYPOTHESIS

In the last decade of the nineteenth century immunologists were confronted in rapid succession by discoveries of a bewildering variety of immune phenomena. Particularly impressive, no doubt, was the extraordinary diversity of activities displayed by a given antiserum. A serum prepared, for example, against the cholera vibrio could 1) protect guinea pigs against an otherwise lethal infection with virulent cholera vibrios, 2) agglutinate a suspension of these organisms, 3) form a precipitate with a filtrate of the broth in which they had grown, 4) specifically enhance their phagocytosis by leukocytes, etc. This wide range of phenomena gave rise to the prevailing **pluralistic** view, according to

which each of these diverse activities was ascribed to a qualitatively different molecular form, named agglutinins, precipitins, opsonins (promoters of phagocytosis), protective antibodies, etc.

With the improved methods of analysis developed in the 1930s, however, this view became clearly untenable. For example, Heidelberger found that all the Ab activities of antiserum to type 3 pneumococci were removed by precipitation with the organism's purified capsular polysaccharide; and the protein subsequently isolated from the precipitate duplicated the diverse activities of the antiserum. Moreover, this capsular polysaccharide is a polymer of cellobiuronic acid (Fig. 15-18); and Avery and

Goebel found that a cross-reacting antiserum, prepared against a conjugated protein substituted with the *p*-azobenzyl ether of cellobiuronic acid, not only precipitated the type 3 polysaccharide and agglutinated type 3 cells, but also protected mice against lethal infection with these organisms.

From these and similar observations there emerged the **unitarian hypothesis,** according to which a given population of Abs will, on uniting with the corresponding ligand, produce any of the diverse consequences of Ab-Ag combination, depending on the state of the ligand and the milieu in which combination takes place: if the ligand is soluble and multivalent, precipitation; if the ligand is a natural constituent of a particle's surface or artificially attached to the surface, agglutination; if the ligand is part of the surface of a virulent bacterium, protection against infection.

These contrasting views may be epitomized by saying that with respect to capacity to elicit the total range of in vivo and in vitro manifestations of Ab-Ag complex formation, the early pluralistic view maintained that a given Ab molecule is **unipotent,** whereas the unitarian view held that the Ab molecule is **totipotent.** While it has been clear since the 1940s that the pluralistic view is not valid, it has also become clear that the unitarian view is a gross oversimplification, e.g., certain Abs do not precipitate their Ags. In subsequent chapters we shall see more striking evidence that among the Ab molecules specific for a given ligand group, some are able to elicit certain reactions (e.g., Anaphylaxis, Ch. 19) and others are not. Though antibodies are multipotent to an impressive degree, they are definitely not totipotent.

APPENDIX

PURIFICATION OF ANTIBODIES

Methods of purifying Abs are based on the dissociability of Ab-ligand complexes. Two stages are usually involved. 1) Abs are precipitated from serum with soluble Ags or adsorbed by insoluble antigenic materials; the latter are often prepared by coupling small haptenic groups or soluble proteins to an insoluble matrix, such as agarose. 2) After extraneous serum is washed away Abs are eluted from the insoluble complexes by specific or nonspecific procedures.

Specific Procedures. With aggregates whose stability depends largely on specific ionic interactions, such as those involving types 3 and 8 pneumococcal polysaccharides (Fig. 15-18), strong salt solutions (e.g., 1.8 M NaCl) elute purified Abs effectively.

When the specific antigenic determinants are simple haptenic groups, such as 2,4-dinitrophenyl, small univalent haptens that encompass the crucial part of the determinant (e.g., 2,4-dinitrophenol) are useful for competitive displacement from the precipitating Ag or adsorbent, yielding soluble Ab-hapten complexes. Depending upon the properties of the Ag, the adsorbent, and the hapten, diverse procedures are then used to isolate the soluble Ab-hapten complexes and finally to separate the hapten from the Ab (e.g., ion-exchange resins, dialysis, gel filtration).

When small univalent haptens are employed for specific elution of Ags it is desirable to use those haptens that are both 1) **weakly bound** by the Ab and 2) **highly soluble.** Highly concentrated solutions of hapten can then be used to elute the Ab in high yield, and the weakly bound hapten is easily sep-

arated from the soluble hapten-Ab complex, e.g., by dialysis or gel filtration.

Nonspecific Procedures. For the isolation of Abs to protein Ags it is usually necessary to expose specific aggregates to conditions that cause reversible denaturation of the Ab, allowing it to dissociate from the Ag. Organic acids at pH 2 to 3 are often effective; various procedures are then used to separate the denatured Ab and Ag, depending upon the properties of the Ag. Since Abs usually regain their native structure on being restored to physiological conditions, neutralization of the Ag-free material yields active Ab, usually without excessive losses due to persistent denaturation.

Yield and Purity. Though Abs can be isolated from serum in high yield (50 to 90%) and with high purity (> 90% of the recovered Abs usually react specifically with Ag) the purified molecules are usually heterogeneous with respect to affinity (see Fig. 15-2) and in many of the physical and chemical properties described in Chapter 16.

FERRITIN-LABELED ANTIBODIES

As noted earlier, fluorescein-labeled Abs provide specific stains for the detection and localization of Ags in the light microscope. For use in the electron microscope Abs must be rendered much more highly electron-scattering than proteins in general, and this can be accomplished by attaching a molecule of ferritin to an Ab molecule. Ferritin, a protein molecule of about the same size as an Ab molecule, has high electron-scattering capacity because of its uniquely high iron content (about

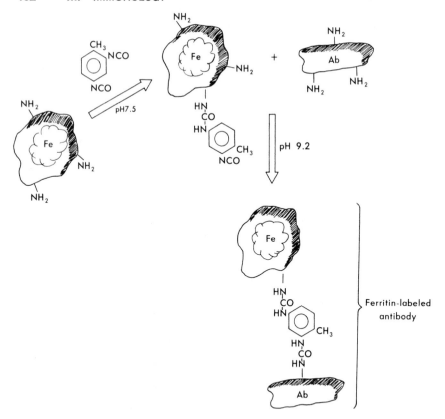

Fig. 15-37. Preparation of ferritin-labeled Ab by reaction with toluene-2,4-diisocyanate. Fe, ferritin. [Based on Singer, S. J., and Schick, A. F. *J Biophys Biochem Cytol 9*:519 (1961).]

20%). Ferritin-Ab conjugates were introduced by Singer, who used a bifunctional reagent to form stable covalent links between the two proteins, as is shown in Figure 15-37.

Ferritin and Hybrid Antibodies. Unmodified ferritin is also useful in conjunction with bivalent "hybrid" Ab molecules in which one combining site is obtained from anti-ferritin Abs and the other site from Abs to an Ag of interest, e.g., a particular cell surface macromolecule. The hybrid Ab can thus link a ferritin molecule (noncovalently) to the Ag target. The preparation of hybrid Abs is described in Chapter 16 and their use with ferritin to stain particular immunoglobulins on mast cells is illustrated in Figure 19-4; the use of hybrid Abs to identify cell surface molecules by light microscopy is given in Chapter 17 (indirect rosettes, Fig. 17-3).

INTRINSIC AND ACTUAL AFFINITIES

The successive steps in the binding of a univalent ligand (L) by a multivalent antibody (B) with n combining sites can be represented by the reactions on the left and their equilibrium constants on the right.

$$B + L \rightleftarrows BL \qquad k_1 = \frac{[BL]}{[B][L]}$$

$$BL + L \rightleftarrows BL_2 \qquad k_2 = \frac{[BL_2]}{[BL][L]}$$

$$\cdots \qquad\qquad \cdots$$

$$BL_{i-1} + L \rightleftarrows BL_i \qquad k_i = \frac{[BL_i]}{[BL_{i-1}][L]} \qquad (10)$$

$$\cdots \qquad\qquad \cdots$$

$$BL_{n-1} + L \rightleftarrows BL_n \qquad k_n = \frac{[BL_n]}{[BL_{n-1}][L]}$$

We wish to find the general expression for the ratio of all bound ligand molecules (L_b) to all Ab molecules (B_t) at equilibrium.

$$L_b = BL + 2BL_2 + 3BL_3 \cdots + iBL_i \cdots + nBL_n, \text{ or}$$
$$= B[k_1 L + 2k_1 k_2 (L)^2 \cdots + ik_1 k_2 \cdots k_i (L)^i \cdots \qquad (11)$$
$$+ nk_1 k_2 \cdots k_n (L)^n]$$

and

$$B_t = B + BL + BL_2 + BL_3 \cdots + BL_i \cdots + BL_n, \text{ or}$$
$$= B[1 + k_1L + k_1k_2(L)^2 \cdots + k_1k_2 \cdots k_i(L)^i \qquad (12)$$
$$\cdots + k_1k_2 \cdots k_n(L)^n]$$

Assume all Ab combining sites are equivalent and independent. Then for the representative step in which the ith site becomes occupied (third step in equation 10), the concentration of vacant Ab sites (S) is:

$$[S] = (n-(i-1)) \, [BL_{i-1}] \qquad (13)$$

and the concentration of occupied sites (SL) is:

$$[SL] = i \, [BL_i] \qquad (14)$$

When equations (13) and (14) are combined, the equilibrium constant for the ith reaction becomes

$$k_i = \frac{n-i+1}{i} \cdot \frac{[SL]}{[S][L]} \qquad (15)$$

[SL]/[S] [L] is defined as K, the **intrinsic association constant**, or the **intrinsic affinity**, for the general reaction in which a representative site binds a ligand molecule (S + L ⇌ SL); i.e.,

$$k_i = \frac{n-i+1}{i} \, K \qquad (16)$$

The constants for the individual steps in equation (10) can thus be expressed in terms of the intrinsic constant (e.g., $k_1 = nK$; $k_2 = (n-1) \, 2 \, K$; $k_n = K/n$; this makes it possible to reduce equations (11) and (12), with the aid of the binomial theorem, to*:

$$L_b = nK[B][L](1 + K[L])^{n-1} \qquad (17)$$

and

$$B_t = [B](1 + K[L])^n \qquad (18)$$

or,

$$\frac{L_b}{B_t} = \frac{nK[L]}{1 + K[L]}$$

Since L_b/B_t is r (moles ligand bound per mole Ab)

and [L] is c (equilibrium concentration of free ligand) we have

$$r = \frac{nKc}{1 + Kc} \qquad (19)$$

which is the same as

$$\frac{r}{c} = Kn - Kr \quad \text{(equation 4)}$$

Intrinsic affinity, K, provides a convenient and rigorous basis for analyzing the function of Ab combining sites and for comparing sites of different Abs with each other and with those of other proteins. However, the multiplicity of binding sites on Ab molecules and on most Ag particles means that for biologically significant Ab-Ag reactions in vivo the actual equilibrium constants can differ greatly from the intrinsic constants. Because most microbes have many identical envelope subunits on their surface, their complexes with Abs probably conform in most instances to Karush's concept of the monogamous complex (above); the equilibrium constants for formation of these complexes can exceed by perhaps 10^5 the intrinsic affinity of their Ab component. The great difference represents a form of statistical cooperativity between sites on the same molecule which is widespread in nature; for example, the bond between a pair of complementary nucleotides (e.g., A-T) is weak but between two polynucleotide strands with many complementary pairs it is enormously greater (Ch. 10).

Even without monogamous binding, actual and intrinsic binding constants are not necessarily the same. For instance, in a reaction that is limited, say by a low level of Ag, to only one site of an Ab molecule that has 2 or 10 sites (lgG vs. lgM, see Ch. 16), the observed equilibrium constant will be 2 and 10 times the respective intrinsic constants (see equation 16). Other things being equal, Ab molecules with more combining sites will form more stable complexes with ligands.

---

* The derivation is due to Dr. B. Altschuler, New York University.

SELECTED REFERENCES

Books and Review Articles

KABAT, E. A. *Kabat and Mayer's Experimental Immunochemistry*, 2nd ed. Thomas, Springfield, Ill., 1961.

KARUSH, F. Immunologic specificity and molecular structure. *Adv Immunol* 2:1 (1962).

LANDSTEINER, K. *The Specificity of Serological Reactions*, rev. ed. Harvard Univ. Press, Cambridge, Mass., 1945. Reprinted by Dover, New York, 1962.

PRESSMAN, D., and GROSSBERG, A. L. *The Structural Basis of Antibody Specificity*. Benjamin, New York, 1968.

WILLIAMS, C. A., and CHASE, M. W. (eds.). *Methods in Immunology and Immunochemistry*, vols I, II, III. Academic Press, New York, 1967, 1968, 1971.

Specific Articles

ARNON, R. A selective fractionation of anti-lysozyme antibodies of different determinant specificities. *Eur J Biochem 5*:583 (1968).

BERSON, S. A., and YALOW, R. S. *Radioimmunoassay: A status Report in Immunobiology*. (R. A. Good and D. W. Fisher, eds.) Sinauer, Stamford, 1971.

EISEN, H. N., and SISKIND, G. W. Variation in affinities of antibodies during the immune response. *Biochemistry 3*:966 (1964).

HAIMOVICH, J., SELA, M., DEWDNEY, J. M., and BATCHELOR, F. R. Anti-penicilloyl antibodies: Detection with penicilloylated bacteriophage and isolation with a specific immunoadsorbent. *Nature 214*:1369 (1967).

HORNICK, C. L., and KARUSH, F. The interaction of hapten-coupled bacteriophage ϕX174 with anti-hapten antibody. *Isr J Med Sci 5*:163 (1969).

KLINMAN, N. R., LONG, C. A., and KARUSH, F. The role of antibody bivalence in the neutralization of bacteriophage. *J Immunol 99*:1128 (1967).

MÄKELÄ, O. Assay of anti-hapten antibody with the aid of hapten-coupled bacteriophage. *Immunol 10*:81 (1966).

PARKER, C. W., GOTT, S. M., and JOHNSON, M. C. The antibody response to a 2,4-dinitrophenyl peptide. *Biochemistry 5*:2314 (1966).

SELA, M., and HAIMOVICH, J. Detection of Proteins with Chemically Modified Bacteriophages. In *Protides of the Biological Fluids*. (H. Peeters, ed.) Pergamon Press, Elmsford, N.Y., 1970.

SELA, M., SCHECHTER, B., SCHECHTER, I., and BOREK, F. Antibodies to sequential and conformational determinants. *Cold Spring Harbor Symp Quant Biol 32*:537 (1967).

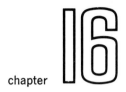

chapter 16

ANTIBODY STRUCTURE: THE IMMUNOGLOBULINS

Though antibodies (Abs) were found early to be a heterogeneous group of proteins (sedimentation constants 7S and 19S), for many years they were regarded simply as "γ-globulins," the class of plasma proteins with least electrophoretic mobility. Thus Tiselius and Kabat showed that the γ-globulin level was increased by intensive immunization and was lowered when Abs were removed from serum by specific precipitation with the corresponding antigen (Ag) (Fig. 16-1). Moreover, purified Abs to various Ags, isolated from specific precipitates, seemed to be indistinguishable from γ-globulins, not only chemically (electrophoretic mobility, solubility, amino acid composition), but also in their reactivity as Ags: for instance, when goats were immunized with γ-globulins from a nonimmune rabbit the resulting antiserum reacted not only with the immunogen but with rabbit Abs of diverse specificities. Some of the electrophoretically faster moving serum proteins also exhibit Ab activity; and many γ-globulins lack activity, probably because they are specific for unidentified ligands. Accordingly, **all proteins that function as antibodies or that have antigenic determinants in common with antibodies are now called immunoglobulins (abbreviated Igs).**

All Igs have a similar structural organization, but they are an immensely diversified family that can be arranged into groups and subgroups on the basis of variations in antigenic properties and amino acid sequences. In this chapter we emphasize the relations between these structural features and the two kinds of functions that are characteristic of every Ab molecule: 1) **specific** binding of one or a few of an almost limitless variety of ligands, and 2) regardless of this specificity, participation in a limited number of **general or effector reactions,** e.g., complement fixa-

tion (Ch. 18), allergic responses (Ch. 19). As we shall see, the two functions are carried out by different parts of the Ab molecule.

Three categories of antigenic determinants are used to classify Igs. 1) Those that differentiate among the main Ig classes are the same in all normal individuals of a given species: they are called isotypic determinants or **isotypes** (Gr. *iso* = same). Various isotypes are associated with different effector functions (see Appendix, Table 16-5), but they are essentially unrelated to ligand-binding activity; thus Abs of diverse Ig classes can be specific for the same antigen (Ag). **Heterologous antisera,** raised in one species against another species' Igs, are used to recognize isotypes (see below).

2) Other Ig determinants reflect regular small differences between individuals of the same species in the amino acid sequences of their otherwise similar Igs. The differences are specified by allelic genes and are called **allotypes** (Gr. *allos* = other). These markers are not associated with particular ligand-binding or effector functions, but they are of great importance in probing the genetic basis for Ab structure and biosynthesis. Allotypes are detected with homologous antiserum or **alloantisera,** which are formed by one individual against Igs with different allotypes from another individual of the same species.

3) Antigenic determinants of a third kind, **idiotypes** (Gr. *idios* = individual), are unique to the Ig molecules produced by a given clone of Ig-producing cells (Ch. 17). These determinants are probably located in or close to the specific ligand-binding sites of Abs, and they are detected with various antisera; e.g., those produced by one individual against an Ab from another individual of the same species and with the same allotypes.

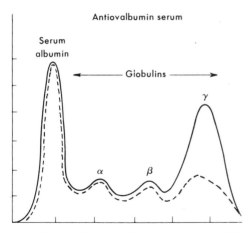

Fig. 16-1. Electrophoresis of serum from a rabbit intensively immunized with ovalbumin, before (——) and after (– – –) removal of Ab molecules by specific precipitation with ovalbumin. [From Tiselius, A., and Kabat, E. A. *J Exp Med 69*:119 (1939).]

CLASSES OF HEAVY CHAINS AND TYPES OF LIGHT CHAINS: ISOTYPES

Heavy-chain Isotypes. Human Igs are divided into five principal classes on the basis of chemical and isotypic properties. The three classes shown in Figure 16-2 are called IgG, IgA, and IgM.* The other two, IgD and IgE,

are present at such low concentrations in normal serum that their detection requires more sensitive methods, e.g., radioimmunoassay for IgE (Chs. 15 and 19).

As will be described later, Ig molecules are made up of small (light) and large (heavy) polypeptide chains. **Each of the five classes has similar sets of light chains but an antigenically distinctive set of heavy chains, which is named with the corresponding Greek letter (γ chains in IgG, μ in IgM, α in IgA, δ in IgD, ε in IgE).** Thus heterologous antisera prepared against human IgG contain Abs specific for heavy chains and others specific for light chains. After absorption with the heavy chains of IgG these antisera, specific for light chains, give reactions of identity with Igs of all classes (Fig. 16-3). In contrast, if the anti-IgG is absorbed with light chains (isolated from any class) the serum becomes monospecific for heavy chains of IgG; i.e., it reacts with Igs only of this class (Fig. 16-3).

Kappa and Lambda Light-chain Isotypes. There are also two main types of light chains,

---

* The main classes are also sometimes referred to as γG, γA, γM, γD, γE. Before 1965 various other designations were used: γ, γ_2, γ_{ss}, 7Sγ for IgG; $\beta_2 A$, $\gamma_1 A$ for IgA; $\beta_2 M$, $\gamma_1 M$, 19Sγ for IgM.

Fig. 16-2. Immunoelectrophoresis of human serum showing IgG, IgA, and IgM. Serum in the center wells (c) was subjected to electrophoresis in agar in 0.1 M barbital, pH 8.6. The rabbit antiserum in the long troughs, parallel to axis of migration of the human proteins, had been prepared against unfractionated human serum. (Courtesy of Dr. C. Kirk Osterland; see also Fig. 13-29, Ch. 13.)

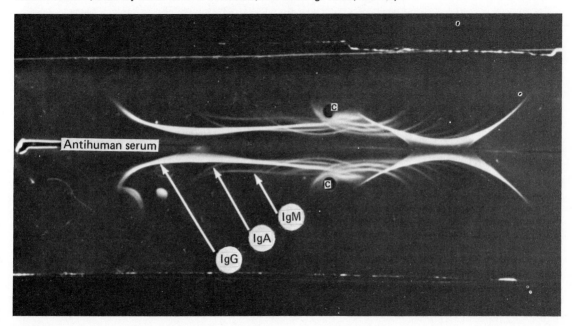

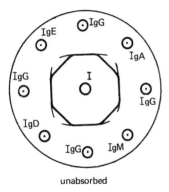 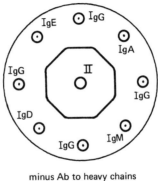 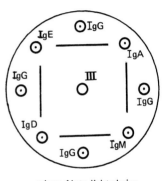

unabsorbed   minus Ab to heavy chains   minus Ab to light chains

Fig. 16-3. Gel diffusion precipitin reactions of human IgG, IgM, IgA, IgD and IgE with rabbit antiserum to human IgG. The antiserum (center wells) was used without absorption (I) or after absorption with heavy (II) or light chains (III) from IgG.

but since they are both present in all Ig classes (Figs. 16-3 and 16-4), they were long indistinguishable. Their distinction became possible only after it was recognized that the **myeloma proteins** secreted by myeloma tumors are Igs. Each of these tumors is a clone of neoplastic cells of the type that normally makes Abs (Ch. 17, Plasma cells); and each clone usually produces a distinctive and homogeneous myeloma protein. These "pathological" proteins have the same basic structure as normal Igs; some of them bind Ags specifically in the same way as ordinary Ab molecules. Some myeloma tumors also secrete homogeneous light chains, called **Bence Jones proteins** (p. 425), and heterologous antisera to individual Bence Jones proteins distinguish two main types of light chains, **kappa (κ) and lambda (λ)**. κ and λ chains differ extensively in amino acid sequences (see below), and **one type or the other is present in every Ig molecule, regardless of its heavy-chain class** (Fig. 16-4). About 60% of human Igs have κ chains and 40% have λ chains; the ratio varies somewhat in different Ig classes (Appendix, Table 16-5).

Igs in other vertebrate species also have κ and λ chains, as defined by homologous amino acid sequences (see below). However, some species have predominantly one type (ca. 95% of all light chains in mice are κ and almost 100% in horses and in birds are λ), while others (e.g., guinea pigs) have nearly equal amounts.

In this chapter we shall first consider the main classes of Igs, then genetic variants, and next individual Igs, whose amino acid sequences will be shown to account for both the unique and common properties of all Igs. The final sections consider the genetic basis for diversity among Igs and the structural basis for the specificity of their combining sites.

Fig. 16-4. Two types of light chains. Antisera to Bence Jones proteins of kappa (κ) and lambda (λ) types were mixed in the center well; κ and λ Bence Jones protein were placed in the lateral wells and normal human γ-globulin in the well at the top.

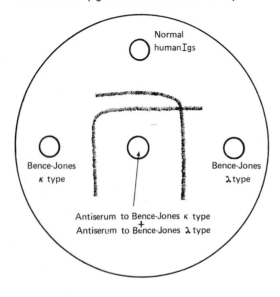

IgG IMMUNOGLOBULINS

These proteins used to be referred to as 7S γ-globulins because their sedimentation coefficient ($S°_{20,w}$) in neutral, dilute salt solution is 6.5 to 6.6 Svedberg units; their molecular weight is 150,000. They constitute over 85% of the Igs in the sera of most normal and hyperimmune individuals; hence they are responsible for many phenomena previously observed with crude γ-globulin fractions.

CHAINS

Multiple Chains. The IgG proteins have 20 to 25 disulfide (S-S) bonds per molecule and the subunit structure was not established until these were split. In 1959 Edelman discovered that reduction of the S-S bonds in human IgG led to a drop in molecular weight, suggesting that multiple chains are linked in the intact molecule by these bonds. The products were soluble only in special solvents (e.g., 8 M urea), probably because many intrachain S-S bonds were also cleaved, and this causes polypeptide chains, in general, to become grossly denatured. Nevertheless, electrophoresis in 8 M urea revealed two components.

Shortly thereafter Fleischman, Pain, and Porter showed that the covalent bridges between chains could be selectively ruptured by scission of only a few S-S bonds (about four). The chains then came apart when the reduced molecule was exposed to an organic acid (acetic, propionic), which broke noncovalent hydrophobic bonds and imposed many positive charges on the chains, leading to their mutual repulsion. By gel filtration two components were then recovered with essentially 100% yield (Fig. 16-5A); the MW of the heavier was about 50,000 and of the lighter was about 25,000. Since recovery was quantitative the arithmetic was simple: on the assumption that each of the fractions was made up of a single kind of chain, **the original molecule of 150,000 daltons consisted of two heavy chains (2 × 50,000) plus two light chains (2 × 25,000).**

Though antigenic and amino acid sequence analyses have revealed a great variety of heavy chains and of light chains, it has been clearly established that **any particular Ig molecule has identical heavy chains and identical light chains** (see Rabbit allotypes, below).

FRAGMENTATION WITH ENZYMES

Early attempts were made to analyze the architecture of Ab molecules by enzymatic frag-

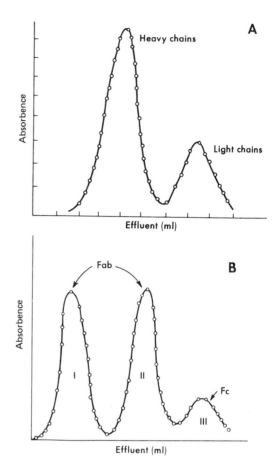

Fig. 16-5. A. Separation of heavy and light chains of IgG. The protein was reduced and alkylated (· · · S-S · · · → · · · SH; + ICH$_2$·COOH → · · · S·CH$_2$·COOH), and subjected to gel filtration in an organic acid (1 M propionic). **B.** Separation of Fab and Fc fragments of IgG. The protein was digested with papain (in presence of cysteine); after dialysis (during which some of the Fc crystallized) the digest was chromatographed on carboxymethylcellulose. [**A** based on Fleischman J. B., Pain, R. H., and Porter, R. R. *Arch Biochem Suppl* 1:174 (1962). **B** based on Porter, R. R. *Biochem J* 73:119 (1959).]

mentation, but this approach contributed little until certain S-S bonds were also cleaved.

Papain Digestion. In 1959 Porter showed that digestion of rabbit IgG with papain, in the presence of cysteine, decreased the sedimentation coefficient from 7S to 3.5S, with loss of only about 10% of the protein as small dialyzable peptides. Ion-exchange chromatography separated the digest into three fractions.

It was subsequently recognized that fractions I and II (Fig. 16-5B) are the same except for small differences in charge, corresponding to differences among the IgG molecules from which the fragments were derived (see Charge heterogeneity, below). When obtained from various purified Abs, these fragments retained the specific combining sites of the parent molecule but were **univalent,** i.e., contained a single ligand-binding site per fragment; and their total yield accounted fully for the ligand-binding activity of the original molecules. These fragments are now called **Fab (antigen-binding fragments).**

The third fragment (III) did not combine with Ags, and it appeared to be uniform in all rabbit IgG molecules, regardless of their specificity as Abs. Moreover, in contrast to intact Ab molecules, this fragment was easily crystallized; hence it is called **Fc (crystallizable fragment).**

Of the total digest prepared with papain, about ⅔ is Fab (MW ca. 45,000) and ⅓ is

Fc (MW 50,000). Hence **an intact, bivalent IgG molecule is made up of two univalent Fab fragments joined through peptide bonds to one Fc fragment.**

Cysteine was added with papain because the activity of the enzyme depends on the reduced state of its SH groups. Subsequently, however, it became clear that the cysteine was performing an additional, critical role, for it also reduced some S-S bonds in the immunoglobulin substrate. Thus fragmentation of IgG molecules into Fab and Fc actually requires two independent reactions, which can be carried out concomitantly or in sequence: 1) hydrolysis of a few peptide bonds (two are sufficient), and 2) reduction of a critical S-S bond (see Pepsin, below).

Other Proteases. Other proteolytic enzymes also split Igs, and **pepsin** has been especially useful: in the absence of cysteine it cleaves from IgG Abs a 5S bivalent fragment, MW ca. 100,000, which can be split by reduction of one S-S bond to yield univalent fragments (Fig. 16-6). The latter are indistinguishable

Fig. 16-6. Schematic diagram of the four-chain structure of IgG, showing some interchain S-S bonds and regions susceptible to proteolytic cleavage (papain, pepsin at arrows). The piece of heavy chain within the Fab fragment is the **Fd piece.** Dots represent noncovalent interchain bonds. The spherical Ag represents an antigen molecule in a ligand-binding site. [Four-chain model from Fleischman, J. B., Porter, R. R., and Press, E. M. *Biochem J 88*:220 (1963). Y-shape at top based on Figs. 16-7 and 16-8. Scheme for pepsin digestion based on Nisonoff, A., Wissler, F., Lipman, L., and Woernley, D. *Arch Biochem 89*:230 (1960).]

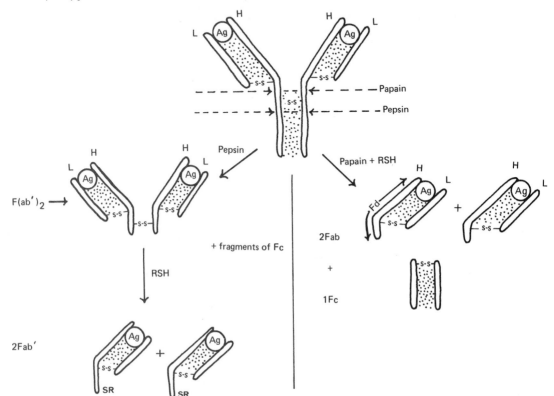

from the Fab fragments prepared with papain with respect to sedimentation constant (3.5S), ligand-binding activity, and antigenicity; but the pepsin fragment has a molecular weight about 10% higher, and it contains some covalently linked carbohydrate. To indicate these small differences the univalent fragment obtained with pepsin is called **Fab'**; the corresponding bivalent fragment is **F(ab')$_2$**. The Fc fragment is not recovered in peptic digests, but is fragmented.

The variety of fragments obtained with various proteases from Igs of many species fit into a coherent pattern: **all IgG Abs have two compact globular domains (corresponding to Fab fragments) joined to a third compact domain (corresponding to the Fc fragment) by connecting regions that are highly susceptible to attack by proteases** (Fig. 16-6).

OVER-ALL STRUCTURE

Relations Between Chains and Fragments. The immunogenicity of the proteolytic fragments made it possible to match fragments with dissociated chains. Thus, goat antisera to the isolated Fc fragment of rabbit IgG form specific precipitates with heavy chains, as well as with Fc, but not with light chains. In contrast, antisera to Fab fragments react with both light and heavy chains (Table 16-1). These findings led Porter to formulate the schematic structure for IgG shown in Figure 16-6, which fits all the information now available.

Shape. A variety of analytical approaches (based on hydrodynamic and fluorescence properties, electron microscopy, and X-ray diffraction) suggest that IgG molecules are **Y-shaped,** with a "hinge" at about the middle of the heavy chain, connecting the two Fab domains with the Fc domain (Figs. 16-7, and 16-8). There may also be **segmental flexibility:** by movement about the hinge, the angle between Fab segments might vary as much as 0 to 180°. But it is not yet clear whether each molecule can assume such a wide variety of angles.

Charge Heterogeneity. IgG migrates in zone electrophoresis as a broad protein band (see Figs. 16-2 and 16-16) because the individual proteins that make up the class vary in net charge (isoelectric points probably range from about 5.0 to 7.5). If IgG is arbitrarily separated by electrophoresis into rapidly and slowly migrating fractions, the heavy chains isolated from each fraction show corresponding differences in mobility. Moreover, each still migrates as a diffuse zone; thus the heavy chains are also inhomogeneous.

The light chains are also heterogeneous. They are small enough to penetrate easily into polyacrylamide gels, where they can be resolved by electrophoresis into many (at least 10) distinct bands, which seem to differ in unit electric charge (Fig. 16-18). Since this heterogeneity is observed in denaturing ("unfolding") solvents, such as 8 M urea, it is due to diversity in covalent structure, and not simply to folding or aggregation (see Amino acid sequences, below).

Carbohydrate Content. Igs are glycoproteins with oligosaccharides covalently linked to the Fc domain of heavy chains. In some IgG molecules carbohydrate is also present in Fab, i.e., on the light chain or the N-terminal half of the heavy chains (Fd piece, Fig. 16-6).

Each of the oligosaccharide substituents has two branches on a central stem, for which, so far, three different sequences have been established (Fig. 16-9). At its base, the stem is linked to an asparagine residue of the heavy chain through a covalent bond with N-acetyl glucosamine. Though a common sequence is present in all branches (galactose $\beta1 \rightarrow 6$ N-acetyl glucosamine $\beta1 \rightarrow 2$ mannose), sialic acid or additional galactose residues are present at some branch termini; and the fucose content of the oligosaccharides is also variable. This "microheterogeneity" has been evident in all samples analyzed, including monoclonal IgG myeloma proteins; the ragged ends probably arise from degradation by glycosidases that act on these proteins as they circulate in blood.

Carbohydrate is less abundant in IgG (3% by weight) than in other Ig classes (Appendix, Table 16-5). Besides having oligosaccharides like the one

TABLE 16-1. Goat Antibodies to Rabbit Fab and Fc Fragments: Precipitation Reaction with Chains Isolated from Rabbit IgG

	Antisera to	
	Fab	Fc
Heavy chains	+	+
Light chains	+	−

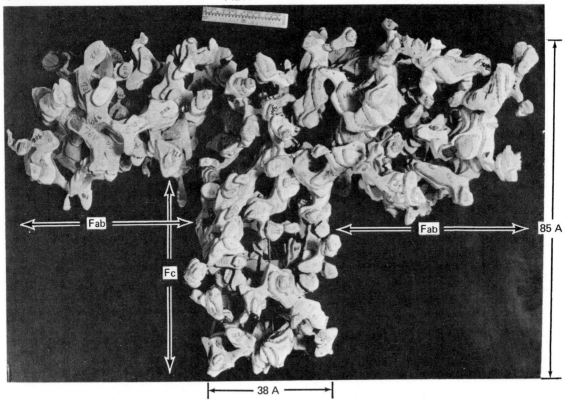

142 A

85 A

38 A

Fig. 16-7. Balsa wood model of an IgG molecule based on a three-dimensional electron density map at 6-A resolution from X-ray diffraction data. The dyad axis relating the halves of the molecule lies in the plane of the paper. The crystallized protein was a human myeloma protein of the IgG-1 subclass (see below). [From Sarma, V. R., Silverton, E. W., Davies, D. R., and Terry, W. D. *J Biol Chem 246*:3753 (1971).]

at the extreme left of Figure 16-9, other Ig heavy chains have additional oligosaccharides, which are distinctive for various classes: α chains (of IgA) have oligosaccharides linked via O- glycosidic bonds to serine OH groups; μ chains (of IgM) have mannose rich groups; ε chains (of IgE) have some that are rich in mannose and others that contain additional galactose residues.

The function of the carbohydrate is unknown: the saccharides could provide binding sites for selective attachment of different Igs to specific receptors on various cells (e.g., IgE on mast cells; see Ch. 19), or the addition of sugar residues during biosynthesis could play a role in the transfer of Ig chains into membranous vesicles, from which they are secreted at the cell surface (Ch. 17).

DISULFIDE BRIDGES

Stability. Proteins of the IgG class are unusually stable. In serum or as purified Abs they can remain unaltered for years at 0°. Moreover, after exposure to denaturing conditions (e.g., 70°, pH 11, pH 2, 8 M urea) they largely recover native structure when returned to dilute salt solution at physiological conditions of pH and temperature. A major factor is the presence of a large number of disulfide (S-S) bonds (20 to 25 per molecule). Three to seven of these S-S bonds link the four chains together; the remainder are distributed within the chains, stabilizing their respective conformations (Figs. 16-6 and 16-20).

In order of increasing resistance to reduction the S-S bonds fall into groups that link: 1) the heavy chains, 2) light to heavy chains, and 3) cysteine residues within chains (intrachain). Hence, under mildest conditions the IgG molecule is split into symmetrical halves, each with one heavy plus one light chain. The halves separate when, at low pH, they acquire large positive charges; they reassociate to form native molecules when returned to neutral pH. Even if their SH groups are blocked chemically, e.g., by treatment with iodoacetic

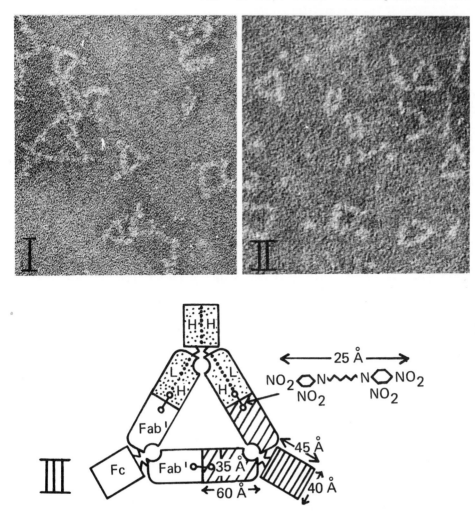

Fig. 16-8. Three IgG anti-Dnp antibody molecules joined in a triangular complex by a ligand with two Dnp groups per molecule [Dnp-NH-(Ch$_2$)$_8$-NH-Dnp; see III]. The ligand is too small to be resolved. The complex in I forms the basis for the diagram in III. The picture in II was obtained after treatment of the complex in I with pepsin, removing the corner projections, which correspond to Fc. I and II, Electron micrograph, ×500,000. [From Valentine, R. C., and Green, N. M. *J Mol Biol* 27:615 (1967).]

acid, the halves can still associate (though without S-S bridges) to form molecules that are essentially indistinguishable from the original in sedimentation properties and antigenicity.

Hybrid Antibodies. When half-molecules (H·L) from purified Abs of a particular specificity are mixed with an excess of half-molecules from nonspecific IgG and allowed to reassociate, most of the Ab behaves in precipitin reactions as though univalent, i.e., as

though formed from one specific plus one nonspecific half-molecule. Thus these "hybrid antibodies" specifically inhibit, rather than contribute to, the corresponding precipitin reaction.

Hybrids can be prepared more easily from the F(ab')$_2$ fragments obtained by pepsin digestion: mild reduction yields Fab' fragments, each with one ligand-binding site and one free SH group. If these fragments are prepared from two purified Abs of different specificity, mixed, and allowed to reoxidize,

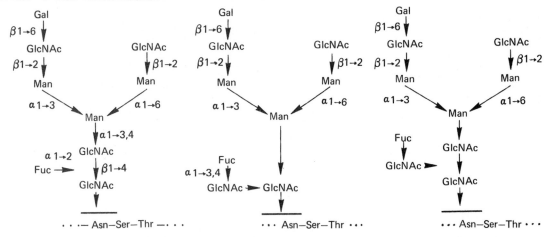

Fig. 16-9. Glycopeptides from three IgG myeloma proteins, showing branched oligosaccharides. The basal N-acetyl glucosamine (GlcNAc) is attached to an asparagine (Asn) residue of the heavy chain. An asparagine or aspartic acid residue in the sequence ··· Asx-X-Thr ··· forms the point of attachment of oligosaccharide in many glycoproteins. Sialic acid groups are attached to the free ends of some branches, but are not shown. Each of the oligosaccharides shown (with 2 sialic acid end groups the MW would be ca. 2500), occurring once per heavy chain, could account for the carbohydrate content of a typical IgG molecule; with 3 to 4 times more carbohydrate on other Ig classes, additional oligosaccharide moieties must be present on IgM, IgA, IgE (see Fig. 16-12). [From Kornfeld, R., Keller, J., Baenziger, and Kornfeld, S. *J Biol Chem* 246:3259 (1971).]

hybrid bivalents appear with a different ligand-binding specificity at each of the two sites (Fig. 16-10). The large proportion of hybrids indicates that the recombination of Fab' fragments is random.

Symmetry. In contrast to the pairs formed in the test tube, **natural IgGs are symmetrical: in any particular molecule the two light chains are identical, as are the two heavy chains, and the two ligand-binding sites are also identical** (Ch. 15). As we shall see later, the symmetry comes about because a given cell makes, at any one time, only one type of light chain and one type of heavy chain (Ch. 17, One cell–one Ig rule).

IgG SUBCLASSES

Careful antigenic analysis with heterologous antisera has revealed that proteins of the IgG class can be differentiated into four subclasses (IgG-1 through IgG-4), each with a distinctive heavy chain, called γ1, γ2, γ3, γ4.

Antisera vary greatly in capacity to differentiate among the four subclasses. Rabbit antisera to the total IgG fraction of human serum do not distinguish among them, while monkey antisera to the same mixture of immunogens can distinguish three of the four. The sharpest serological distinctions are

made with antisera against the individual, homogeneous Igs produced by different clones of neoplastic plasma cells (see Myeloma and Bence Jones proteins, below). Adsorption of such an antiserum by appropriate myeloma proteins of other IgG subclasses make it monospecific for the subclass of its immunogen, i.e., it reacts only with Igs whose heavy chains belong to the same subclass (Fig. 16-11).

With the aid of monospecific antisera, the subclasses have been detected in all normal human sera: IgG-1, -2, -3, and -4 make up about 70, 19, 8, and 3%, respectively, of the IgG proteins. Their characteristic determinants (Isotypes, above) are localized in their Fc segments. The subclasses also differ in their general effector functions and in several other properties (Appendix, Table 16-5). Fundamental differences in their amino acid sequences and patterns of interchain S-S bonding are described later (Amino acid sequences and Fig. 16-20, below).

Four subclasses of IgG have also been identified in the mouse, the only other species in which many myeloma proteins are available for the preparation of subclass-specific antisera. But fewer subclasses have been recognized in other species (e.g., two in the guinea pig and in the rat), perhaps because homogeneous Igs have not yet been obtained from them and the only IgG subclasses recognized are

Fig. 16-10. Formation of hybrid bivalent Ab fragments. **Top.** F(ab′)$_2$ fragments prepared from anti-O and anti-● were reduced to Fab′ fragments, then mixed and allowed to reoxidize. For precipitation of hybrid F(ab′)$_2$ fragments it was necessary to have both Ag O and Ag ● present (Ch. 15, Fig. 15-13). **Bottom.** Dual specificity of hybrid Ab fragments revealed by mixed hemagglutination. The Fab′ fragments were obtained from rabbit Abs specific for chicken ovalbumin (Ea) or for bovine γ-globulin (BγG). Human red cells (small, spherical, nonnucleated) were coated with Ea, and duck red cells (large, oval, nucleated) were coated with BγG. In **a** reoxidized F(ab′)$_2$ fragments prepared exclusively from anti-Ea clumped only the human cells. In **b** the reoxidized fragments prepared exclusively from anti-BγG clumped only the duck cells. In **c** a mixture of the two F(ab′)$_2$ fragments of **a** and **b** formed separate clumps of human and of duck cells. In **d** hybrid F(ab′)$_2$ fragments formed mixed clumps, with both human and duck cells. [From Fudenberg, H., Drews, G., and Nisonoff, A. *J Exp Med 119*:151 (1964).]

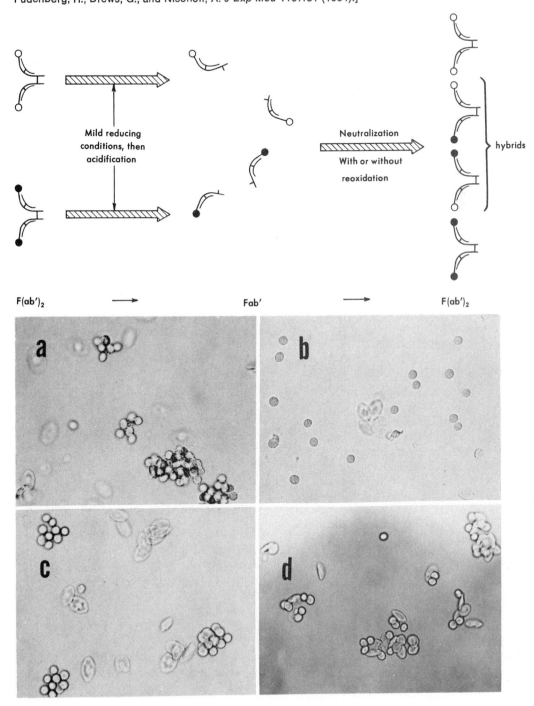

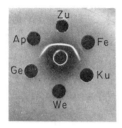
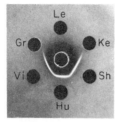

Fig. 16-11. IgG subclasses. Twelve IgG myeloma proteins (each from a human with a myeloma tumor) were tested with monkey antiserum to the protein from patient Zu, after the antiserum had been absorbed with Igs of other subclasses. Five additional proteins were precipitated (Ap, Fe, Vi, Hu, Sh); hence they belong to the same subclass as Zu (IgG-3). The six nonreacting IgGs belong to other subclasses. [From Grey, H. M., and Kunkel, H. G. *J Exp Med 120*:253 (1964).]

those that happen to be relatively abundant and to differ substantially in electrophoretic mobility (Fig. 19-6, Ch. 19).

Antigenic differences among subclasses are less pronounced than among classes. For example, after Abs to light chains are removed, antisera prepared against IgG-1 cross-react with IgG-2, IgG-3, IgG-4 but not with Igs of the other classes (IgM, IgA, etc.). Amino acid sequence data (below) confirm these relations by revealing greater homologies among heavy chains of the γ subclasses than among those of diverse classes (Fig. 16-23).

OTHER IMMUNOGLOBULIN CLASSES

IgM

The first Abs studied in the ultracentrifuge (Heidelberger and Pedersen) had high sedimentation values (predominantly 19S). Obtained from horses immunized with pneumococci, they appeared at first to be curiosities, because most other Abs (made in other species to other Ags) subsequently proved to be 7S IgG molecules. However, hemagglutination and other sensitive assays then revealed that 19S Abs are formed in almost every immune response, though nearly always early and only at low levels; they are usually soon overshadowed by larger amounts of IgG Abs to the same Ag (Ch. 17).

Now called IgM (M, macroglobulin), its molecular weight of about 900,000 is accounted for by five tetrameric subunits linked

through S-S bonds between cysteine residues near the hinge region of the heavy chains (Fig. 16-12A). Under mild reducing conditions, which cleave only interchain S-S bonds, IgM molecules dissociate into 7S subunits which yield (after treatment with acetic or propionic acid) light and heavy chains in the same proportion as from IgG molecules (Fig. 16-5A). However, the IgM heavy chains (μ chains) are ca. 20% longer and have more oligosaccharide branches and a higher carbohydrate content (ca. 10%); their molecular weight is accordingly higher (ca. 70,000 compared with 50,000 for the γ chains of IgG).

IgM is split by papain at 37° into a variety of heterogeneous fragments, unlike IgG which yields well-defined Fab and Fc fragments under these conditions. However, Fab and Fc can be derived from the IgM molecule under special conditions (trypsin at 56 to 60°). The Fab fragment resembles that of IgG (one light chain plus one Fd piece), but the Fc is a decamer, with 10 heavy-chain fragments joined by S-S bonds (Fig. 16-12A). The presence of 10 Fab domains and a correspondingly large number of combining sites per molecule probably accounts for the relatively high avidity of IgM antibodies for Ags (Ch. 15). The high avidity is notable especially because IgM Abs generally have much lower intrinsic affinities (per site) than IgG Abs of the same specificity.

The 7S subunits (IgM$_s$) derived by mild reduction do not give agglutination reactions even though their combining sites seem to be unaltered (as shown by equilibrium dialysis measurements of ligand binding; Ch. 15). The dependence of agglutinating activity on more than two sites could be due to low intrinsic affinity (per site) or to unknown steric factors that interfere with effective function of both sites on the 7S subunit. Whatever the reason, IgM can be distinguished from IgG Abs by the loss of agglutinating activity after reduction with 2-mercaptoethanol. The test is useful but not infallible, because Abs of other classes (IgA, IgE) can also lose agglutinating activity after mild reduction (below).

Besides heavy and light chains, IgM immunoglobulins have one additional polypeptide, called J, per 10 light chains. The **J chain** (MW ca. 20,000) differs antigenically and in amino acid composition from the other

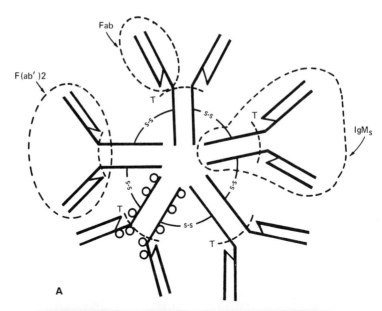

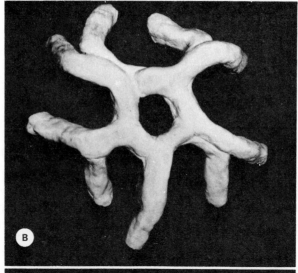

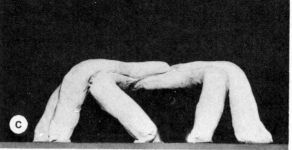

Fig. 16-12. A. Structure of IgM. Five four-chain 7S subunits (IgM$_s$) are joined by S-S bridges. The subunits might be linked directly, as shown, or indirectly through an S-S bond between each heavy chain and the J chain, which is not shown. Trypsin (at 60°) cleaves at the dotted lines (T), yielding 10 Fab fragments and an Fc decamer. The positions of oligosaccharide groups (O) are shown only in the IgM$_s$ subunit at 7 o'clock. B and C. Models of an IgM molecule, based on electron microscopy. B. Molecule in top view displaying flexible subunits. C. Profile view of the molecule bound at multiple sites to the surface of an Ag [A based on Miller, F., and Metzger, H. J Biol Chem 240:4740 (1966), and on Shimizu, A., Putnam, F. W., Paul, C., Clamp, J. R., and Johnson, I., Nature 231:73 (1971). B and C from Feinstein, A., and Munn, E. A. Nature 224:1307 (1969); also Svehag, S. E. Bloth, B., and Seligmann, M. J Exp Med 130:691 (1969).]

chains. Its function is not known; it could be the glue that stabilizes multimeric Igs (see also IgA, below).

IgA

Immunoelectrophoresis of human serum led to the identification of IgA (Fig. 16-2), whose basic structural unit corresponds to the four-chain molecule shown in Figure 16-6. Unlike IgM, which is a pentamer, and IgGs, which are uniformly monomers, IgA occurs in a variety of polymeric forms: monomer (7S), dimer (9S), trimer (11S), and even higher multimers (ca. 17S). The various multimers are evidently S-S linked monomers, because mild reduction is necessary (and sufficient) for their dissociation into 7S molecules. As with IgM, the reduced 7S molecules are defective in cross-linking activity though they retain two combining sites with unaltered affinity for small ligands.

IgA is normally present at about ⅕ the concentration of IgG in human serum (Table 16-5). But in man and in some other mammalian species **IgA is the principal Ig in exocrine secretions (milk, respiratory and intestinal mucin, saliva, tears).** The cells that produce IgA are concentrated in the subepithelial tissue of exocrine glands and respond to Ags that enter locally (e.g., by ingestion, inhalation, via the conjunctivae, etc.). The secreted IgA Abs seem to be important in protecting mucosal surfaces from invasion by pathogenic microbes. About as much IgA as IgG is synthesized per day in man, but loss in exocrine secretions probably accounts for its relatively low level in serum.

Human serum IgA occurs mostly as the monomer, while exocrine IgA is largely a dimer. After cleavage of S-S bonds, all forms of IgA yield heavy and light chains in the same proportions as IgG and IgM. Multimeric IgA also yields one **J chain** per four light chains. Exocrine IgA has, in addition, a fourth polypeptide chain, **secretory piece** (MW ca. 60,000), whose function is not known; it may be responsible for the unusual resistance of exocrine IgA to proteolysis, and hence contribute to its persistence in intestinal and other secretions.

As in the IgG class, antisera to human myeloma proteins of the IgA class differentiate subclasses, IgA-1 and IgA-2, with antigenically distinctive α chains (α1, α2). About 11% of normal IgA and of IgA myeloma proteins belong to the IgA-2 subclass (Appendix, Table 16-5).

IgD

These Igs were discovered not as Abs but as rare myeloma proteins that failed to react with specific antisera to IgG, IgM, and IgA. These myeloma proteins, and the antigenically similar normal immunoglobulins, are called IgD. They are found in normal sera at about 1/50 the level of IgG (Appendix, Table 16-5).

IgE

Though present in normal human sera at only about 1/25,000 the level of IgG, the IgE proteins are responsible for severe, acute, and occasionally fatal allergic reactions (Ch. 19). IgE was discovered by the Ishizakas, who suspected its existence because the Abs that mediate acute allergic skin reactions in man are inactivated by rabbit antisera to crude mixtures of human Igs, but not by monospecific antisera for IgG, IgM, IgA, IgD (see Ch. 19, Reagins).

Like μ chains of IgM, ε chains of IgE are longer than γ and α chains (of IgGs and IgAs) by about 100 amino acid residues, suggesting that they have an additional domain (Amino acid sequences, below). Though other Igs are remarkably heat-stable, when IgE is heated for 4 hours at 56° it loses the ability to sensitize skin, but retains the capacity to bind Ags. Both activities are lost on reduction and alkylation of S-S bonds (Ch. 19).

Several other mammalian species have Igs that resemble IgE; i.e., they are also present in serum in trace amounts, are labile to heat and S-S splitting reagents, and have skin-sensitizing activity (Ch. 19, Homocytotropic Abs and reagins). Abs with these properties from several species (man, rat, rabbit, monkey) also cross-react antigenically.

The cells that produce IgE are relatively abundant in mucosa of the respiratory and intestinal tracts, and Abs of the IgE class are also found in exocrine secretions. Though present here also only in trace amounts, they probably play an important role in localized allergic reactions, e.g., hay fever, asthma.

Some properties of various classes and sub-classes of human Igs are summarized in the Appendix (Table 16-5).

GENETIC VARIANTS: ALLOTYPES

Though animals only rarely form Abs to components of their own tissues, some substances derived from one individual are regularly immunogenic in certain other individuals of the same species (**isoantigens** or **alloantigens**). Oudin showed that some Igs behave in this manner and introduced the term **allotypes** for their various forms (see above). Other alloantigens, on cell surfaces, determine host responses to blood transfusions and organ transplants; they are discussed at length in Chapter 21.

HUMAN ALLOTYPES

A chance observation led to the discovery of genetic variants of human Igs. Serum from persons with rheumatoid arthritis often contains **rheumatoid factors**, which are Igs (generally IgM) that react with pooled human IgG; for example, they specifically agglutinate human red blood cells (RBC) coated with human anti-RBC Abs of the incomplete type (Ch. 15, Blocking Abs; Fig. 19-20; Ch. 21, Rh system). In studying these reactions Grubb observed that some patients' rheumatoid factors reacted only with cells that had been coated with Abs from certain persons. Moreover, any particular agglutination reaction could be specifically inhibited by serum only from particular individuals, whose Igs presumably carried the same antigenic determinants as the Ab molecules adherent to the red cells and therefore competed for the same rheumatoid factor (Fig. 16-13).

Some normal sera also contain Igs that agglutinate particular Ab-coated RBC. Called SNaggs (for serum normal agglutinators), they discriminate more sharply among related IgG variants than do most rheumatoid serum agglutinators (Raggs), but both are valuable reagents for typing human Igs.

At least some of the agglutinating activities in normal sera are probably due to maternal-fetal incompatibilities. In about 10% of human pregnancies mothers have Ig allotypes their babies lack. With transfer of maternal Ig across the placenta about half of these babies are stimulated to make antiallotype Abs. Detected with the sensitive hemagglutination assay (Fig. 16-13), these Abs generally reach peak titers at about 6 months of age (after the large amount of maternal Ig present in the infant's blood at birth has been eliminated; see Ch. 17, Ontogeny). Antiallotypes are also detected in about 1% of normal adults. Antiallotypes are also frequently formed in persons who receive multiple blood transfusions (for chronic anemias, open-heart surgery, etc.), because donors often have allotypes foreign to recipients.[*]

Through the reactions of Raggs and SNaggs with sera from thousands of persons, many human allotypes have been identified and classified into several groups, of which the principal ones are *Gm* (for gamma) and *Inv* (for inhibitor of the reaction with serum from patient V). These groups are specified by independently segregating genes and they are located on different chains. **The Gm markers are on γ (heavy) chains, and thus found only in IgG; the Inv markers are on light chains of κ type, and occur in all Ig classes.**

Gm Allotypes. The nomenclature of Gm allotypes has grown increasingly cumbersome as more varieties have been recognized. Hence a numerical system, resembling those used for Rh blood factors and *Salmonella* Ags (Chs. 21 and 29), has recently been adopted. Agglutinating sera of a given specificity are designated by number. An Ig that reacts, or fails to react, with a particular agglutinator receives the corresponding positive or negative number; for instance, an Ig with allotype Gm(1,-4) reacts with anti-Gm(1) but not with anti-Gm(4) (the absence of other numbers in this example would mean that the Ig was not tested with other agglutinators). As is conventional with other systems, alleles are italicized, their products are not: e.g., the allele *Gm⁵* specifies a γ chain of allotype Gm(5).

Over 20 Gm allotypic determinants have

---

* Most human Abs to IgG allotypes appear to have low affinity, and transfusions of blood with foreign allotypes of this class rarely cause allergic reactions (Chs. 19 and 21), even in recipients with high titers of the corresponding antiallotype. Severe reactions have occurred, however, when the discordant allotype is IgA, some of which is polymeric and may form more stable complexes with its antiallotype (Ch. 15, Multivalent binding).

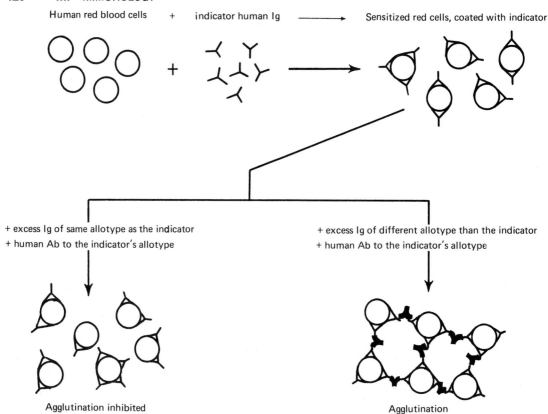

Human red blood cells   +   indicator human Ig   ⟶   Sensitized red cells, coated with indicator

+ excess Ig of same allotype as the indicator
+ human Ab to the indicator's allotype

+ excess Ig of different allotype than the indicator
+ human Ab to the indicator's allotype

Agglutination inhibited

Agglutination

Fig. 16-13. Agglutination-inhibition assay for human allotypes. In the assay for Gm and Inv allotypes the indicator Ig is nonagglutinating Ab specifically bound to red cells (anti-Rh on Rh+ red cells; see Ch. 21). In the assay for some other allotypes the indicator Ig is adsorbed nonspecifically on CrCl₃-treated red cells. [Based on Grubb, R., and Laurell, A. B. *Acta Pathol Microbiol Scand 39*:195,390 (1956).]

been recognized. Each IgG subclass has its own group of allotypes (Table 16-2), specified by codominant* alleles at a complex autosomal (i.e., not sex-linked) locus. Hence a given allotypic determinant may be present on all or on approximately half the molecules of its subclass, depending on whether the individual is homozygous or heterozygous. Moreover, allotypic markers on myeloma proteins have shown that the chain specified by one allele can have several allotypic determinants, as expected from the multiplicity of antigenic determinants on protein chains in general (Ch. 15). Thus some IgG-1 molecules are Gm (1, 17): their γ1 chains have the Gm(1) marker on Fc and the Gm(17)

marker on the Fd piece (Table 16-2). Some γ1 chains in certain ethnic groups have three markers: Gm(1), Gm(4), and Gm(22) (Table 16-3 and Fig. 16-14).

The inheritance of allotypes follows mendelian rules. For example, a *Gm¹⁷* homozygous mother [whose γ1 chains and IgG-1 molecules are all Gm(17)] and a *Gm²²* homozygous father [whose γ1 chains and IgG-1 molecules are all Gm(22)] invariably have heterozygous children, *Gm¹⁷/Gm²²*, with each marker on about half their IgG-1 molecules. The Gm allotypes are of considerable value in population genetics and in anthropology, and in cases of disputed paternity they are accepted as legal evidence in some countries (Norway, France).

The alleles for Gm markers are linked in complexes that differ conspicuously in diverse racial groups; for example, a common

---

* Alleles in a heterozygous diploid individual are codominant when both are expressed more or less equally.

TABLE 16-2. Allelic Groups of Gm Allotypic Markers on Heavy Chains of IgG Subclasses

Subclass	Heavy chain	Gm allotype	Molecular local-ization*	Comments
IgG-1	γ1	1 2 17	Fc Fc Fd	Probably represent one allele; they are found on the same chains, but (2) is detected less often than (1). Present in ca. 60% of Western Europeans (and their descendents) and in ca. 100% of all others.
		3 4 22	Fd Fd Fc	Probably represent one allele; (3) and (4) are detected only when the γ1 chain is associated with light chain, and (3) is detected less often than (4). Present in >90% of Caucasians and Chinese, but in only 13% of Japanese.
IgG-2	γ2	23	Fc	Present in ca. 50% of Caucasians, 90% of Chinese, ca. 0% of Negroes. An antiserum is lacking for Gm (−23), the allelic product.
IgG-3	γ3	5 6 10 11 13 14	Fc Fc Fc Fc Fc Fc	A family of γ3 determinants present in ca. 100% of Negroes, 90% of Europeans and Chinese, and absent in Australian aborigines. When (6), (10), (11), (13), (14) are detected, they are nearly always associated with Gm(5).
		21	Fc	Allelic with the Gm(5) family.
IgG-4	γ4	4a 4b	? ?	Agglutinators of (4a) react with all IgG-1 and IgG-3 molecules. Agglutinators of (4b) react with all IgG-2 molecules.

Based on summary by Grubb, R. *The Genetic Markers of Human Immunoglobulins*, Springer, New York, 1970. Data for IgG-4 from Kunkel, H. G., Joslin, F. G., Penn, G. M., and Natvig, J. B. *J Exp Med 132*:508 (1970).

* See Figure 16-31 for amino acid substitutions associated with some of these markers.

heritable complex in caucasoids is 22,4,23,5 (Table 16-3). Each of these complexes behaves as a stable heritable unit. For example, a person who is heterozygous for γ1 and γ3 genes (with, say, the following allotypes— γ1: 1, 17, 4, 22; γ3: 21, 5) would have inherited one set of genes from one parent (γ1: 1, 17; γ3: 21) and the second set from the other parent (γ1: 4, 22; γ3: 5).

Surveys of large populations have shown that the crossover frequency between genes for γ1, γ2, and γ3 is extremely low; indeed, these genes may be adjacent, and probably represent the most closely linked human genes recognized so far.* However, a few pedigrees

have provided evidence for recombination, yielding the order of genes shown in Figure 16-14. An ancient crossover event probably accounts for the combination of markers on some γ1 chains in mongoloid populations (Fig. 16-14).

Some relations among allotypes suggest that genes for certain γ subclasses might have arisen in evolution by duplication of preexisting alleles of an older subclass (see below, Evolution of immunoglobulins). Thus some heavy-chain markers that are allelic in one γ subclass are uniformly present (i.e., nonallelic) in certain other γ subclasses: e.g., one allelic variant of γ4—Gm(4a)—occurs on all γ1 and γ3 chains and another γ4 variant—Gm(4b)—occurs on all γ2 chains. Hence an ancient γ4a allele might have given rise by duplication to genes that evolved into those of present-day γ1 and γ3 and

* Rare individuals have normal levels of IgG but fail to react with any of the known Gm agglutinators, suggesting that there are additional Gm alleles. However, in some Gm-less persons the γ chains were "hybrids," with the Fd piece of γ3 type, and Fc of γ1 type. This unusual chain probably arose from crossover between γ3 and γ1 genes: it is Gm-less

because Gm markers are not known for the Fd of γ3 and are lacking in the Fc of some γ1 chains. (This γ chain resembles the "hybrid Lepore type" hemoglobin chain, which is half β chain and half δ chain.)

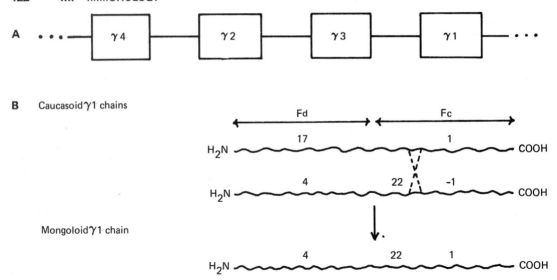

Fig. 16-14. A. Order of linked genes for γ chains of human IgG. The position for γ4 is still tentative. **B.** Alignment of allotypic markers in common γ1 chains. Recombination (dashed lines) between alleles for the caucasoid chains could account for the markers in a mongoloid γ1 chain. [Based on Natvig, J. B., Kunkel, H. G., and Litwin, S. D. *Cold Spring Harbor Symp Quant Biol* 32:173 (1967).]

an ancient γ4b allele might have similarly given rise to γ2; through subsequent mutation-selection the duplicated products would have eventually evolved their own allelic variants while retaining the imprint of the γ4 allele from which they originated.

Amino acid residues associated with Gm and other allotypic markers are given later (see Fig. 16-24).

TABLE 16-3. Common Gene Complexes in Different Human Populations*

Racial group	IgG-1	IgG-2	IgG-3
Caucasoid	·····1, 17	·····−23	·····21·····
	·····22, 4	····· 23	····· 5·····
Negroid	·····1, 17	·····−23	····· 5·····
Mongoloid	·····1, 17	·····−23	····· 5·····
	·····1, 17	·····−23	·····21·····
	···1, 22, 4	····· 23	····· 5·····

* The gene complexes are aligned horizontally; see Figure 16-14 for the order of linked genes. Data for the racial distribution of IgG-4 allotypes are not yet available.

Based on Natvig, J. B., Kunkel, H. G., and Litwin, S. D., *Cold Spring Harbor Symp Quant Biol* 32:173 (1967); and on Muir, W. A., and Steinberg, A. G., *Semin Hematol* 4:156 (1967).

Am Allotypes. Genetic variants of IgA were discovered through reactions to blood transfusions (footnote, p. 419, and Ch. 21): recipients who lack an IgA variant can suffer severe reactions when transfused more than once with blood that contains it. (The first transfusion induces formation of the anti-allotype, which reacts with that allotype in subsequent transfusions.) With these human antiallotypes and the hemagglutination assay described above (Fig. 16-13), two heritable variants of α2 chains have been detected in IgA-2, the minor subclass of IgA; by analogy with Gm allotypes of IgG they are called Am(1) and Am(2).

Inv Allotypes. Two allelic variants of κ light chains, differing in a single amino acid (at position 191; see sequences below) are distinguished by agglutinating sera. Kappa chains with leu-191 are called Inv(1,2) and those with val-191 are Inv(3).

The remarkably discriminating agglutinators (Fig. 16-13) for these allotypes thus distinguish between light chains on the basis of a single -CH_2- group (in a leucine vs. a valine residue). Moreover two kinds of antisera to Inv(1,2) have been recognized: anti-Inv(1) and anti-Inv(2). They might recognize subtle modifications of the allotypic marker due to pairing of kappa with different heavy chains (see Light chain–heavy chain interaction, below).

Rare individuals are Inv(-1,-2,-3), suggesting additional Inv alleles. The geographical and ethnic distribution is as uneven for Inv as for Gm alleles (Table 16-2): e.g., Inv(1,2) is present in 10 to 20% of Europeans and in >90% of Venezuelan Indians.

Allotypic variants of human λ light chains have not yet been definitely identified.

RABBIT ALLOTYPES

Careful experiments by Oudin in France revealed genetic variants of rabbit Ig chains at the same time that human allotypes were disclosed in Sweden by Grubb's chance observation. Though the principles are the same in man and in rabbit, studies of the experimental animal contributed additional important insights.

Rabbit allotypes were first recognized by precipitin reactions with antisera from rabbits immunized with Abs of other rabbits.* Examination of rabbit populations with a variety of these antisera eventually disclosed three distinct sets of allotypes, each associated with a different Ig chain: three *a* allotypes (a1, a2, a3) on heavy chains, three *b* allotypes (b4, b5, b6) on κ chains (which make up about 80% of rabbit light chains), and two *c* allotypes (c7, c21) on λ chains. Each of these sets is specified by an autosomal locus with codominant alleles. Studies of pedigrees have shown that **the three loci (for heavy, κ, and λ chains) are completely unlinked: they segregate independently, as though located on different chromosomes.**

Rabbit allotypes played a key role in establishing the concept that each Ig chain is coded for by two genes (below), and they were also instrumental in establishing the

---

* Unlike the sensitive hemagglutination assay for human allotypes (Fig. 16-13), precipitin reactions require high titers of Ab (Table 15-5, Ch. 15). Since soluble Igs are poor immunogens, antiallotype sera are produced by immunizing rabbits with other rabbits' aggregated Abs (cross-linked by an Ag), usually incorporated in Freund's adjuvant; the adjuvant is too irritating for use in humans (Ch. 17, Adjuvants).

identity of heavy chains and the identity of light chains in any given molecule, even when synthesized in a heterozygous animal. For example, successive additions of anti-b4 and anti-b5 precipitate 50 and 30%, respectively, of the Ig molecules in serum from a heterozygous b4,b5 rabbit. When the order of additions is reversed (anti-b5 then anti-b4) the amounts precipitated by each antiallotype are unaltered. Thus anti-b4 does not precipitate molecules with the b-5 marker and anti-b5 does not precipitate those carrying b-4 (Fig. 16-15). Similar findings with pairs of antisera to *a* allotypes and with anti-κ and anti-λ, reinforced by amino acid sequence analyses (below), established that **despite the great diversity of Ig chains synthesized in an individual, any particular Ig molecule has identical heavy chains and identical light chains.** The basis for this principle is that Ig-producing cells synthesize, at any one time, only one kind of heavy chain and one kind of light chain; the chains become irreversibly associated in the cell before they are secreted (Ch. 17).

MOUSE ALLOTYPES

Recognition of allotypes in mice has been simplified by the existence of inbred strains, whose individual members are isogenic (i.e., have essentially the same genome) and are homozygous at virtually all loci. Accordingly, allotype-specific antisera are easily produced by immunizing mice of one strain with Igs from another. A pair of allotypes for each of three IgG subclasses, and three allelic variants of α chains (IgA) have been identified.

Not a single recombinant has been detected in about 2000 progeny of crosses and F_2 back-crosses between inbred strains with different allotypes for heavy chains. Thus genes for γ and α chains appear to be tightly linked, as with the various γs in man (see Fig. 16-14). Allotypes for mouse light chains have not been identified.

UNIQUE DETERMINANTS OF INDIVIDUAL IMMUNOGLOBULINS: IDIOTYPES

Unlike particular isotypes and allotypes, which are found on many Igs, a given idiotype is essentially restricted to a particular Ab in a

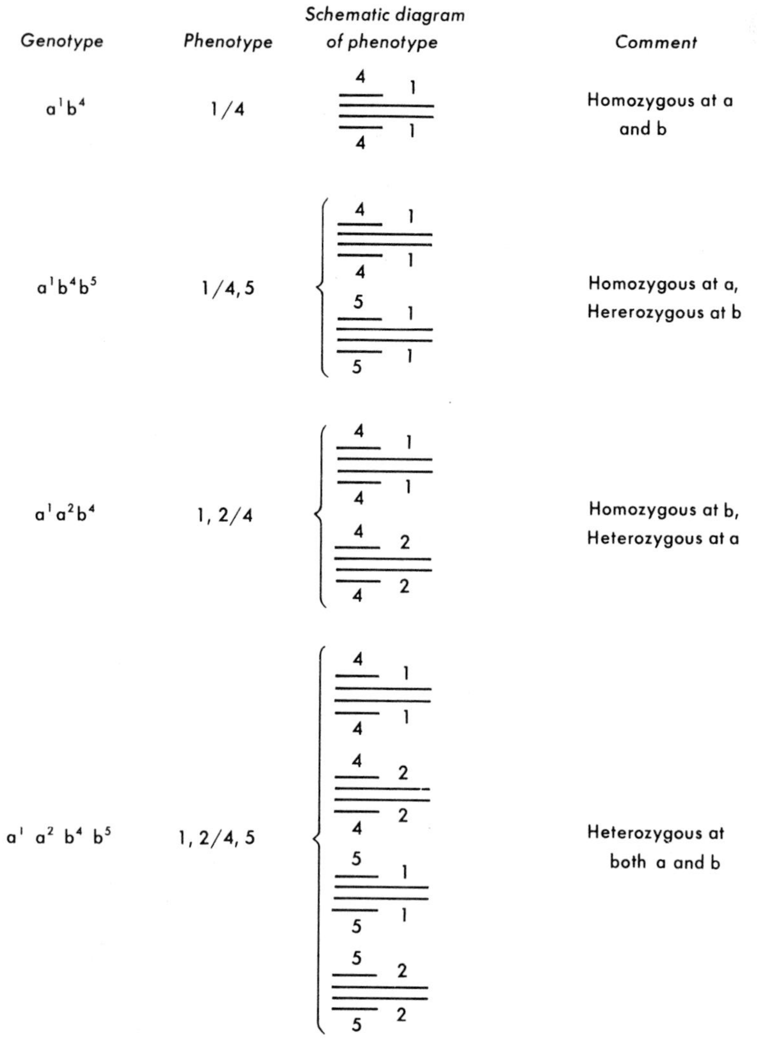

Genotype	Phenotype	Schematic diagram of phenotype	Comment
a^1b^4	1/4		Homozygous at a and b
$a^1b^4b^5$	1/4,5		Homozygous at a, Hererozygous at b
$a^1a^2b^4$	1, 2/4		Homozygous at b, Heterozygous at a
$a^1 a^2 b^4 b^5$	1, 2/4, 5		Heterozygous at both a and b

Fig. 16-15. Some allotypes of rabbit IgG. [Based on Dray, S., and Nisonoff, A. *Proc Soc Exp Biol Med 113*:20 (1963).]

particular individual.* Idiotypes were discovered by Oudin, who injected anti-*Salmonella* Abs from one rabbit (donor) into recipient rabbits with the same allotypes as the donor. Some recipients formed Abs (antiidiotypes) that reacted specifically with the immunogen but not with other Igs from the donor or to a significant extent with anti-

Salmonella Abs from other rabbits. It was found later, moreover, that each idiotype-specific antiserum recognizes only a particular subset of Ab molecules in the heterogeneous population of Abs used as immunogen. Idiotypes on some relatively homogeneous human Abs (e.g., to dextrans) have also been identified with rabbit antisera formed against the purified Abs from one person and then absorbed with all the other Igs from the same individual.

Idiotypes are confined to Fab fragments, where they appear to be localized at the ligand-binding sites. Thus, haptens can block competitively the reaction of an antihapten Ab with its antiidiotype. Idiotypes are also

---

* With certain inbred (genetically uniform) strains of mice identical or similar idiotypes are present in some of the Abs (of a given specificity) formed by various members of the strain. With outbred animals, in contrast, there are virtually no idiotypic cross-reactions among Abs of the same specificity from different individuals.

dependent on the singular conformation of appropriately combined light and heavy chains: when the isolated inactive chains reassociate, the antiidiotype usually reacts only with those correctly reconstituted molecules that recover the original Ag-binding activity.

Antigenic properties and amino acid sequences of myeloma proteins, considered in the following sections, reinforce the view that idiotypes are associated with those amino acid residues that are responsible for the uniqueness of each Ab.

HOMOGENEOUS IMMUNOGLOBULINS

MYELOMA AND BENCE JONES PROTEINS

Certain human diseases provide anomalies that are crucial for understanding normal structures and mechanisms, just as microbial mutants play a vital role in elucidating the physiology of wild-type organisms. Long apparent for the endocrine and nervous systems, this generalization has come more recently to apply to the immune response, especially through studies of the Igs secreted by the neoplastic plasma cells in patients with **multiple myeloma.** These **myeloma proteins** have been indispensable in revealing fundamental patterns of amino acid sequences and in the discovery of various light chain types, IgE, IgD, and the subclasses of IgG and IgA. A similar proliferative disease of lymphoid cells that produce IgM is called **Waldenström's macroglobulinemia.** Because the tumor in each patient appears to be a single clone, the homogeneous Ig it secretes is often called a **monoclonal** or **M protein.**

Similarly homogeneous Igs are also produced in occasional older individuals without obvious neoplastic or other proliferative disorders of lymphoid cells (ca. 2% of persons over 70). Mouse plasma cell tumors that secrete M proteins (IgG, IgA, IgM) are of great experimental value, as they can be readily induced in certain inbred strains (BALB/c, NZB) by intraperitoneal injections of mineral oil or implants of lucite shavings.

Many individuals with plasma cell tumors also excrete in the urine a peculiar **Bence Jones** protein, named after the physician who first studied it in the mid-nineteenth century. This protein has unusual thermosolubility

properties (in man, but not in mice): it precipitates on being heated to 45 to 60°, redissolves on boiling, and precipitates again on cooling. In contrast, serum Igs, like most other proteins, are coagulated irreversibly on boiling. These urinary proteins came under intensive study after Edelman and Gally and Putnam *et al.* showed that the Bence Jones protein excreted by a patient is nearly always identical with the light chain of his myeloma protein.

Myeloma and Bence Jones proteins are particularly valuable for antigenic and chemical analyses: not only is each homogeneous, but many are also available in large quantities. For example, a patient may have serum levels of a myeloma protein as high as 10 gm/100 ml, and may excrete up to 2 gm of a Bence Jones protein per day in his urine.*

Studies with labeled amino acids show that Bence Jones proteins are synthesized independently of myeloma proteins, rather than derived from them by cleavage. With mouse myeloma tumors, cells that secrete only light chains (Bence Jones protein) arise as frequent variants (possibly mutants) from tumor cells that produce complete myeloma proteins (Ch. 17).

COMPARISON BETWEEN "PATHOLOGICAL" AND NORMAL IMMUNOGLOBULINS

The fundamental identity of pathological and normal Igs has been established not only by their structural similarity but by the finding that some myeloma proteins bind ligands specifically, in the same way as authentic Abs (e.g., at one site per Fab fragment). Moreover, in response to certain immunization procedures occasional animals form Abs that appear to be as homogeneous as myeloma proteins (see below). It is now clear that **normal Igs and conventional Abs are mixtures of many individual proteins, each resembling a myeloma protein in its homogeneity and individuality.**

Homogeneity. The contrast between normal Igs and myeloma proteins can be epitomized by considering an individual whose myeloma

---

* The production of normal Igs and Abs is correspondingly poor, and these patients are sometimes detected clinically because they suffer from repeated bacterial infections.

tumor produces an IgG-1 protein. His normal IgG-1 will have κ and λ chains (Fig. 16-4) and, if he is heterozygous at loci for heavy and light chains, it will contain many allotypes—e.g., Gm(1), Gm(22), Inv(1,2), Inv(3). In contrast, the heavy chains of his myeloma protein will be **either** Gm(1) or Gm(22), its light chains will be **either** κ or λ, and if κ **either** Inv(1,2) or Inv(3). The myeloma protein's light chains would, like the Bence Jones protein he might excrete, appear in acrylamide gel disc electrophoresis as one

or two bands (monomer and dimer forms of the same chain), not the many bands observed with the light chains of his normal IgG-1 (Fig. 16-18). In addition, with conventional zone electrophoresis the normal Ig would form a broad ("polyclonal") band, whereas the myeloma protein would probably migrate as a compact ("monoclonal") peak (Fig. 16-16). The singularity of the amino acid sequences of a myeloma protein's heavy and light chains (below) also shows that in a given four-chained Ig molecule both light chains are identical, as are both heavy chains.

Though homogeneous in amino acid sequence some myeloma proteins are polydisperse in charge and in sedimentation velocity; this is especially common with IgA myeloma proteins, in which dimers, trimers, and higher multimers of the 7S monomer are formed by the same tumor. Electrophoretic inhomogeneity probably also arises from erratic losses of amide groups from glutamine and asparagine residues, perhaps from the action of plasma amidases.

Fig. 16-16. Electrophoresis of human sera on a cellulose acetate film. **A.** Normal serum. **B.** Serum with elevated, heterogeneous Igs (polyclonal hypergammaglobulinemia). **C–E.** Sera from three patients with multiple myeloma. Each myeloma protein (arrow) is a compact band (monoclonal Ig); note their different mobilities. **F, G.** Sera from children with virtual absence of immunoglobulins (agammaglobulinemia, see Ch. 17). Serum albumin is the compact dark band at left. (Courtesy of Dr. C. Kirk Osterland.)

Individuality. Like other Igs, myeloma proteins have isotypic antigenic markers, corresponding to the class (or subclass) of their heavy chain and the type of their light chain, and also allotypic markers, in accord with the genotype of the person or mouse in whom the tumor arose. Moreover, antisera to individual myeloma proteins reveal that each also has individual (idiotypic) antigenic peculiarities, recognized as spurs in gel diffusion tests. These idiotypic reactions can be blocked competitively, like the idiotypic reactions of conventional Abs, by ligands that are bound specifically by the myeloma protein.

When a pool of normal Igs is used to absorb an antiserum to a myeloma protein, the Abs to its isotypic and allotypic determinants are readily removed, but antiidiotypes are removed, if at all, by enormous amounts (e.g., 100 mg/ml antiserum). Hence the unique determinants in the ligand-binding regions of many individual myeloma proteins, like those of conventional Abs, are each represented at exceedingly low levels (if at all) in normal serum Igs.

HOMOGENEOUS ANTIBODIES

The homogeneity and high serum levels of myeloma proteins have been matched by Abs

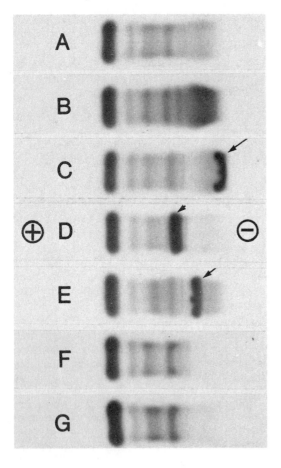

to bacterial capsular polysaccharides produced by animals after intensive immunization with streptococcal or pneumococcal vaccines (Figs. 16-17 and 16-18). In many of these animals serum Ab levels of 20 to 50 mg/ml are attained, and the Abs are of **restricted heterogeneity,** i.e., they are separable into two or three distinctive, homogeneous Abs.

A rare animal may produce a massive amount of a single Ab, as homogeneous as a myeloma protein, but unlike actual myeloma tumors, production depends on continued administration of immunogen. A clinical analogy is seen in occasional elderly persons with a benign form of Waldenström's macroglobulinemia who produce, without known immunization, two to four monoclonal IgM proteins, some of which react specifically with bacterial polysaccharides. It is possible that these individuals are subjected to prolonged antigenic stimulation by one of their own cryptic microorganisms or perhaps by cross-reacting "self" Ags (see Ch. 17, Tolerance; Ch. 20, Autoimmune disease). Ags that ordinarily elicit highly heterogeneous Abs (such as Dnp-proteins in the production of anti-Dnp Abs) appear to elicit Abs of restricted heterogeneity in animals of certain highly inbred strains, suggesting that genetic control, not just the nature of the Ag, determines **clonal dominance,** the ability of one or

a few clones of Ab-forming cells to overgrow others (Ch. 17, Clonal selection).

AMINO ACID SEQUENCES: THE BASIS FOR IMMUNOGLOBULIN DIVERSITY

Since Abs are highly diverse with respect to ligand-binding activities their combining sites must have diverse shapes. How can this variability be reconciled with the limitations imposed by the over-all structural uniformity described above? The cogency of this question is emphasized by the contrast with enzymes of diverse specificities, which are conspicuously dissimilar in structure (Table 16-4). A general answer emerged from analyses of amino acid sequences, which also established a chemical basis for the distinctions among isotypes, allotypes, and idiotypes, and brought into focus fundamental genetic issues underlying the diversity of Abs and their evolutionary development.

Most preparations of purified Abs are mixtures of many kinds of Ig molecules. Accordingly, the most extensive sequences have been established for myeloma and Bence

Fig. 16-17. Homogeneous antibody (arrow) raised in a rabbit. Serum samples were analyzed by electrophoresis on a cellulose acetate membrane. **A.** Before immunization. **B.** After 16 injections (4 weeks) of streptococcal vaccine (group C); the sample had about 40 mg Ab per milliliter serum. **C.** After absorption of the sample in **B** with purified envelope carbohydrate of group C streptococci. Compact, dark bands of serum albumin are at the right. [From Eichmann, K., Lackland, A., Hood, L., and Krause, R. M. *J Exp Med 131*:207 (1970).]

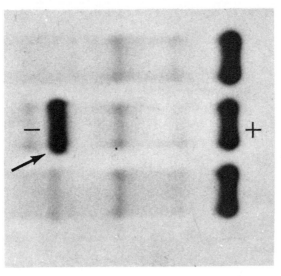

A preimmune

B 4th week   —   +

C abs with CHO

TABLE 16-4. Contrast Between Structural Diversity of Enzymes and Gross Structural Uniformity of Antibodies

Enzymes	Molecular weight	No. of chains	IgG antibodies specific for	Molecular weight	No. of chains
E. coli alkaline phosphatase	80,000	2	Diphtheria toxin	150,000	4
Pancreatic RNase	13,700	1	Bacteriophage T2	150,000	4
Phosphorylase a	495,000	4	Lysozyme	150,000	4
Yeast enolase	67,000	1	Azophenyl-β-lactoside	150,000	4
Glutamic acid dehydrogenase	336,000	6	2,4-Dinitrophenyl	150,000	4

Jones proteins, which are homogeneous. Similar (but less extensive) sequences have been determined for Igs from normal serum, and especially Abs of restricted heterogeneity [elicited by certain bacterial polysaccharides in outbred rabbits (genetically highly diversified) and by hapten-protein conjugates in inbred strains of guinea pigs].

GENERAL FEATURES OF LIGHT AND HEAVY CHAIN SEQUENCES: DOMAINS

Light chains vary slightly in length (211 to 217 residues). Heavy chains are twice as long: γ and α chains have about 450 residues, while μ and ε chains have about 550 residues. All chains consist of linearly repeating, similar

Fig. 16-18. Light chains from purified rabbit antibodies to pneumococcal polysaccharide (type 8) examined by polyacrylamide disc electrophoresis. **A.** From a rabbit with heterogeneous (polyclonal) Abs. **B–D.** From a rabbit after the first **(B)**, second **(C)**, and third **(D)** courses of immunization. Virtually homogeneous (monoclonal) Ab was obtained after the second course **(C)**. Bence Jones proteins and light chains from a myeloma protein migrate as one band (or sometimes as two due to presence of a dimeric form of light chain). [From Pincus, J. H., Jaton, J.-C., Bloch, K. J., and Haber, E. *J Immunol 104*:1149 (1970).]

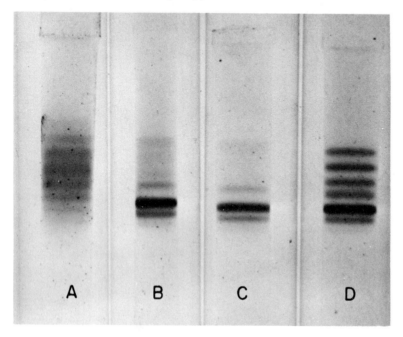

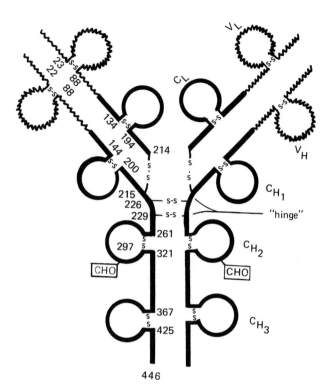

Fig. 16-19. Linear periodicity in amino acid sequences suggests that light (L) and heavy (H) chains have repeating domains, each with about 110 amino acid residues and an approximately 60-membered S-S bonded loop. Domains with variable sequences are represented by jagged lines (V_L, V_H); those with invariant sequences in a given class of H or type of L are represented by smooth lines (C_L, C_{H1}, C_{H2}, C_{H3}; see Fig. 16-21). Numbered positions refer to cysteinyl residues that form S-S bonds, or to the point of attachment of an oligosaccharide (CHO). For other arrangements of interchain S-S bonds see Figure 16-20. [Based on Edelman, G. M. *Biochemistry* **9**:3197 (1970).]

(but not identical) segments of about 110 residues: in each segment an S-S bond establishes an approximately 60-membered loop. Similarities in sequence suggest that each segment may be folded into a compact globular **domain,** stabilized by the S-S bond (Fig. 16-19). Adjacent domains are evidently linked by less tightly folded regions: thus pepsin can cut isolated light chains into halves, just as it cleaves between two heavy chain domains in intact Ig molecules in the production of Fab′ fragments (Fig. 16-5). Light chains contain two such domains, and heavy chains contain four (γ and α chains) or five (μ and ε chains). (Occasional domains have additional, smaller S-S bonded loops.)

Other cysteine residues form the interchain S-S bonds that link chains within molecules. The interchain bonds differ in number and position in different classes and subclasses of heavy chains (Fig. 16-20) and types of light

chains; e.g., the light-heavy interchain S-S bond involves a cysteine that is C-terminal in κ chains and penultimate in λ chains (see Fig. 16-23).

VARIABLE (V) AND CONSTANT (C) SEGMENTS

The first two Ig chains that were sequenced (human κ chains by Hilschmann and Craig and by Putnam *et al.*) revealed a remarkable pattern that has since been found consistently in all others. The two chains had different amino acid residues at many positions; but, strikingly, the differences were all clustered in the **amino-terminal half** of the chain, now called the variable or V segment or V_κ (Fig. 16-21). In the carboxyl half of the chain, called the constant or C segment (or C_κ), the sequences were identical except at position 191, where leucine and valine occur as

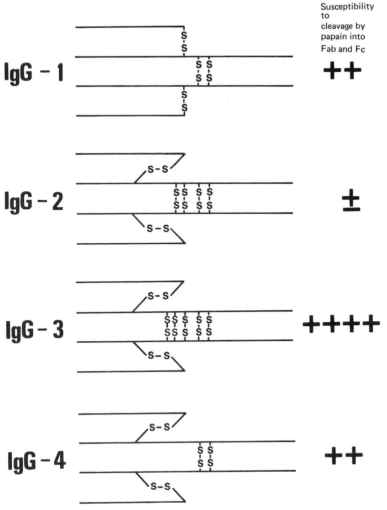

Susceptibility to cleavage by papain into Fab and Fc

IgG – 1   ++

IgG – 2   ±

IgG – 3   ++++

IgG – 4   ++

Fig. 16-20. Interchain S-S bridges in different IgG subclasses. The variations contrast with the virtual constancy of intrachain S-S bonds (Fig. 16-19). The heavy-heavy interchain bridges are in the hinge region, and their variations may be related to other differences among IgG subclasses, e.g., in susceptibility to papain digestion (Table 16-2). The heavy-chain cysteinyl residue forming the heavy-light S-S bridge in IgG-2,-3,-4 is about 100 residues closer to the amino terminus than in IgG-1 (left). [Based on data from Frangione, B., Milstein, C., and Pink, J. R. L. *Nature 211*:145 (1969).]

heritable variants (see Inv allotypes, above). A similar pattern is evident among human λ light chains, which also differ at many positions in the amino-terminal domain (V_λ), but have essentially the same sequence in the carboxy-terminal domain (C_λ).

Alternatives are found at two positions in the C_λ domain of λ chains: 153, ser-gly, and 190, lys-arg. Antisera can differentiate between λ chains with arg-190 and those with lys-190 (called Oz+ and Oz−, respectively, after the patient whose Bence Jones protein elicited the distinguishing antiserum). All of the variants at positions 153 and 190 have been found, in various combinations, among the peptides in proteolytic digests of light chains from

each of the 30 persons tested. Hence the C_λ variants are probably isotypes (i.e., present in all individuals), rather than allotypes like the Inv variants of C_κ.*

Heavy chains also differ extensively in sequence in the amino-terminal domain (V_H), but within a class or subclass the sequence in the remainder of the chain is identical (C_H segment), except for a few substitutions

---

* If the C_λ variants were allotypes the homozygous state (e.g., corresponding exclusively to λ_{arg} or to λ_{lys}) ought to have been observed even in a sample as small as 30 individuals.

that correspond to allotypic markers. The V_H segments are slightly longer than those of V_κ and V_λ (ca. 115 as compared with ca. 107 residues).

Though many positions in V segments are variable many others are invariant (or show little variation) within a given type (V_κ, V_λ, or V_H; see Fig. 16-21). For instance, the amino terminus of most V_λ segments is a cyclized glutamine residue (pyrrolidone carboxyl) without a free NH_2 group, whereas all V_κ sequences begin with a free amino group (usually of glu or asp). **The V_κ sequences are always associated with C_κ, and V_λ with C_λ. In contrast, the V_H sequences are not restricted to particular classes or subclasses of heavy chains.** The significance of these strict V-C associations is considered later in this chapter.

The over-all characteristics of amino acid sequences of Igs, derived initially from partial sequences of many chains, has been firmly established by Edelman *et al.*, who determined the complete sequences of both light and heavy chains of a myeloma protein (Fig. 16-22). Sequences that distinguish diverse chains and allotypic variants are illustrated in Figures 16-23 and 16-24.

V SUBGROUPS AND HYPERVARIABLE REGIONS

Comparison of many chains has revealed that sequence variability in V segments is dis-

Fig. 16-21. Variable (V) and constant (C) segments illustrated by selected amino acid sequences from some human light chains (named SH, etc., for the myeloma patient from whom the protein was derived). Sequences are aligned for maximal homology. At some positions in V segments the residues seem to be invariant in all light chains, including those from mice (e.g., Thr-6, Tyr-93, Gln-7, Phe-107, Gly-108, Gly-110, Thr-111). Amplitude of the jagged line above represents extent of variability. (Based on references in Dayhoff, M. ed. *Atlas of Amino Acid Sequence and Structure,* vol. 5. National Biomedical Research Foundation, Silver Spring, Md., 1972.)

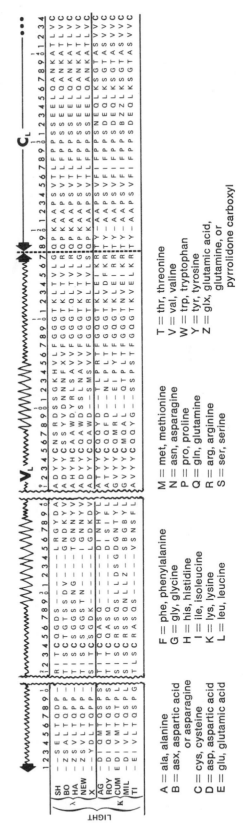

A = ala, alanine
B = asx, aspartic acid or asparagine
C = cys, cysteine
D = asp, aspartic acid
E = glu, glutamic acid
F = phe, phenylalanine
G = gly, glycine
H = his, histidine
I = ile, isoleucine
K = lys, lysine
L = leu, leucine
M = met, methionine
N = asn, asparagine
P = pro, proline
Q = gln, glutamine
R = arg, arginine
S = ser, serine
T = thr, threonine
V = val, valine
W = trp, tryptophan
Y = tyr, tyrosine
Z = glx, glutamic acid, glutamine, or pyrrolidone carboxyl

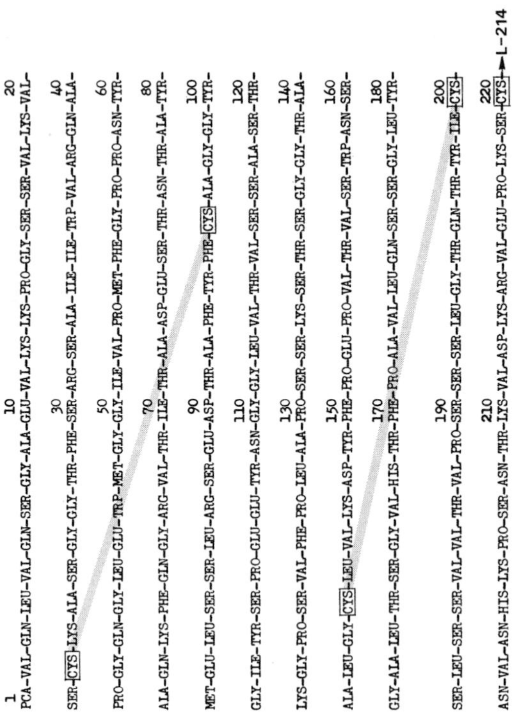

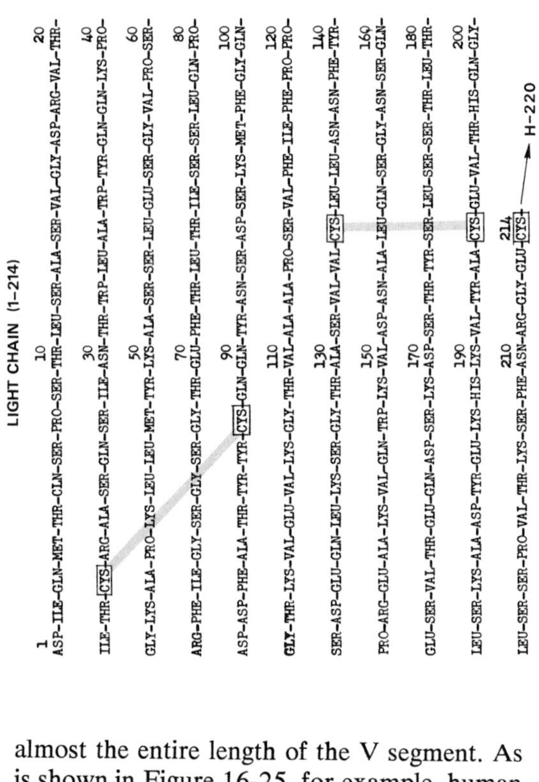

Fig. 16-22. Complete amino acid sequence of the light (κ) and heavy (γ1) chains of a human IgG1 myeloma protein (EU). Intrachain SS bonds are indicated by shaded bands and the interchain SS bridge between heavy (H) and light (L) chains by arrows. CHO is an oligosaccharide attached to the Asx residue (aspartic acid or asparagine) at position 297 (see Fig. 14-9). [Based on Edelman, G. M. *Biochemistry* 9:3197 (1970).]

tributed in a remarkable pattern, with two important features. First, those of a given type (V_κ, V_λ, V_H) can be arranged into sets, or **subgroups,** each of which is characterized by distinctive amino acids at certain positions, dispersed at unequal intervals throughout almost the entire length of the V segment. As is shown in Figure 16-25, for example, human V_κ sequences fall into three subgroups; five subgroups have similarly been recognized in human V_λ and three in human V_H. V segments that belong to the same subgroup differ in about 10 to 15 of their approximately 110 residues; those from different subgroups of the same type (e.g., $V\kappa_I$ vs. $V\kappa_{II}$) differ in about 25 to 35 residues. V segments of a given subgroup can be arranged in a genealogical order, as though the structural genes coding for them were derived sequentially by a series of single-step mutations (Fig. 16-26). Though divisions into subgroups are somewhat arbitrary, these sets are of considerable importance for theories concerned with the genetic basis for the diversity of Igs (see below).

The second important feature is that variability is especially pronounced at a few restricted regions, of which there are three in light chains (24-34, 50-55, 89-97), and four in heavy chains at approximately homologous positions (31-37, 50-65, 86-91, 101-109) (Fig. 16-27). When V segments of various chains are aligned for comparison it is necessary to introduce gaps (or insertions) into some of them in order to achieve maximal sequence homology, and the gaps also tend to cluster in the hypervariable regions. Chemical studies of the combining sites suggest that they are formed by the hypervariable regions (Affinity-labeling, below).

THE HINGE

Near the middle of heavy chains a special stretch of about 15 residues includes all the cysteines that form the heavy-heavy interchain S-S bonds. This region probably corresponds to the "hinge" in the Y-shaped molecule (Figs. 16-6 to 16-8). Amino acid **sequences at the hinge are distinctive for each class and subclass of heavy chains** (Fig. 16-28); **they are not homologous with other**

COOH ENDS

Human γ1 ...	Z	K	S	L	S	L	S	P	G
Human γ2 ...	Z	K	S	L	S	L	S	P	G
Human γ3 ...	Z	K	S	L	S	L	S	P	G
Human γ4 ...	Z	K	S	L	S	L	S	L	G
Human α ...	M	A	E	V	D	G	T	C	Y
Human μ ...	M	S	B	T	A	G	T	C	Y
Human κ ...	K	S	F	N	R	G	E	C	
Human λ ...	K	T	V	A	P	T	E	C	S
Mouse α ...	M	S	E	G	D	G	T	C	Y
Mouse κ ...	K	S	F	N	R	N	E	C	
Mouse λ1 ...	K	S	L	S	R	A	D	C	S
Mouse λ2 ...	K	S	L	S	P	A	E	C	L

Fig. 16-23. Representative C-terminal nonapeptides illustrating differences between heavy-chain classes and subclasses, and between κ and λ light chains. The cysteine that is C terminal in κ and penultimate in λ chains contributes to the S-S bonds that link light and heavy chains (see Fig. 16-22). For abbreviations, see legend, Figure 16-21. (Based largely on references in Dayhoff, M., ed., *Atlas of Amino Acid Sequence and Structure*, vol. 5. National Biomedical Research Foundation, Silver Spring, Md., 1972.)

parts of light or heavy chains. Diversity of sequences in the hinge region may be associated with some of the different biological properties of different Ig classes, e.g., in natural half life (see Appendix, Table 16-5).

	Allotypes	Amino acid substitutions	Position of substitution	Domain
Fig. 16-24. Amino acid substitutions associated with some allelic allotypes. Each substitution can be accounted for by a single base difference in the corresponding codon (e.g., Phe → Tyr is UU^U_C → UA^U_C). (Based on references in Grubb, R. *The Genetic Markers of Human Immunoglobulins*, Ch. 3. Springer, New York, 1970.)	Gm(1) Gm(-1)	··· Arg–**Asp**–Glu–**Leu**–Thr ··· ··· Arg–**Glu**–Glu–**Met**–Thr ···	356,358	C_{H3} of γ1
	Gm(4) Gm(-4)	··· Asp–Lys–**Arg**–Val–Glu ··· ··· Asp–Lys–**Lys**–Val–Glu ···	214	C_{HI} of γ1
	Gm(5) Gm(21)	··· Arg–**Phe**–Thr–Gln–Lys ··· ··· Arg–**Tyr**–Thr–Gln–Lys ···	Ca. 436	C_{H3} of γ?
	Inv(1, 2) Inv(3)	··· Lys–**Leu**–Tyr–Ala–Cys ··· ··· Lys–**Val**–Tyr–Ala–Cys ···	191	$C_κ$

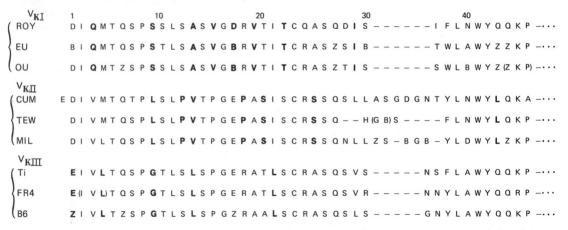

V_{KI}

	1				10					20				30				40

ROY   D I **Q** M T **Q** S P **S** S L S **A** S V G D R V T I **T** C Q A S Q D I S − − − − − I F L N W Y Q Q K P −···

EU   B I **Q** M T **Q** S P **S** T L S **A** S V G B R V T I **T** C R A S Z S I B − − − − − T W L A W Y Z Z K P −···

OU   D I **Q** M T Z S P **S** S L S **A** S V G B R V T I **T** C R A S Z T I S − − − − − S W L B W Y Z (Z K P) −···

V_{KII}

CUM   E D I V M T Q T P **L** S L **P** V T P G E **P A S** I S C R **S** S Q S L L A S G D G N T Y L N W Y **L** Q K A −···

TEW   D I V M T Q S P **L** S L **P** V T P G E **P A S** I S C R **S** S Q − − H (G B) S − − − − F L N W Y **L** Q K P −···

MIL   D I V L T Q S P **L** S L **P** V T P G E **P A S** I S C R **S** S Q N L L Z S − B G B − Y L D W Y **L** Z K P −···

V_{KIII}

Ti   **E** I V L T Q S P **G** T L S **L** S P G E R A T **L** S C R A S Q S V S − − − − N S F L A W Y Q Q K P −···

FR4   **E** (I V L) T Q S P **G** T L S **L** S P G E R A T **L** S C R A S Q S V R − − − − − N N Y L A W Y Q Q R P −···

B6   **Z** I V L T Z S P **G** T L S **L** S P G Z R A A **L** S C R A S Q S L S − − − − − G N Y L A W Y Q Q K P −···

Fig. 16-25. V_κ subgroups. Amino acid sequences at N-terminal region of some human κ chains demonstrate three subgroups. Subgroup-specific residues are in boldface. Alignment maximizes homology; dashes (gaps) represent deletions (or insertions). Residues in parentheses are known by peptide composition, and not actually sequenced. See Figure 16-21 for abbreviations. [Data are from several laboratories, reviewed by Hood, L., and Prahl, J. *Adv Immunol 14*:291 (1971).]

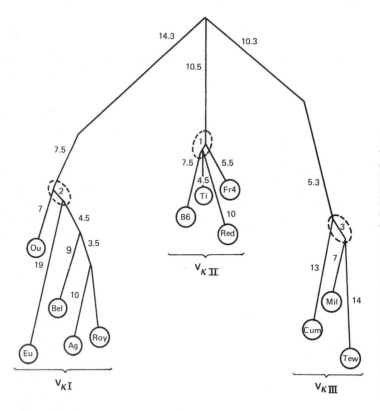

Fig. 16-26. A genealogical tree for human V_κ domains, based on residue-by-residue comparison of several κ chains. The numbers alongside each branch represent the average number of nucleotide differences required after each nodal point to code for the observed amino acid differences. Divergences of uncertain order are enclosed in a dashed line. Similar genealogies are characteristic of families of proteins that arise in evolution by successive mutations (Ch. 12). The circled name or number identifies the sequenced Bence Jones protein. [Based on Smith, G. P., Hood, L., and Fitch, W. M. *Annu Rev Biochem 40*:969 (1971).]

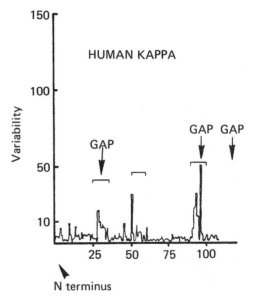

Fig. 16-27. Hypervariable regions in V segments of human κ chains. Variability (v) is defined as the number (n) of different amino acids at a given position in the chains under comparison divided by the frequency (f) of the most common amino acid at that position (v = n/f). Variability can range from 1.0 (no variation) to 400. Regions with greatest variability are 89 to 97 in V_L and 95 to 102 V_H domains. [From Kabat, E. A., and Wu, T. T. *Ann NY Acad Sci 190*:382 (1971).]

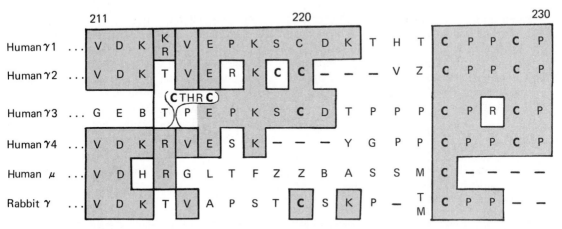

Fig. 16-28. Hinge region of some heavy chains. Shaded residues are identical with γ1. Cys in boldface form interchain heavy-heavy S-S bonds (see Fig. 16-20); cys not in boldface (220 in human γ1) forms interchain heavy-light S-S bonds. The alternatives at 214 in human γ1 and at 225 in rabbit γ are associated with allotypes (Fig. 16-26). The sequences are aligned with an insertion in γ3 and gaps in other chains in order to maximize homology with γ1. Other than the differences shown, the various human γ chains (subclasses) seem to be identical at almost all other positions in their respective C regions (e.g., Fig. 16-23). For abbreviations, see legend, Figure 16-21. (Based on references in Dayhoff, M., ed., *Atlas of Amino Acid Sequence and Structure,* vol. 5. National Biomedical Research Foundation, Silver Spring, Md. 1972.)

In γ chains the hinge region contains an unusual abundance of proline and hydrophilic residues (lysine, aspartic), which promote the exposure of this region, without tight folding, to solvent. This feature is probably related to the susceptibility of this region to attack by proteases, and to the apparent flexibility of the Fab arms of the Y-shaped molecule. The hinge region of μ chains is not rich in proline; instead it has an attached oligosaccharide, which might similarly promote exposure to solvent.

GENETIC BASIS OF IMMUNOGLOBULIN STRUCTURE

TWO GENES—ONE CHAIN

The finding that chains of the same type have identical sequences in the C domain but different sequences in the V domain seemed difficult to reconcile with the doctrine that every polypeptide chain is coded for by one gene. The mendelian inheritance of C-region allotypes implies that each C sequence is coded for by a **single** structural gene. But there must be **multiple** V genes, for each V subgroup must be specified by at least one gene. Otherwise, many parallel and independent somatic mutations would be required to generate the many members of each subgroup in each individual, and this seems most unlikely. The generally accepted solution (based on an early suggestion by Dreyer and Bennett) is that any one of many V genes can be associated with a single C gene in the synthesis of an Ig chain: i.e., **each immunoglobulin chain seems to be coded for by two genes, one for the V segment and one for the C segment.**

The following observations support this hypothesis:

1) In addition to the a allotypes (Rabbit allotypes, above) the γ chains of rabbit IgG contain genetic markers $d11$ and $d12$, determined by alleles at the d locus. Markers a and d are linked but can separate in out-breeding populations (by recombination?), and mutations in a and d alter different parts of the same γ chain. The residues associated with various a markers seem to be localized in the V_H domain and appear to occupy several (ca. 15) widely dispersed positions near the amino terminus, whereas the single residue associated with the d marker (a methionine for $d11$ and a threonine for $d12$) is located near the middle of the chain (position 225; Fig. 16-28).* Thus one gene seems to code for the amino terminal section (about 115 residues) and the other gene for the remainder of the chain; and somehow they become associated in specifying a complete chain. The finding that the **same** a allotypic markers, located in the N-terminal section, can occur on various classes of heavy chains (γ, μ, α, ε; the Todd phenomenon) also supports the two genes–one chain hypothesis, and, indeed, first prompted its serious consideration.

2) About 1% of patients with multiple myeloma form two distinct myeloma proteins. In one patient with such a "biclonal" tumor the IgM and IgG myeloma proteins had the same idiotype, which became understandable when it was later found that the μ and γ chains of the two proteins had the same V_H sequence and were associated with the same light chain.

TRANSLOCATION HYPOTHESIS

If it is true that two genes specify one polypeptide chain, how do they cooperate? Do the genes fuse, or are their separate products joined in cells at the level of mRNA or polypeptide? Suggestive evidence for fusion at the DNA level is provided by rare patients who produce unusually short heavy chains ("heavy-chain disease"). Secreted in urine, these chains (γ and α) lack some of the carboxyl (internal) end of the V_H segment and some of the adjacent amino end of the C_H segment. They can be understood as the product of an aberrant recombination between a V and a C gene with a large internal deletion (for which there is ample genetic precedent). The alternatives would not only require a novel mechanism for joining mRNA or polypeptide molecules, but would require that the mechanism be able to function without the ends that are normally ligated.

The fusion of V and C genes is also con-

---

* The association of several different amino acid residues with each a allotype is an exception to the rule that allelic polypeptide chains generally differ from each other in only one or two residues per 100; e.g., normal and sickle cell α hemoglobin chains, Inv allotypes of human κ light chains (above).

sistent with evidence that in Ab-forming cells (pulse-labeled with radioactive amino acids) the nascent Ig chains elongate continuously from the amino terminus, without interruption, as do proteins in general. In addition, the RNA for an Ig light chain has been found to be large enough to code for the complete chain.

As noted before, there are stringent limitations to the association between V and C segments: i.e., V_κ sequences are always associated with C_κ, and V_λ sequences with C_λ. V_H sequences, however, are not differentiated among the various C_H classes (C_γ, C_μ, C_α, etc.). A basis for this rule has been suggested by the finding that the genes for κ light chains, those for λ light chains, and the set of closely linked genes for the diverse classes of heavy chains segregate independently and hence are probably on separate chromosomes. **This separateness could**

account for the V-C restrictions if only V and C genes on the same chromosome can fuse to code for a given chain (Fig. 16-29A,B).

Supporting evidence for this view is provided by a study of two pairs of allelic markers in different parts of the same heavy (γ) chains of rabbit IgG: *a1* and *a3* in the V_H segment, *d11* and *d12* in the $C\gamma$ segment. When homozygous rabbits were crossed (a1,d11 × a3,d12) the doubly heterozygous progeny had the expected variety of markers, but their individual γ chains were almost exclusively of parental type: i.e., **either** a1,d11 **or** a3,d12. (As noted above, however, genetic recombination between the *a* and *d* markers must occur occasionally, because various combinations are found in large outbreeding populations; e.g., a1,d12 and a3,d11.)

One scheme for joining separate V and C genes is shown in Figure 16-29B, which depicts a chromosome with a linear array of

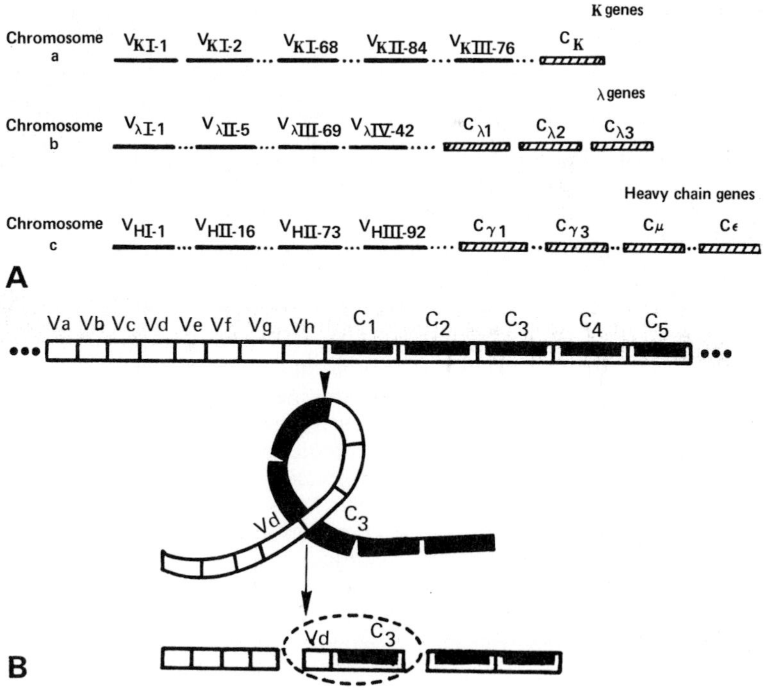

Fig. 16-29. A. Studies with allotypic markers show that the three families of V and C genes (κ, λ, heavy) segregate independently, as though located on different chromosomes (a, b, c). **B.** Scheme for translocation of a V to a C gene, forming a complete structural gene ($V_d \cdot C_3$) for an Ig chain.

The Ig genes of a given chromosome constitute a "translocon"; see p. 440. [**B** derived from Dreyer, W. J., and Bennett, J. C. *Proc Nat Acad Sci USA 54*:864 (1965), and Gally, J. A. and Edelman, G. M. *Ann Rev Genet 6*:1 (1972).]

linked V_H and C_H genes. One of many V_H genes is presumed to move next to and join a C_H gene further along on the same chromosome by crossover at a region of homology, as in the integration of a temperate phage into the bacterial chromosome. [This crossover might recognize nucleotide sequences at positions corresponding to the ends that become ligated: thus the N-terminal 3 to 4 amino acid residues of C_{HI} segments are the same in γ, μ and α chains.]

ORIGIN OF DIVERSITY

In any particular species the number of different C segments is limited: in man there are 4 or 5 for C_L and about 10 for C_H, and where allotypic variants of these sequences are known they are inherited as uncomplicated mendelian alleles. It appears therefore that each C segment is coded for by a single structural gene, and transmitted from generation to

generation in the germ line. With V segments, however, the number of distinctive amino acid sequences is enormously greater: any individual must be able to synthesize thousands of different V_L and V_H sequences in producing an immense variety of Abs. Figure 16-30 summarizes the main theories that try to account for the origin of this great multitude of V sequences.

Germ Line Theory. According to this theory germ cells carry structural genes for all the V_L and V_H sequences an individual can synthesize. These genes would have arisen during evolution through conventional mechanisms for gene duplication, mutation, and selection. The germ line theory not only provides an explanation within the known framework of molecular genetics but also readily accounts for the genealogical relation among V sequences (Fig. 16-26) and their orderly, though arbitrary, arrangements into sub-

Fig. 16-30. Theories of origin of diversity of immunoglobulin V genes. (Based on Edelman, G. M. In Neurosciences, Second Study Program, F. O. Schmitt (ed.), Rockefeller Univ. Press, N.Y., 1970.)

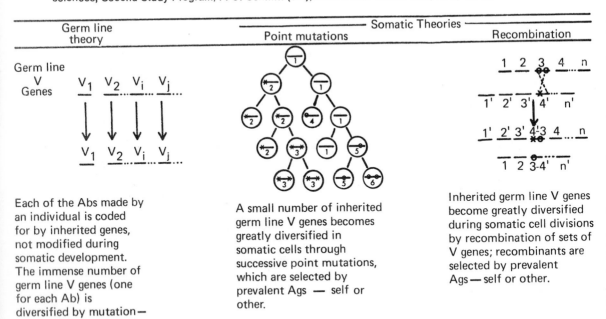

groups. Moreover, the required number of V genes could easily be accommodated in the vertebrate genome.

A typical diploid mammalian cell has about 10^{-11} g DNA, which could code for about 4×10^9 amino acid residues in proteins.* Hence as many as 1×10^4 V genes (each coding for 110 residues) would occupy only about 0.025% of the genome (e.g., $1 \times 10^4 \times 110/4 \times 10^9$). If the number of V_L and V_H genes were approximately equal and their products could pair at random, and if each paired V_L-V_H sequence established a unique, specific combining site, this number of genes could generate about 1×10^8 different Abs—or perhaps 1×10^7 if only 10% of the V_L-V_H pairs resulted in stable Ig molecules (see Reconstruction of combining sites, below). This number is probably sufficient to account for the apparently limitless diversity of antigenic determinants to which an individual can make an immune response.

There are, however, difficulties with the germ line theory. Foremost, perhaps, is the implication that the preservation and diversification of thousands of germ line V genes throughout evolution is governed, like that of other genes, by selection for survival value and loss by genetic drift: it is difficult to see how this mechanism would provide Abs to Ags that probably never existed in the past history of a species, such as those of recently synthesized organic chemicals (e.g., benzenearsonate). The preservation of so many unused genes during eons of evolution seems impossible unless a given Ig can react specifically with many structurally dissimilar ligands, and such strange cross-reactions have not been generally found. However, some do occur: e.g., between anti-Dnp Abs and a 1,4-naphthoquinone (menadione) that resembles the vitamin K-like molecules produced by common intestinal bacteria.

Another difficulty is that a few positions have the same residues in all V sequences of a given type in a particular species (species-specific residues) or in a given allotype. It is difficult to see how such invariant species-specific and allotype-specific codons can be present in thousands of independent germ line V genes, for this development would seem to have required a highly unlikely series of parallel, independent mutations plus exceedingly strong selective pressure for these residues. Moreover, if the same allotype-specific residues are present in thousands of V sequences, recombination among the multitude of similar alleles in heterozygous individuals must somehow be prevented. Otherwise these allotypes would not be recognizable as distinct mendelian markers.

Though severe, these difficulties may not be insurmountable. Hood has suggested that sets of V genes might undergo rapid expansion and contraction in evolution through preferential duplication of particular genes in a set, and that this process could lead to the appearance of species-specific or allotype-specific residues. Moreover, a precedent exists for the absence of recombination among genes of certain chromosomes, e.g., in male *Drosophila*.

Somatic Mutation Theory. This theory maintains that a small number of germ line genes become highly diversified through mutation in somatic cells, yielding differentiated clones of immunologically competent cells (Ch. 17, Lymphocytes) that differ in V genes. Though the number of V genes per somatic cell is presumed to be as small as in germ cells, their variety in the individual animal could be immense if there were a sufficient number of different cells (lymphocytes).

The severest problem faced by this theory is that of accounting for the accumulation of a vast number of different sequences during the period between fertilization of an egg and acquisition of immunological competence by the embryo (Ch. 17, Ontogeny). Special mechanisms have been proposed for increasing mutation rates in cells destined to make Abs, but they seem unnecessary: even with ordinary mutation rates (ca. 10^{-7}/base pair/cell division) the mutation rate per V gene might well be about one per 10^5 cell divisions, since there are ca. 330 nucleotide base pairs per V gene and perhaps 10% of the mutations would be compatible with a functional Ig chain. It is likely that many (e.g., 1000) immunologically competent cells with V gene mutations could arise each day among the special sets of rapidly dividing lymphocytes of even so small an animal as the mouse (e.g., the ca. 1×10^8 cells of the thymus; see Ch. 17). However, to account for the observed diversity of V sequences the cells with mutations would have to be selected for, relative to the vastly greater number of cells with unmutated germ line V genes.

The effects of an immunogen on the corresponding Ag-sensitive cell (Ch. 17) suggest that if a cell expressing a particular mutant V gene should happen to encounter the appropriate Ag the cell would be stimulated to proliferate (**positive selection**). The need for a large number and variety of selective Ags during ontogeny is bypassed in Jerne's proposal

---

* On the basis of a triplet code and a weight of 600 daltons for each nucleotide pair, 1×10^{-11} g DNA/$3 \times 600 = 6 \times 10^{-15}$ moles amino acid equivalents; and $6 \times 10^{-15} \times 6 \times 10^{23}$ (Avogadro's number) $= 36 \times 10^8$ amino acid residues in proteins.

for **negative selection:** germ line V genes are assumed to code for V domains that are specific for certain self-Ags (histocompatibility Ags on cell surfaces, Ch. 21), leading to suppression of the cells that express these anti-self genes, as part of the normal mechanism for maintaining self-tolerance (Ch. 17). Hence cells with V gene mutations coding for Igs that are specific for *anything* other than self-Ags would be preferentially preserved. The resulting selection would thus operate in favor of mutations in hypervariable regions (which determine Ab specificity, see below), without requiring the fortuitous presence of the corresponding Ags. Random mutations in C genes and in relatively invariant regions of V genes probably also occur but would not accumulate, either because they are selected against (if, for instance, they are incompatible with a functional Ig molecule) or because they are neutral and not subject to any selective pressure.

Somatic Recombination of Germ Line Genes. According to this theory, diversity arises in somatic cells through recombination among a limited number of germ line V genes for each subgroup. If there are a different codons at each of n positions, unlimited recombination could yield a^n sequences. If, for example, there were several germ line V genes for a given subgroup with 12 variable positions and 4 different codons represented at each of these positions, unlimited recombination could result in 4^{12}, or about 10^7, different sequences in this V subgroup. The germ line V genes are assumed to have been selected in evolution for ability to generate highly diverse somatic recombinants rather than for ability to determine V regions of a particular specificity. Thus this theory avoids the necessity of either preserving through eons of evolution a large number of germ line genes for Ags that have yet to come into existence (like the germ line theory) or of generating through successive point mutations a large repertoire of useful mutations during embryonic development (like somatic mutation theory).

The hypothetical recombination in somatic cells is postulated to occur among V genes of the same chromosome (see "translocon," Fig. 16–29). Recombination between homologous chromosomes would require their pairing, which is exceedingly rare in mitosis (unlike its regular occurrence during meiosis in formation of gametes). So far, V sequences have not yielded evidence for recombination. But relatively few V sequences are completely known and recombination would be difficult to detect if the number of recombining genes were large (e.g., 100).

Other, more unconventional suggestions include the proposal that episomes coding for hypervariable regions might be inserted into V genes in chromosomal DNA. If the variability were present in the episomes its origin would still have to be explained; if it were generated during the insertion process (e.g., by incision and repair errors) it is not clear why those chains that differ more in the hypervariable regions also differ more in the less variable parts of the V segments. Another proposal, without known precedents in other genetic structures, suggests that the vertebrate chromosome contains parallel, interconnecting networks of DNA strands that are transcribed by a polymerase that can switch back and forth among the strands, generating a large number of different mRNAs for V segments.

A firm decision between germ line and somatic theories cannot be made on available evidence. But preliminary results from hybridization of radioactive mRNA for an Ig light chain to homologous DNA suggest that the mouse genome probably has between 40 and 500 genes for light chains; the smaller number, if valid, would certainly rule out the germ line theory.

EVOLUTION OF IMMUNOGLOBULINS

Homologies Among Chains. Because serological analyses are sensitive to small antigenic variations they are particularly valuable for revealing differences among Ig chains. Amino acid sequences, in contrast, are especially useful for revealing similarities among chains, including those that do not cross-react at all serologically. The relatedness of two chains is apparent from the frequency with which corresponding positions are occupied by the same amino acid. A more searching comparison determines the minimum number of mutations necessary to change from one chain to the other. Both approaches give essentially the same result, and for both it is usually necessary to introduce occasional gaps in one or another chain, corresponding to genetic deletions, to bring out the full extent of their homology.

The sequences shown in Figures 16-21, 16-23, and 16-28 illustrate variations in homology, and the matrix of Figure 16-31 summarizes homology relations among a number of C segments. Extensive analyses of this kind lead to the following generalizations:

1) Homology is greater between the C_κ sequences of different species (man and mouse), and between

Fig. 16-31. Matrix comparison of frequencies of identical amino acid residues in homologous positions of the constant (C) regions of various Ig chains, expressed as identities per 100 residues (%). The most striking homologies (>60%) are encircled. Because there are 20 amino acids, 5% identity is the background level expected when randomly chosen chains are compared. (In fact, when the first 110 residues of the human hemoglobin α chain are compared with the above Ig chains identities range from 4 to 8%.) (Based on sequences and references in Dayhoff, M. D., ed. *Atlas of Protein Sequence and Structure*, vol. 5. National Biomedical Research Foundation, Silver Spring, Md., 1972.)

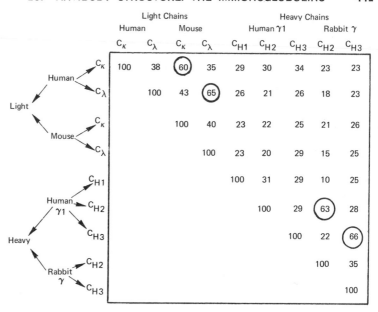

| | | Light Chains | | | | Heavy Chains | | | | |
| | | Human | | Mouse | | Human γ1 | | | Rabbit γ | |
		C_κ	C_λ	C_κ	C_λ	C_{H1}	C_{H2}	C_{H3}	C_{H2}	C_{H3}
Human	C_κ	100	38	(60)	35	29	30	34	23	23
	C_λ		100	43	(65)	26	21	26	18	23
Mouse	C_κ			100	40	23	22	25	21	26
	C_λ				100	23	20	29	15	25
Human γ1	C_{H1}					100	31	29	10	25
	C_{H2}						100	29	(63)	28
	C_{H3}							100	22	(66)
Rabbit γ	C_{H2}								100	35
	C_{H3}									100

the C_λ sequences of different species, than between C_κ and C_λ of the same species.

2) Successive domains in the constant part of heavy chains of a particular class (C_{H1}, C_{H2}, C_{H3} of γ chains) have extensive homology with each other, with the corresponding domains of other species (cf. human and rabbit γ), and also with C_κ and C_λ sequences.

3) Hardly any homologies are detectable between V and C sequences, even when those of the same chain are compared.

4) In spite of variations among different molecules, there is more homology **within** each of the V_κ, and V_λ, and the V_H sets than among these sets (Fig. 16-21). Nevertheless, discernible low-level homology among all V sequences sets them apart from all the C sequences.

5) The V_H and V_L sequences of the same molecule may have no more homology than those from different molecules.

Order of Evolution. From these observations it has been suggested that structural genes for present-day Igs evolved from a primordial gene coding for a polypeptide with the general characteristics of V and C segments, viz., about 110 amino acids with two cysteine residues that form an approximately 60-membered S-S loop. The small degree of homology between V and C sequences suggests that as one of the earliest events duplication of the primordial gene probably gave rise to the primitive precursors of V and C genes. Genes for constant segments of diverse heavy chains could have arisen from unequal ("illegitimate") crossover, yielding duplicated C genes (Fig. 16-32). The light chains in immuno-

globulins of sharks (among the most primitive existing vertebrates) appear to be only of the κ type. This finding and the extensive homology between avian and mammalian λ chains, suggest that C_κ is the more primitive C_L gene and that it probably gave rise by duplication to the C_λ gene some time before birds and mammals diverged, about 250 million years ago. Present day μ chains are assumed to correspond most closely to primordial heavy

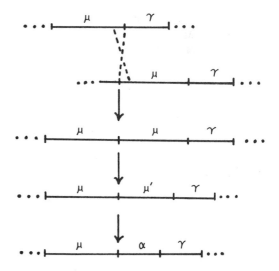

Fig. 16-32. Illegitimate crossing over could generate additional genes, whose occasional missense mutations could be selected for, leading eventually to the appearance of new Ig classes or subclasses (e.g., μ → α).

chains, because sharks and teleost fish have only one class, resembling μ of higher forms. Chains resembling γ are present only in amphibia and higher vertebrates; hence C_γ may have arisen from C_μ (with a deletion). Recognized clearly so far only in mammals and in birds, α chains probably arose by a still later duplication, most likely of the μ gene, since μ and α are more alike than either is like γ, at least near the C-terminus (see Fig. 16-23). This order of evolution (Fig. 16-33) is in accord with the successive appearance of Igs during embryonic development and infancy (IgM first, then IgG, finally IgA), and with the principle that ontogeny recapitulates phylogeny. Ontogeny and phylogeny of the immune response are considered further in Chapter 17.

COMBINING SITES: THE BASIS FOR ANTIBODY SPECIFICITY

The biological activity of an Ab molecule centers on its ability to bind ligands specifically. As noted before, binding studies reveal two combining sites per four-chain molecule, one in each Fab region (see Ch. 15, Equilibrium dialysis, and above, this chapter), while Fc fragments have other sites that engage in general effector reactions (Table 16-5; also see Ch. 18, Complement Fixation; Ch. 19, Allergic Responses). After an Fab fragment is completely unfolded (e.g., in 7 M

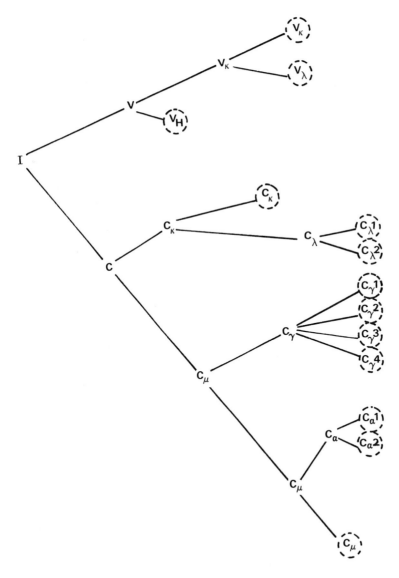

Fig. 16-33. Possible order of evolution of contemporary Ig genes (in dashed circles) from a primitive precursor (I) over approximately 4×10^8 years. δ and ε are not included as too little is known of their structure.

guanidine-HCl) and has had all its S-S bonds cleaved by reduction, it can spontaneously regain some of its original activity following air oxidation (2SH→S-S) and annealing (refolding) in dilute solution under physiological conditions of pH and ionic strength. Hence, just as with enzymes, **the amino acid sequences of Ig chains determine the shape, composition, and specificity of the Ab molecule's combining site.**

COMPOSITION OF COMBINING SITES

A number of elegant methods have been devised to identify the amino acid residues that form the active site. In the widely used method of **affinity-labeling** chemically reactive small molecules serve as univalent haptens. In reacting with the corresponding Ab, these reagents are first bound specifically in the active site by noncovalent bonds, and then form stable covalent bonds with susceptible amino acids in or close to the site. For example, Abs to the 2,4-dinitrophenyl group bind *m*-nitrobenzenediazonium salts, which can form azo derivatives of tyrosine, histidine, or lysine residues. The derivatives are stable during separation of the chains and their cleavage into peptides, making it possible to establish the position of the labeled residue

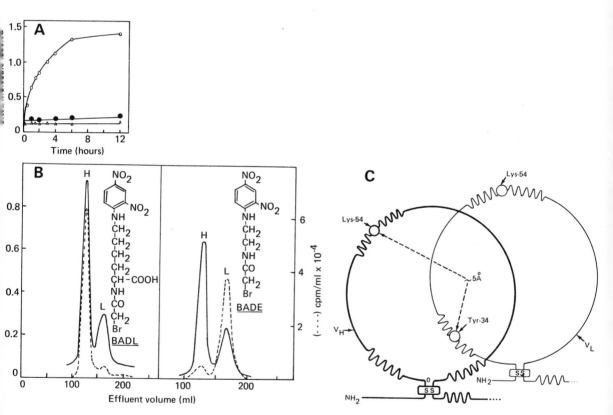

Fig. 16-34. Affinity-labeling of a mouse myeloma protein with antihapten activity (anti-Dnp). **A.** Rate of labeling the combining sites of the myeloma protein (O) with a bromoacetyl-Dnp reagent (BADE; structure shown in right panel of **B**). The presence of excess ε-Dnp-L-lysine specifically blocked the binding and reaction of BADE (●) ("hapten protection"). In a control test BADE did not label nonspecific mouse Ig (△). **B.** Separation of heavy (H) and light (L) chains of the myeloma protein after reaction with ^{14}C-BADL, which labeled only the H chain, or with ^{14}C-BADE, which labeled only the L chain. **C.** Localization of labeled residues in hypervariable regions (jagged lines) of V_L (light lines) and V_H (heavy lines) domains. A bifunctional Dnp reagent with bromoacetyl groups at two positions (ca. 5 Å apart), one resembling its position in BADL and the other its position in BADE, labeled **both** Lys-54 on V_H and Tyr-34 on V_L, cross-linking H and L chains (dashed lines). A second myeloma protein with anti-Dnp activity was specifically labeled by BADE in Lys-54 of V_L domain. [Based largely on Haimovich, J., Eisen, H. N., Hurwitz, E., and Givol, D. *Biochemistry 11*:2389 (1972).]

in a chain. The specificity of the labeling reaction can be vertified by **hapten protection,** in which an excess of a conventional hapten (which cannot form a covalent bond) specifically blocks the covalent reaction (Fig. 16-34A).

Because of their homogeneity, myeloma proteins with combining sites of known specificity are especially useful for affinity-labeling, furnishing labeled peptides in high yield. From studies of these proteins and of conventional, heterogeneous Abs it is clear that amino acid residues of **both** heavy and light chains of a single Ig can be specifically labeled, and that **the labeled residues fall within the hypervariable regions of the V_L and V_H segments** (Fig. 16-34). However, the residues that become labeled are sometimes common to many chains (conserved amino acids) and are not unique to Abs of a particular specificity. Hence the labeled residue is useful in locating regions involved in the combining site, but it is not necessarily of singular importance in establishing the unique structure of that site.

The close approximation of hypervariable regions of both V_L and V_H in the combining site is emphasized by the specific reaction of a bifunctional affinity-labeling reagent, with which it has been possible to label covalently **two** amino acid residues in the same site, one in a hypervariable part of V_H and the other in a hypervariable part of V_L. From

the dimensions of the reagent it is clear that substituted residues in hypervariable V_L and V_H are within 8 A in the intact molecule (Fig. 16-34).

Comparison of sequences of selected Igs provides independent evidence that hypervariable regions determine the specificity of combining sites. Thus several Abs with the same ligand-binding specificity have had virtually identical residues in hypervariable regions of their V_L and V_H segments (Fig. 16-35); moreover, some of the identical residues are rarely present in the corresponding regions of chains from randomly selected Igs.

SIZE OF COMBINING SITES

The dimensions of the combining sites have been estimated primarily from binding studies (Ch. 15). Abs to dextran (poly-D-glucose) bind with increasing strength glucose oligosaccharides of increasing size up to a maximum of about six or seven residues (Fig. 16-36). Similar results have been obtained with Abs to polythymidylic acid or to polyalanine, where binding also appears to be maximal with oligomers of four, five, or six residues. If the combining sites for these ligands were shaped as an invagination that encompassed an extended four- to six-membered oligomer, about 20 of the approximately 220 amino acid residues of the V_L and the V_H segments of an antibody molecule might make contact with the ligand. (A similar number of contact residues have been demonstrated by X-ray diffraction to constitute the active site of

Fig. 16-35. Evidence that variable residues, especially in hypervariable regions, are associated with specificity of combining sites. Sequences from N terminal to position 40 for light (κ) chains of three human monoclonal antibodies (Dav, Fin, Lay; specific for IgG), are compared with Bence Jones κ chains of V_{K_1} subgroup, of which protein AG is the prototype. Listed above the AG sequence are the substitutions, and their approximate frequencies, in other light chains of V_{K_1} subgroup. The identity of Dav and Fin is impressive but Lay, with the same specificity, is somewhat different, showing that various sequences are compatible with a given specificity. Variability is pronounced at the hypervariable region (30 to 32 and 34), but it is certainly not limited to that region. See Fig. 16-21 for abbreviations. [Based on Capra, J. D., Kehoe, J. M., Winchester, R. J., and Kunkel, H. G. *Ann NY Acad Sci* 190:371 (1971); AG is due to Titani, K., Whitley, E., Avogardo, L., and Putnam, F. W. *Science* 149:1090 (1965); for sources on substitutions above AG see refs. in Wu, T. T. and Kabat, E. A. *J Exp Med* 132:211 (1970).]

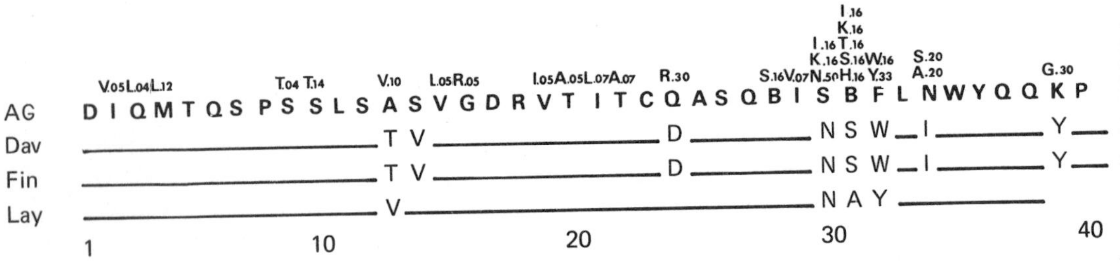

	$V_{.05}L_{.04}L_{.12}$			$T_{.04}$ $T_{.14}$		$V_{.10}$	$L_{.05}R_{.05}$			$L_{.05}A_{.05}L_{.07}A_{.07}$		$R_{.30}$			$S_{.16}V_{.07}N_{.50}H_{.16}$ $Y_{.33}$	$I_{.16}$ $K_{.16}$ $I_{.16}T_{.16}$ $K_{.16}S_{.16}W_{.16}$	$S_{.20}$ $A_{.20}$			$G_{.30}$	
AG	D I Q M T Q S	P S	S L S A S	V G D R V T	I T C Q A S Q	B I	S B F	L N W Y Q Q K P
Dav	————————————	T V	————————	———————	————— D	——	N S W — I	———— Y —
Fin	————————————	T V	————————	———————	————— D	——	N S W — I	———— Y —
Lay	————————————	V	————————	———————	—————	——	N A Y	————————
	1		10			20			30				40

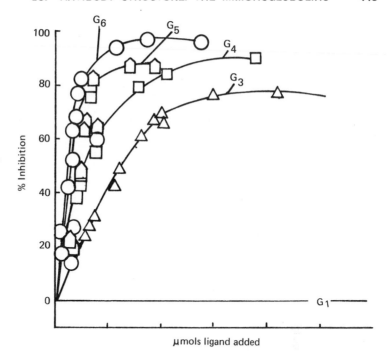

Fig. 16-36. Estimate of size of Ab combining sites. Inhibition of the dextran:antidextran precipitin reaction with a homologous series of polyglucose (G_n) oligosaccharides of increasing size: G_3 (Δ), G_4 (□), G_5 (□), G_6 (o). Isomaltoheptaose (G_7) was no more inhibitory than isomaltohexaose (G_6) with four of five antidextran sera, but inhibited marginally more with a fifth antiserum. G_1(glucose) was not inhibitory. [From Kabat, E. A. *J Immunol* 77:377 (1956); *84*:82 (1960).]

lysozyme, an enzyme that binds a hexasaccharide.) Additional variable residues of V segments probably also play a vital role in determining specificity by modulating the three-dimensional positions of the "contact" amino acids.

Among the Ab molecules of a given specificity some exhibit maximal binding with smaller ligands than others. This means that active sites vary in size or shape (or both) in different Ab molecules. These variations are consistent with the diversity of affinities observed among Abs of a given specificity (Ch. 15).

RECONSTRUCTION OF COMBINING SITES

Light Chain–Heavy Chain Interaction. Though interchain S-S bonds stabilize the native Ig molecule, they are not indispensable for the characteristic structure. Thus when heavy and light chains are separated, and the SH groups that constituted their S-S links are chemically blocked (e.g., with iodoacetate), they can reassociate through noncovalent bonds, spontaneously forming four-chain molecules that closely resemble native 7S Abs in physical, chemical, and antigenic properties; they even yield Fab fragments when

treated with papain. Chains derived from different Igs, and even from different species, also pair and form 7S molecules (e.g., human light with rabbit heavy chains). It is significant nonetheless that when a mixture of light chains from diverse Igs compete for a limiting amount of heavy chain from one Ig, the homologous pairs (derived from the same molecule) usually recombine more readily with each other than with heterologous chains (from different Igs).

The mutual affinity of all light and heavy chains probably derives from invariant sequences in C domains while the preferential binding of homologous chains probably is due to additional interaction between some residues in V_H and V_L domains. (Indeed an Ig cleaved by pepsin between V_L and C_L and between V_H and C_H domains yielded a stable fragment (called Fv) that consisted essentially of V_L plus V_H linked entirely by noncovalent bonds; this fragment retained all the ligand-binding activity of the intact Ig from which it was derived.) It is nevertheless possible that many light chains might pair equally well with a given heavy chain, and that many heavy chains might pair equally well with a particular light chain. Hence the number of different Ig molecules that could be assembled from *l* light and *h* heavy chains could be about (0.1) (*l* × *h*), if 10% of all chain combinations formed stable molecules (Origin of diversity, above).

Activity of Recombined Chains. The heavy chains isolated from an Ab can bind the corresponding ligand, though much less strongly than the original molecule. The isolated light chains bind far less well. Nevertheless, the light chains must make a profound and specific contribution to the combining site, because 7S molecules reconstituted from the chains of a given Ab have much greater affinity for ligand than those formed from the same heavy chain and other light chains.

The 7S molecules reconstituted from the chains of a homogeneous Ab (e.g., a myeloma protein with active sites) are fully as active as the native molecule. However, when recombination is carried out with chains from conventional Ab preparations, which are nearly always heterogeneous populations of molecules, the reconstituted molecules have far less activity for the test Ag than the native ones, probably because many mismatched heavy-light pairs are formed and lack appreciable affinity for the original ligand. It seems likely, though, that many of the mismatched pairs possess their own unique combining sites, specific for other (unknown) ligands.

APPENDIX

TABLE 16-5.   Some Properties of Classes and Subclasses of Human Immunoglobulins

Property	IgG-1	IgG-2	IgG-3	IgG-4	IgA-1	IgA-2	IgM	IgD	IgE
Sedimentation coefficient (S)	7	7	7	7	7–13	7–13	18–32	7	8
Molecular weight ($\times 10^{-3}$)	150	150	150	150	150–600	150–600	900	?	190
Heavy chains	$\gamma 1$	$\gamma 2$	$\gamma 3$	$\gamma 4$	$\alpha 1$	$\alpha 2$	μ	δ	ε
Light chains: κ/λ ratio	2.4	1.1	1.4	8.0	1.4	1.6	3.2	0.3	?
Carbohydrate (%, approx.)	3	3	3	3	7	7	12	13	11
Average concentration in normal serum (mg/ml)	8	4	1	0.4	3.5	0.4	1	0.03	0.0001
Half life in serum (days, in vivo)	23	23	8	23	6	(6?)	5	3	2.5
Heavy chain allotypes	Gm	Gm	Gm	Gm		Am			
Earliest Ab usually detected in primary immune responses*							+		
Most abundant Ab in most late immune responses*	←——— + ———→								
Conspicuous in mucinous exocrine secretions					+	+			+
Transmitted across placenta*	+	±	+	+	0	0	0	?	0
Effector Functions:									
Active in complement fixation†	++	+	++	0‡	0‡	0‡	++	?	0‡
Sensitizes human mast cells for anaphylaxis (homocytotropic)§	0	0	0	0	0	0	0	0	+
Sensitizes guinea pig mast cells for passive anaphylaxis (heterocytotropic)§	+	0	+	+	0	0	0	?	0
Binds to macrophages‖	++	+	++	±			0		

* Chapter 17.
† Chapter 18.
‡ Can activate complement via bypass mechanism (Ch. 18).
§ Chapter 19; IgE molecules are reagins and responsible for atopic allergy.
‖ "Cytophilic" Abs (Ch. 20).

SELECTED REFERENCES

Books and Review Articles

DORRINGTON, K. J., and TANFORD, C. Molecular size and conformation of immunoglobulins. *Adv Immunol 12*:333 (1970).

EDELMAN, G. M., and GALL, W. E. The antibody problem. *Annu Rev Biochem 38*:415 (1969).

GREEN, N. M. Electron microscopy of the immunoglobulins. *Adv Immunol 11*:1 (1969).

GRUBB, R. *The Genetic Markers of Human Immunoglobulins.* Springer, New York, 1970.

KOCHWA, S., and KUNKEL, H. G. (eds.). Immunoglobulins. *Ann NY Acad Sci 190*:1 (1971).

KRAUSE, R. M. The search for antibodies with molecular uniformity. *Adv Immunol 12*:1 (1970).

LENNOX, E. S., and COHN, M. Immunoglobulins. *Annu Rev Biochem 36*:365 (1967).

METZGER, H. Structure and function of γM macroglobulins (IgM). *Adv Immunol 12*:57 (1970).

NATVIG, J. B., and KUNKEL, H. G. Human Immunoglobulins: Classes, subclasses, genetic variants, and idiotypes. *Adv Immunol 16*:1 (1973).

OUDIN, J. Genetic regulation of immunoglobulin synthesis. *J Cell Physiol 67 (Suppl. 1)*:77 (1966).

POTTER, M. Immunoglobulin producing tumors and myeloma proteins of mice. *Physiol Rev 52*:631 (1972).

SMITH, G. P., HOOD, L., and FITCH, W. M. Antibody diversity. *Annu Rev Biochem 40*:969 (1971).

TOMASI, T. B., and BIENENSTOCK, J. Secretory immunoglobulins (IgA). *Adv Immunol 9*:2 (1968).

Two genes–One polypeptide chain: A symposium. *Fed Proc 31*:177 (1972).

Specific Articles

BRIDGES, S. H., and LITTLE, J. R. Recovery of binding activity in reconstituted mouse myeloma proteins. *Biochemistry 10*:2525 (1971).

BRIENT, B. W., and NISONOFF, A. Inhibition by specific haptens of the reaction of anti-hapten antibody and anti-idiotypic antibody. *J Exp Med 132*:951 (1970).

HAIMOVICH, J., EISEN, H. N., HURWITZ, E., and GIVOL, D. Localization of affinity-labeled residues on the heavy and light chains of two myeloma proteins with anti-hapten activity. *Biochemistry 11*:2389 (1972).

HOOD, L., and TALMAGE, D. Mechanism of antibody diversity: Germ-line basis for variability. *Science 168*:325 (1970).

KINDT, T. J., MANDY, W. J., and TODD, C. W. Association of allotypic specificities of group *a* with allotypic specificities A11 and A12 in rabbit immunoglobulins. *Biochemistry 9*:2028 (1970).

JERNE, N. K. The somatic generation of immune recognition. *Eur J Immunol 1*:1 (1971).

MORRISON, S. L., and KOSHLAND, M. E. Characterization of the J chain from polymeric immunoglobulins. *Proc Nat Acad Sci USA 69*:124 (1972).

OUDIN, J., and MICHEL, M. Idiotypy of rabbit antibodies: I and II. *J Exp Med 130*:595, 619 (1969).

TOSI, S. L., MAGE, R. G., and DUBISKI, S. Distribution of allotypic specificities among IgG molecules. *J Immunol 104*:641 (1970).

WANG, A. C., WILSON, S. K., HOPPER, J. E., FUDENBERG, H. H., and NISONOFF, A. Evidence for the control of synthesis of the variable regions of the heavy chains of IgG and IgM by the same gene. *Proc Nat Acad Sci USA 66*:337 (1970).

WOFSY, L., METZGER, H., and SINGER, S. J. Affinity-labeling: A general method for labeling the active sites of antibody and enzyme molecules. *Biochemistry 1*:1031 (1962).

WU, T. T., and KABAT, E. A. An analysis of the sequences of the variable regions of Bence Jones proteins and myeloma light chains and their implications for antibody complementarity. *J Exp Med 132*:211 (1970).

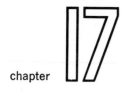

chapter 17

ANTIBODY FORMATION

CELLULAR BASIS FOR ANTIBODY FORMATION

This chapter is concerned with the sequence of events that begins with entry of antigen (Ag) into the body and culminates in the appearance in serum of the corresponding antibodies (Abs). In the past 70 years, the general framework for viewing this process has undergone several radical transitions, which have assigned different roles to the immunogen.* According to **selective** theories the immunogen stimulates certain cells to make greater amounts of the Ab molecules that they already make at a low level in advance of immunization. **Instructive** theories, in contrast, assume that the immunogen is an obligatory participant in the formation of the corresponding Ab, providing essential information for determining its structure.

The first detailed theory, proposed by Ehrlich in 1900, was selective. Cell surfaces were supposedly covered by a variety of Ab-like receptors; in combining with matching ones the immunogen was supposed somehow to stimulate selectively their further synthesis and secretion by the cells. This theory was abandoned by the 1920s when recognition of the enormous variety of immunogenic substances, including newly synthesized organic chemicals, suggested that the diversity of Ags is almost limitless: it seemed beyond belief that the corresponding Abs could all preexist.

In its place an instructive "antigen-template" theory (suggested by Pauling, Breinl and Haurowitz, and by others) came to be widely favored in the 1940s and 1950s. According to this view the specificity of an

Ab molecule was determined not by its amino acid sequence but by the process of molding the nascent molecule around the immunogenic determinant; the immunogen would act as a template at the site of protein synthesis, creating a complementary conformation at the combining sites of the Ab. However, this model became untenable when the specificity of the Ab molecule was shown to be determined by its amino acid sequence (Ch. 16), for alteration of the corresponding messenger RNA sequence could hardly have been immediately acquired from the encounter with Ag. Identification of the cells forming a specific Ab also contributed: with highly radioactive Ag it could be shown that these cells contained no detectable Ag (less than 10 molecules per cell).

Clonal Selection. Even before the antigen-template theory had to be discarded Burnet proposed a **clonal selection** theory, based on the success of mutation-selection in explaining microbial adaptations. According to this theory an immunologically responsive cell (lymphocyte, see below) can respond to only one Ag (or a few related ones), and this capacity is somehow acquired before the Ag is encountered (see Ch. 16, Origin of diversity). Accordingly, an individual's lymphocytes are an immensely diversified pool of cells—some capable of responding to one Ag, others to a second, etc. When an immunogen penetrates the body it binds to an Ab-like receptor on the surface of the corresponding lymphocyte, which is then somehow stimulated to proliferate and generate a clone of differentiated cells. Some of these (plasma cells, see below) secrete Abs, while others circulate through blood, lymph, and tissues as

---

* In this and in subsequent chapters "immunogen" is used as a synonym for "antigen" when emphasizing its function in inducing immune responses (Ch. 14).

an expanded reservoir of Ag-sensitive "memory" cells. The same immunogen encountering these cells months or years later evokes a more rapid and copious secondary response.

Older theories are contrasted with clonal selection in Figure 17-1. Several lines of evidence support the clonal hypothesis. 1) A given Ag is bound specifically by only a small proportion of an individual's lymphocytes, whose stimulation results in production of the corresponding Abs; inactivation of these cells eliminates ability to form these Abs. 2) Immunoglobulin (Ig)-forming cells make only one kind of Ig molecule, at least at one time; and in an animal stimulated with two Ags, or even with an Ag that has two distinguishable determinants (A and B) some cells make anti-A, others make anti-B, and none make both.

It has been known since the 1950s that the **principal Ab-producing cells are plasma cells** (see below). However these cells become prominent in tissues only several days after antigenic stimulation, and little was known of the early cellular events until several major developments in the past decade. Gowans' use of purified cell populations established that the **Ag-sensitive cells** with which the immunogen reacts initially are **small lymphocytes,** and these cells were later recognized (largely from immunological defects following extirpation of thymus or bursa of Fabricius) as being of two types: **T cells,** which are derived from the thymus, and **B cells,** which are thymus-independent and are derived from the bursa of Fabricius in birds and possibly from bone marrow in mammals. As we shall see, the full immunogenic activity of many Ags depends upon cooperation between B and T cells and on ancillary support from large phagocytic cells: motile **macrophages** and sessile **reticular** cells. Other, "T-independent" immunogens (especially those of high molecular weight with repeating antigenic determinants) can stimulate B cells without any assistance from T cells and macrophages. The mystery surrounding the earliest events has also begun to lessen with the demonstration that specific receptors on Ag-sensitive B lymphocytes are Igs, linking the structural characteristics of Ab molecules (Ch. 16) and the principles of the Ab-Ag reaction (Ch. 15) with the initiation of cellular events in the induction of Ab formation.

Before describing the cells involved in Ab formation (B and T lymphocytes, plasma cells, and macrophages), we review briefly the main methods used to study the consequences of Ag reaction with these cells.

METHODS FOR STUDYING ANTIBODY FORMATION AT THE CELLULAR LEVEL

Immunofluorescence, introduced by Coons (see Ch. 15, Fig. 15-34), can be used to identify individual cells that contain Abs. **Killed cells,** in which the cell interior is accessible, are stained by the "sandwich" technic, which amplifies the method's sensitivity: the cells (usually in a tissue section) are incubated with multivalent antigen X and then with fluorescein-labeled Ab against X. The cells that contain anti-X bind the Ag, and each molecule of bound Ag can then bind many molecules of fluorescent anti-X (Fig. 17-2).

With **living cells,** whose surface membrane is not penetrated by extracellular Ab molecules, the membrane-bound Ab molecules that serve as Ag-binding receptors can be detected on the cell surface with fluorescent anti-Igs, whose specificity also helps identify the receptor's heavy-chain class, light-chain type, and allotype (Fig. 17-2).

Ag-binding receptors on lymphoid cells can also be detected by **direct rosette formation:** red cells (or Ag-coated red cells) bind to lymphocytes or plasma cells whose membrane contains the corresponding receptor (Fig. 17-3). **Indirect rosettes** are formed with the aid of bridging "hybrid" Ab molecules (Ch. 16): one site binds to the cell-bound Ig and the other to an Ag on the erythrocyte.

Ab production by individual cells can be detected in small **microdrops** (ca. 10^{-6} ml) of dilute cell suspensions; some drops contain a single cell. Ab produced in such microdrops (kept under mineral oil to prevent evaporation) can be measured by sensitive technics, such as specific immobilization of motile *Salmonella* or neutralization of bacteriophages (see Ch. 15, Rates of reaction).

The **hemolytic plaque assay,** introduced by Jerne, is a particularly useful method for counting Ab-forming cells. In a typical test spleen cells from a mouse immunized with sheep erythrocytes (SRBC) are plated in agar with the SRBC. During the following in-

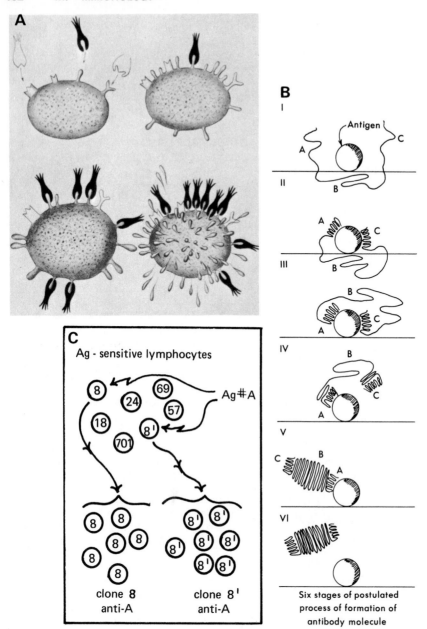

Fig. 17-1. Comparison of selective and instructive theories of Ab formation. **A.** Ehrlich's selection hypothesis, showing multiplication and shedding of a cell receptor following its specific combination with an immunogen; each cell was assumed to be able to combine with any Ag. **B.** Antigen-template theory: immunogen reacts with the nascent Ig chain, A-B-C, causing it to acquire sites that are complementary to determinants of the immunogen. **C.** Burnet's clonal selection hypothesis resembles **A,** but with the important difference that the population of reactive cells is diversified and each cell can respond to only one or a few immunogens. [**A** from Ehrlich, P. *Proc R Soc Lond, Biol 66*:424 (1900). **B** from Pauling, L. *J Am Chem Soc 62*:2643 (1940). **C** based on Burnet, F. M. *The Clonal Selection Theory of Acquired Immunity.* Vanderbilt Univ. Press, Nashville, 1959.]

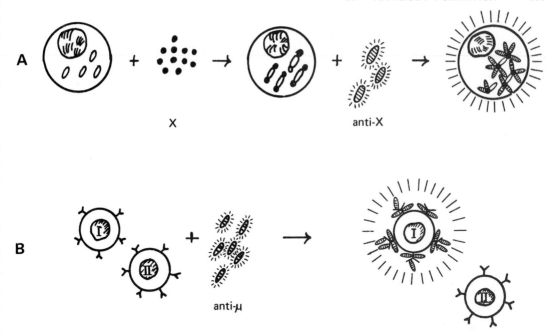

X anti-X

anti-μ

Fig. 17-2. Identification by immunofluorescence of Ab-producing cells **(A)** and Ag-sensitive cells with Igs on the surface membrane **(B).** In **A** cells (e.g., plasma cells) are killed, rendering Ab at sites of synthesis inside the cell accessible to the test reagents (sandwich technic): multivalent ligand X and fluorescein-labeled Ab (anti-X) (see Fig. 17-24B). In **B** the cells (e.g., small lymphocytes) are living and only their surface Ig molecules are accessible for reaction with labeled Ab. Assume that the surface Igs are IgM in cell I and IgG in cell II; with fluorescein-labeled anti-μ only cell I would be stained, and with labeled anti-γ only II would be stained (for aggregation of surface Igs see Fig. 17-10).

cubation some of the lymphoid cells synthesize and secrete Abs that lyse surrounding SRBC when complement is added (Ch. 18). This leaves clear plaques, resembling those produced by lytic phage on a lawn of susceptible bacteria, with the Ab-secreting cell in the center of each plaque (Fig. 17-4). By using red cells with various covalently attached haptens and Ags this method can be extended to detect cells forming a wide variety of Abs.

The unmodified ("direct") plaque technic counts cells that produce IgM Abs, but not those that produce IgG Abs. The reason is that lysis of an Ab-coated red cell by complement requires only a single IgM molecule on the erythrocyte's surface, while a pair of adjacent IgG molecules is necessary (Ch. 18): with relatively few Ab molecules secreted by a single cell, the close packing of bound Ab molecules is likely to be infrequent, especially if spacing of the red cell's antigenic determinants are unfavorable. However, cells that secrete Abs of the IgG class can be counted by the "indirect" technic: addition of an antiserum to IgG results in clusters of anti-IgG

Abs on each molecule of bound anti-red-cell Ab, and the red cell can then be lysed by complement (Fig. 17-4). If the added antiserum is specific for a particular allotype it is possible to recognize cells that produce that allotype; antiserum to IgA, which does not fix complement (Ch. 18), similarly allows "indirect" enumeration of cells that produce Abs of the IgA class.

Transplantation is extensively used to analyze the types of cells needed for Ab production. In transfers of living lymphoid cells* from one animal to another **(adoptive immunity)** the recipient is usually first heavily irradiated (e.g., 750 rad) and sometimes the thymus gland is also removed; by eliminating essentially all the recipient's functional lymphoid tissue these procedures convert it into a

---

* The term "lymphoid cells" is used to emphasize that the cell suspensions ordinarily isolated from lymph node, spleen, blood, etc., are highly heterogeneous mixtures of lymphocytes (themselves highly diversified), macrophages, rare plasma cells, and some granulocytes and erythrocytes.

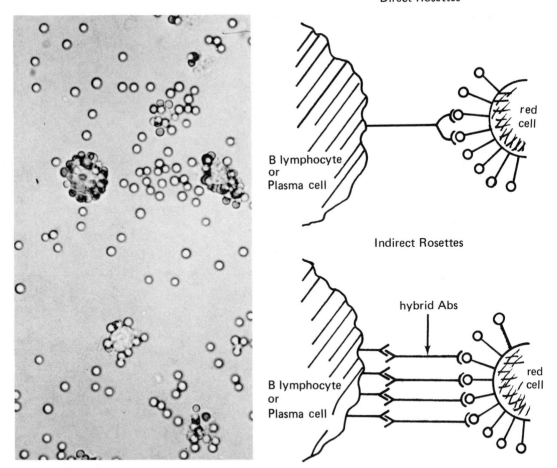

Fig. 17-3. Identification of surface Igs by rosette formation. Rosettes formed by the indirect method (using hybrid Abs with one combining site for the B cell's surface Ig and one for a ligand on red cells) are more stable than those formed by the direct method, because many more bonds can be formed between B cells and red cells. The photograph shows direct rosettes formed with trinitrophenyl (Tnp)-coated red cells and a myeloma cell whose surface Ig has anti-Tnp combining sites. (Courtesy of Drs. K. Hannestad, M. S. Kao, and R. G. Lynch.)

"walking tissue culture." In addition, donor and recipient are generally chosen from the same inbred strain to avoid complications that would otherwise arise from an immune attack by the host against histocompatibility Ags on the surface of the donors cells or vice versa (Ch. 21).

The principles governing survival or rejection of transplanted cells are considered in detail in Chapter 21. It is useful to realize here that histocompatibility Ags are **alloantigens** (Gr. *allos* = different): like immunoglobulin allotypes (Ch. 16), they segregate genetically and various ones are thus present in some and absent in other members of a given species. An animal almost invariably destroys transferred cells carrying histocompatibility Ags that it lacks. However, members of a highly inbred strain are essentially identical genetically **(syngeneic)** and antigenically: they accept grafted cells freely from each other, while rejecting genetically different (allogeneic) cells from other inbred strains of the same species.

Cell Separations. Lymphoid cells differ in various physical properties and, most importantly, in the specificity of their Ag-binding surface receptors. **Velocity sedimentation** at unit gravity (1 g) sepa-

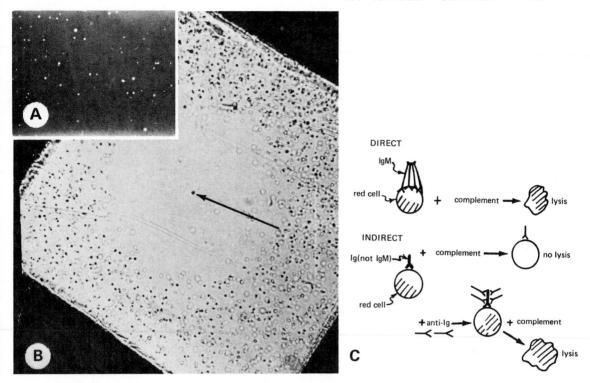

Fig. 17–4. Hemolytic plaque assay for Ab-producing cells. **A.** Multiple plaques in a petri dish. ca. ×15. **B.** A single plaque with its central Ab-secreting cell (arrow). Though these cells are only rarely observed in mitosis, ca. 40% of those stimulated by Ag appear to have arisen from a recent mitotic division (based on ^{3}H-thymidine content in DNA). Some representative plaque-forming cells are shown in Figure 17–11. (ca. ×100). **C.** Contrast between **direct plaques,** which reveal cells that secrete Abs of IgM class, and **indirect plaques** which require appropriate anti-Igs to obtain complement-dependent lysis of the red cells. [**A** courtesy of Dr. L. Claflin; **B** from Harris, T. N., Hummeler, K., and Harris, S. *J Exp Med 123*:161 (1966).]

rates cells of different size (large cells sediment faster than small ones). **Density-gradient centrifugation** separates cells of different densities; the centrifugation is carried out in a medium whose different densities are either distributed continuously in a gradient or discontinuously in multiple layers.

Macrophages adhere to glass, and passage through a column of fine glass beads removes these cells from populations of lymphoid cells. B cells also tend to adhere to glass and nylon surfaces, but are more efficiently removed on glass beads that are coated with anti-Igs. In a form of "affinity chromatography," columns of glass or polyacrylamide beads coated with Ag retain cells with the corresponding Ag-binding surface receptors, and a few of the retained cells can even be recovered (though with difficulty) by elution with Ag at high concentration.

In an automatic **"cell-sorting" machine** a stream of microdrops containing single cells is monitored for particular cell-surface markers (by binding fluorescein-labeled Abs); microdrops with fluorescent living cells are collected, yielding particular subsets from heterogeneous cell populations.

Induction of Ab Formation in Cell Culture. Incubation with Ag induces cells in cultured fragments of spleen to produce Ab. However, dispersed cell suspensions are not consistently induced unless they are given highly enriched media and allowed to reaggregate into small clusters. The importance of cell aggregation in culture probably reflects the need for cooperative interactions among several cell types (two kinds of lymphocytes, macrophages; see below). In contrast to bacterial cells, which usually function well as solitary individuals, many functions of lymphoid and other animal cells require cell–cell interactions (as though animal cells, like animals, have societal needs). With sheep red cells as

Ag, the incidence of plaque-forming cells induced in short-term primary cultures of dispersed spleen cells (5 to 7 days) is close to that found in the spleen of an immunized animal (e.g., $500/10^6$ nucleated spleen cells).

Living vs. Dead Cells. Lymphoid cells (especially lymphocytes, see below) are fragile. Many are killed inadvertently during isolation, or deliberately by cytotoxic immune reactions of their surface Ags (Ch. 18; Ch. 20, Cytotoxic assays). Permeability to anionic dyes (such as trypan blue) is commonly used to distinguish dead from living cells: the dyes penetrate into and stain dead cells, while living cells remain unstained.

Living and dead cells can also be separated by centrifugation through a dense solution of polyglycol and sodium triiodobenzoate: dead cells are denser and sediment to the bottom while live cells accumulate at the surface.

LYMPHOCYTES

B AND T CELLS

Lymphocytes are relatively small (5 to 15 μm diameter), round, nondescript cells that are ubiquitous in blood, lymph, and connective tissues. As is described below, the two funda-

mentally different kinds, B and T cells, differ in origin, in surface macromolecules, in circulation patterns, and above all, in the mode and consequences of their interaction with Ags.

The induction of Ab formation by many immunogens requires specific interaction with both B and T cells, with the T cells somehow regulating the proliferation and differentiation of B cells into Ab-secreting plasma cells. Thus, in working with recipient mice that were both thymectomized and irradiated (to destroy virtually all lymphocytes), Claman *et al.* found that the amount of Ab formed against sheep red cells in recipients of bone marrow and thymus cells exceeded by far the sum of the amounts formed in recipients of either one alone (Table 17-1): **the cooperation of both populations was evidently necessary to restore ability to make an optimal Ab response.**

Subsequent studies showed that the active cells in bone marrow and thymus are precursors of B and T cells, respectively (see below), and that the **Ab-secreting cells are derived from the marrow and not from the thymus cells.** For instance, when marrow and thymus cells were obtained from donors that differed in Ig allotype but were otherwise syngeneic (see Ch. 21, Congenic strains) the

TABLE 17-1. Cooperation Between Thymus and Bone Marrow Cells in Induction of Antibody Synthesis*

Donor cells	Recipients	
	% Spleen fragments secreting antibody	Serum antibody activity†
None	0.8	None detected
Bone marrow (1 $\times$ 10⁷)	1.3	None detected
Thymus (5 $\times$ 10⁷)	12.3	0.2
Bone marrow (1 $\times$ 10⁷) + Thymus (5 $\times$ 10⁷)	53.7	2.1

* X-irradiated (800 r) mice were injected with the indicated numbers of thymus or bone marrow cells (or both, or neither) from normal donors, and the recipients were then given sheep red cells (SRBC) as Ag. Eleven days later Ab production was determined by measuring the serum Ab titer and the percentage of spleen fragments that secreted hemolytic anti-SRBC Abs in culture.

† Log₂ hemolysin titer.

Based on Claman, H. N., Chaperon, E. A., and Triplett, R. F. *J Immunol* 97:828 (1966).

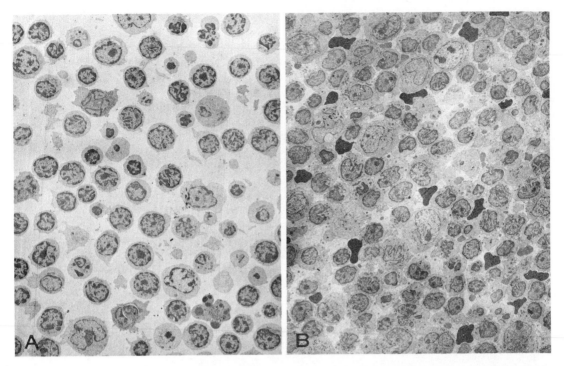

Fig. 17-5. Heterogeneity of lymphocytes in lymph from thoracic duct of rat **(A)** and human **(B)**. Most of the cells are of T lineage (Table 17-2). Some have well developed rough endoplasmic reticulum; others lack these organelles. Dark, irregular forms in **B** are erythrocytes. **A**, ×2400; **B**, ×1200. [From Zucker-Franklin, D. *Seminars in Hematology* 6:4–27 *(1969)* **(A)**; *J Ultrastruct Res* 9:325–339 *(1963)* **(B)**.]

allotype of the Ab produced was always that of the bone marrow donor.

Appearance and Generation Times. B and T lymphocytes look alike and both are motile, nonphagocytic cells of varying size (Fig. 17-5). In the smallest ones (5 to 8 μm diameter) mitochondria are scanty, ribosomes are single, and no endoplasmic reticulum is discernible; in the light microscope the cytoplasm forms a barely perceptible rim around the dense nucleus (Fig. 17-6). Specific binding of Ag by membrane-bound receptors on the cell surface can stimulate transformation of small lymphocytes into larger ones (up to 15 μm diameter), whose more abundant cytoplasm contains endoplasmic reticulum and a prominent Golgi apparatus, and is richer in mitochondria and in polysomes (Fig. 17-6). In accord with the appearance of a secretory system (endoplasmic reticulum, Golgi apparatus) some of the large lymphocytes (of B type) secrete Abs (see Fig. 17-11). The large cells also divide more

rapidly (generation time ca. 6 to 48 hours), and some of those of B lineage differentiate into mature plasma cells, the most active of all lymphoid cells in synthesis and secretion of Igs (Figs. 17-6 and 7-11). Many large lymphocytes also revert back eventually into small ones, which probably function as "memory" cells (see Secondary response, below). Small lymphocytes rarely divide unless stimulated by Ag (for important exceptions in the thymus and bursa of Fabricius, see below).

Even after 40 days' continuous infusion of ³H-thymidine into mice and rats the DNA remains unlabeled in most of the small lymphocytes in blood.

Another approach has shown that these cells also survive for long periods in man without dividing. After intensive X-ray therapy chromosomes in many lymphocytes become badly damaged; the cells can survive but they are unable to complete a mitotic division. When blood lymphocytes are subsequently treated with certain mitosis-stimulating plant proteins (mitogens, see below) and forced to

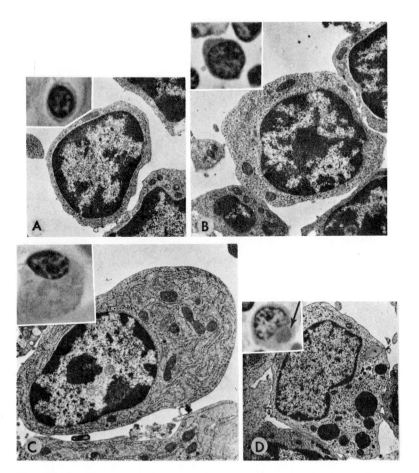

Fig. 17-6. Principal cells involved in antibody formation. **A,** Small lymphocyte; **B.** large ("transitional") lymphocyte; **C,** plasma cell; **D,** macrophage. The macrophage contains a phagocyted red cell (arrow, inset **D**), corresponding to the larger of the dark cytoplasmic inclusions in the associated electron micrograph. The plasma cell (inset, **C**) has its secretory vesicles distended with immunoglobulin. Electron micrographs are: **A,** ×7500; **B,** ×6600; **C,** ×6600; **D,** ×5500. Light microscope photographs of the corresponding cells (upper left insets) stained with toluidine blue. Magnifications are approximately: **A,** ×4000; **B,** ×3000; **C,** ×3000; **D,** ×2000. (Courtesy of Dr. R. G. Lynch.)

undergo mitosis, cytological examination reveals some cells with such pronounced chromosomal aberrations that they are unlikely to have divided once since incurring their X-ray damage. From the decreasing incidence of such cells with time after irradiation it has been estimated that the mean generation time of circulating small lymphocytes (B and T cells) in man is about 5 years; some small lymphocytes seem to survive 10 years without division, which might account for the long persistence of immunological memory (below).

Differences Between B and T Cell Surfaces. B cells have abundant surface membrane-bound Ig molecules (ca. 100,000/cell), which are restricted in a given cell to molecules of a particular allotype and isotype, and probably also restricted to one idiotype, accounting for the cell's selective response to a given Ag (see One cell–one antibody rule, below). T cells in contrast, seem to have far fewer surface Igs (perhaps 1000-fold less per T cell than B cell);

TABLE 17-2.   Comparison of Mouse B and T Lymphocytes

Properties	B cells	T cells
Differentiation (from uncommitted Ag-insensitive "stem" cells to Ag-sensitive cells) in:	Bursa of Fabricius (in birds) or as yet unknown equivalent in mammals	Thymus
Ag-binding receptors on the cell surface:	Abundant Igs, (restricted to 1 isotype, 1 allotype, 1 idiotype per cell)	Nature of specific receptors is un-certain; Igs are sparse
Cell surface antigens:*		
θ	−	+
TL	−	+
Ly	−	+
PC	+ (plasma cells)	−
H-2 transplantation Ags	+	+
Approximate frequency (%) in:		
Blood	15	85
Lymph (thoracic duct)	10	90
Lymph node	15	85
Spleen	35	65
Bone marrow	Abundant	Few
Thymus	Rare	Abundant
Functions		
secretion of antibody molecules	Yes (large lym-phocytes and plasma cells)	No
Helper function (react with "carrier" moieties of the immunogen)	No	Yes
Effector cell for cell-mediated immunity	No	Yes
Distribution in lymph nodes and spleen:	Clustered in follicles around germinal centers	In interfollicular areas
Susceptibility to inactivation by:		
X-irradiation	++++	+
Corticosteroids	++	+
Antilymphocytic serum (ALS)	+	++++

* θ occurs at high levels in thymus and in brain. Two allotypes are known: θ-AKR (in AKR and a few other inbred mouse strains), and θ-C3H (in C3H, BALB/c, and most other mouse strains).

TL is present on normal thymus cells of only some mouse strains (TL+), but is present on leukemic lymphocytes of TL+ and TL− strains.

Ly is present on thymus cells and circulating lymphocytes, but absent from all nonlymphoid cells. There are two loci: Ly-A and a second one with linked Ly-B and Ly-C; two alleles are known at each.

PC is present on plasma cells (including myeloma cells).

H-2 histocompatibility Ags (see Ch. 21). B and T cells also differ in ability to adsorb Igs: B cells, but not T cells, bind Ab·Ag·complement (C) complexes through surface sites that are specific for activated third component of C (C3, see Ch. 18). Other sites on B cells bind aggregated Igs (cross-linked, for instance, by Ag), probably through specific reaction with the Fc domains of the aggregated molecules.

though predominantly IgM molecules, it is not certain that they are restricted in idiotype.

B and T cells also differ in other surface macromolecules. In mice, where they are best characterized, T cells have a variety of heritable alloantigens (θ, TL, Ly; Table 17-2) that are lacking in B cells. Like other **alloantigens** (see Ch. 16, Ig allotypes, and especially Ch. 21), these differ in various inbred mouse strains and are thus recognizable by **alloantisera,** raised in a strain that lacks the alloantigen by injecting appropriate cells from mice that possess it.

The most important of the T cell alloantigens is θ, which is defined by antisera raised in AKR mice against T cells from C3H mice. After absorption with various C3H cells (other than T cells), to remove Abs to histocompatibility Ags, the resulting antiserum reacts specifically with T cells of C3H and of other strains of mice with the same θ allotype. In conjunction with complement (Ch. 18), anti-θ destroys T cells selectively in a simple procedure that is widely used to determine whether various properties of a population of lymphocytes are due to its T cells or to its B cells. Though useful, this approach is not foolproof because circulating T cells (in blood, lymph, lymph nodes, spleen) have less θ on their surface than those in the thymus; and some are not killed by anti-θ (plus complement) but can be eliminated by antisera to other distinctive surface antigens (Table 17-2).

B and T cells also differ in the areas they occupy in lymphatic organs (see Fig. 17-8), and in susceptibility to inactivation by certain immunosuppressive agents (see Table 17-2 and Suppression by antilymphocytic serum, below).

Origin of B and T Cells. Transplantation experiments in chickens have shown that B cells arise from migrant bone marrow stem cells (primitive precursors of hematopoietic and lymphoid cells) that lodge in the bursa of Fabricius (see below) where they begin to synthesize Igs (Fig. 17-7). In mammals, which lack a bursa, it is not certain where the B cell precursors become committed to synthesize a particular Ig: this could happen in the bone marrow itself or in lymph nodes or in gut-associated lymphoid structures, such as appendix or tonsils.

T lymphocytes also originate from bone marrow stem cells, which migrate to the thymus where they divide rapidly (generation time about 8 hours). Most of the rapidly

dividing cells die without leaving the thymus; the survivors, mature T cells, differ from entering stem cells in several important properties that are acquired in the thymus, or possibly in other tissues under the aegis of a thymus hormone (see below). 1) They develop characteristic surface Ags (Table 17-2); theta (θ) is particularly useful for detecting and tracing these cells (see above). 2) They can react specifically with one or a few Ags, i.e., they become Ag-sensitive ("immunologically committed") lymphocytes. 3) Besides acquiring the capacity to regulate B cell responses to Ags, specifically reactive T lymphocytes can become specific effector cells for cell-mediated immune responses: they can destroy tumor cells, cause rejection of allografts, and promote the differentiation of resting macrophages into highly bactericidal cells capable of destroying microbial pathogens (Chs. 20 and 21). T cells are heterogeneous and it is likely that T cell effectors of cell-mediated immune reactions (Ch. 20) differ from those that regulate the differentiation of B cells into Ab-secreting cells (see below).

Circulating T cells also differ from thymus cells in having more histocompatibility Ags. About 25 to 50 times fewer circulating T cells than thymus cells are necessary to support cell-mediated immune responses (e.g., Ch. 21, Graft-vs.-host reaction), perhaps because mature T cells in the thymus (ca. 5% of the total) are diluted by the more abundant immature ones.

Circulation of B and T Cells. Lymphocytes circulate through blood, lymph, and peripheral lymphatic tissues (lymph nodes, spleen, Peyer's patches of intestinal wall, etc.), where the T cells tend to congregate in special interfollicular T-cell areas while B cells cluster in adjacent follicles (see Figs. 17-8, 17-15, 17-16). Lymphocytes subsequently leave these areas via efferent lymph channels that eventually fuse to form the thoracic duct, through which lymphocytes return to blood and recirculate. **The majority of circulating lymphocytes are T cells** (Table 17-2), except in rare disorders affecting the thymus and T cells (see Immunodeficiency diseases, below) and in some individuals with chronic lymphocytic leukemia.

Separation of B and T Cells. Separation of these cells is necessary for evaluating their respective

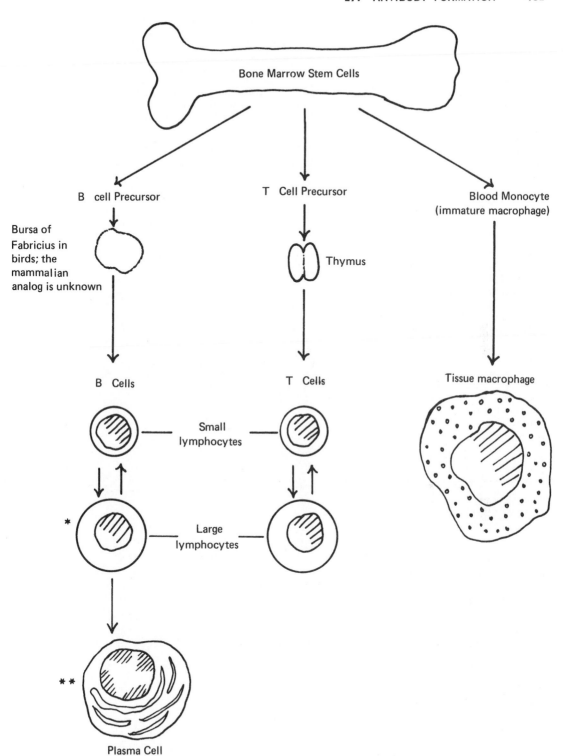

Fig. 17-7. Maturation pathways of the principal cells in the immune response. Antibody molecules are secreted by large lymphocytes (∗) and especially by plasma cells (∗∗) in the B-cell lineage. Lymphocytes of B and T lineages are morphologically indistinguishable.

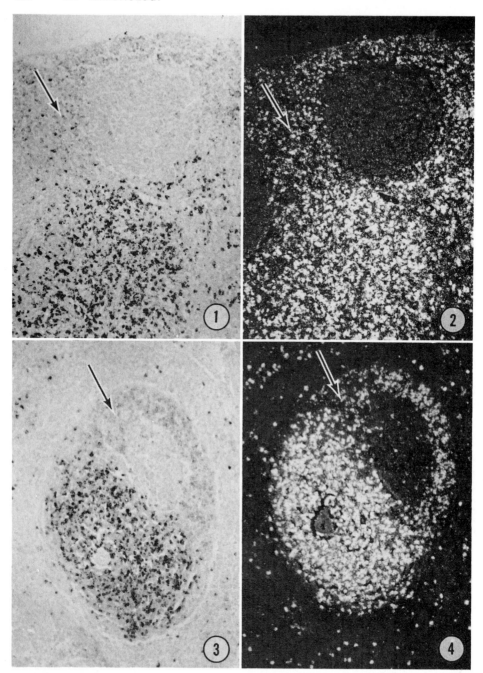

Fig. 17-8. B and T zones in secondary lymphatic organs. The T cells are highly radioactive (because of ^{3}H-ribonucleoside incorporation into RNA) and are concentrated in interfollicular and deep cortical areas of lymph nodes **(1,2)** and in periarteriolar areas of white pulp of spleen **(3,4).** B cells (arrows) are clustered around germinal centers of lymph node **(1,2)** and spleen white pulp **(3,4).** (For reasons that are not clear the B cells incorporate much less ^{3}H-ribonucleoside into RNA and are less radioactive than the T cells.) See also Figures 17-15 and 17-16. Bright- and dark-field views of the same field of a lymph node **(1,2)** and of spleen **(3,4).** [From Howard, J., Hunt, S., and Gowans, J. *J Exp Med 135*:200 (1972).]

properties. The following are some experimental procedures.

1) Thymus cells are injected into heavily irradiated recipients (ca. 800 r). If an Ag is administered at the same time, or is present as an alloantigen on the recipient's own cells (e.g., a histocompatibility Ag lacking in the donor), the corresponding thymus cells proliferate, yielding an enriched population of Ag-stimulated or "educated" T cells.

2) Repeated passage of heterogeneous lymphoid cell populations over glass beads coated with anti-Igs removes B cells (and macrophages), yielding a T-cell suspension.

3) Treatment of heterogeneous populations with anti-θ sera and complement destroys almost all T cells, leaving lymphocytes of predominantly B type.

4) Virtually all lymphocytes of mutant "nude" mice with defective development of the thymus are B cells (see Thymus, below).

MACROPHAGES

These large, highly phagocytic cells (15 to 20 μm diameter) do not form Abs. However,

the following indirect evidence suggests that they have an important accessory role, co-operating with T cells in aiding the response of B cells to many immunogens.

1) Ags, especially in particulate form, are conspicuously taken up by macrophages.

2) Trace amounts of Ag bound to the macrophage surface are far more potent immunogenically than the same amount of free, unbound Ag.

3) Macrophages adhere to glass and plastic surfaces; and in spleen cell cultures most Ags can induce B lymphocytes to differentiate into Ab-secreting plasma cells only in the presence of both adherent cells and T cells (see Cell cooperation, below, and Fig. 17-9).

The action of macrophages on Ags has long seemed paradoxical. The cell's sticky surface binds Ags, which are then endocytized and degraded (see below). Cleavage of covalent bonds of soluble Ags usually reduces or destroys immunogenicity (see Ch. 15, Conformational antigenic determinants). Yet Ags associated with macrophages are more im-

Fig. 17-9. Evidence that induction of Ab synthesis by certain (T-dependent) Ags requires three cells. **A.** Induction of Ab formation to sheep erythrocytes by cultured mouse spleen cells, which were separated into adherent (predominantly macrophages) and nonadherent (lymphocyte) populations. By adding one cell population in excess and titrating with graded amounts of the other, the dependence of induction on the number of titrated cells indicated (from slopes, b) that one adherent and two nonadherent cells were needed to induce the appearance of one Ab-secreting cell. With unseparated spleen cells, the slope was 2.6, or close to 3. Induction was measured by the number of plaque-forming cells (PFC) that appeared. **B.** Some hypothetical inductive complexes. Evidence in **A** favors a 3-cell model (B-T-macrophage). [**A** from Mosier, D. E. and Coppelson, L. W. *Proc Natl Acad Sci USA* 61:542 (1968).]

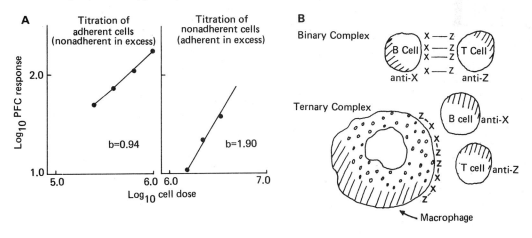

munogenic than unbound Ag. It was thought that an intermediate level of degradation ("processing") might be the solution, but it now appears that while the internalized Ag is indeed destroyed, the unmodified Ag on the sticky surface is exceedingly immunogenic: removing it with trypsin or blocking it with Abs eliminates the immunogenicity of macrophage-associated Ag. However, with complex Ags, such as bacterial cells, phagocytosis and digestion by macrophages might contribute to immunogenicity by releasing internal molecules that would not otherwise become free to react with lymphocytes.

Macrophages wander through tissues. Together with reticular cells that are immobilized on reticulum fibers and other phagocytic cells in the endothelial lining of vascular, sinus-like spaces (of spleen, lymph nodes, liver, etc.), they constitute the scavenger **reticuloendothelial system** which traps, ingests, and degrades foreign particulate matter (bacteria, many viruses, aggregated macromolecules). The degradative activity is due to effective phagocytosis plus abundant cytoplasmic vesicles **(lysosomes)** that are filled with various hydrolytic enzymes: proteases, RNase, DNase, lipase, esterases, lysozyme, phosphatases, etc. When coated with opsonizing Abs and fragments of activated complement (C3b and C5b, see Ch. 18), foreign particles adhere to the sticky cell membrane and are then ingested into a phagocytic vacuole **(phagosome)** that fuses with lysosomes to form the **phagolysosome,** in which degradative enzymes attack the ingested material.

"Cytophilic" antibodies stick to the macrophage surface and help bind the corresponding Ags to the cell; for example, red cells form rosettes around macrophages that have been incubated in antiserum to red cells. The use of myeloma proteins established that **only certain Ig classes are cytophilic** (e.g., human IgG-1 and IgG-3; see Ch. 16), doubtless through binding sites in the Fc domain. Though these Abs dissociate from macrophages at 37°, and thus have questionable activity in vivo, they seem to promote destruction of some target tumor cells in vitro (Ch. 20, cytotoxic mechanisms).

Macrophages can divide, but they probably survive for only a short time in acute inflammatory lesions (due to infection, irritants, or adjuvant mixtures with Ag), where they arise by differentiation of monocytes carried to the lesion via blood. The blood monocytes (which derive from "promonocytes" in bone marrow) are less active as phagocytes and have fewer lysosomes (Figs. 17-6 and 17-7). The life span of mature tissue macrophages is not known, but they can survive many weeks in tissue culture. In some chronic inflammatory lesions macrophages differentiate further into epithelioid cells and into multinucleated giant cells (Chs. 22 and 35).

An additional role of macrophages in cell-mediated immunity will be discussed in Chapter 20: Ags react specifically with T lymphocytes and cause release of factors that stimulate macrophages to differentiate into "angry" cells, which have greatly increased numbers of lysosomes and are more actively phagocytic.

CELL COOPERATION IN INDUCTION OF ANTIBODY FORMATION

As noted above, both thymus and bone marrow cells are needed for optimal restoration of responsiveness in thymectomized-irradiated mice. Cooperation between cell populations is also evident from the "carrier effect," which provides hints about how the cells interact.

Carrier Effect. When an animal is injected once ("primed") with a hapten-protein conjugate, such as Dnp-bovine γ-globulin (Dnp-BγG), and then given the same immunogen many weeks later, anti-Dnp Abs are formed rapidly and copiously (Secondary response, below). However, if the second injection is made with Dnp attached to certain other carrier proteins, say ovalbumin (EA), a substantial antihapten response is usually not elicited unless the animal has also been previously primed with EA itself. This suggests that recognition of both hapten and carrier contributes to the secondary response.

The same result can be obtained by adoptive transfer: an irradiated recipient of spleen cells from a mouse primed with hapten-protein I does not make significant amounts of antihapten Ab in response to hapten-protein II, unless it is also given "helper" spleen cells from a second mouse primed with protein II. The helpers are T cells: their effect is eliminated by treatment with antisera to θ (plus complement).

The requirement for carrier recognition seems, however, not to be absolute: it can be bypassed by giving a large amount of hapten-protein II or by preparing it from special proteins (e.g., hemocyanin). Other measures that bypass the carrier requirement are described below (see Allogeneic effect, also soluble factors released by T cells; Ch. 20).

The distinction between hapten and carrier determinants also applies to natural immunogens (proteins, red cells), some of whose determinants (hapten-like) bind the elicited Abs (formed by B cells), while others (carrier-like) react with helper T cells in the induction of the B cells. For instance, a brisk secondary response in formation of non-cross-reacting Abs to both *a* and *b* subunits of tetrameric lactic acid dehydrogenase (porcine) could be elicited in rabbits primed with the a_2b_2 form of the enzyme and then boosted with a_2b_2, but no Abs to either subunit were formed in animals boosted with b_4, as though b were a hapten-like subunit requiring the carrier effect of the a subunit. Though distinguishable functionally, the structural distinctions between haptenic and carrier determinants of natural Ags are completely obscure.

T-cell Function. How do T cells promote induction of B cells? According to Mitchison's **focusing hypothesis,** simultaneous binding of an Ag by B and T cells provides additional bonds, which stabilize its binding by membrane receptors of the B cell (Fig. 17-9). Stabilization would be especially helpful for those Ags that have only a single copy of a given determinant per molecule, such as serum albumin and other proteins with one chain per molecule (Ch. 15). In these Ags, moreover, different determinants would have to react with the T and B partners, requiring different specificities of the cooperating cells. This prediction is in accord with the carrier effect, and also with the rule that **T-dependent immunogens have more than one kind of determinant per particle:** the haptenic or hapten-like determinants react with B cells and the carrier determinants with T cells ("associative recognition"). **Thus haptens are not immunogenic unless attached to a carrier;** and proteins are especially effective as carriers (and as immunogens) because they have a great variety of potential carrier determinants per particle, facilitating the engagement of many helper T cells.

T cells seem to exercise their effects both through contact with B cells and the release of diffusible factors that act at short range on nearby B cells. Thus T cells can aid B cells when they react at the same time, and in the same locale, with **separate** immunogenic particles, and even when the cooperating cells are separated by an artificial membrane that is permeable to macromolecules but not to cells. Nevertheless, the highest Ab yields are obtained when the cooperating B and T cells are specific for determinants on the **same** immunogenic particle. Indeed, there seem to be two diffusible factors: a low-molecular-weight (dialyzable) nonspecific substance that enhances the response of B cells of any specificity, and a high-molecular-weight (nondialyzable) specific factor that augments only those B cells that can react specifically with the same immunogen that activated the T cell's release of the factor. It has been suggested that the specific factor might be an Ig of a special class (8S IgM) that

moves from the carrier-activated T cell to the surface of a macrophage where its specific binding of multiple Ag units would facilitate their binding to and activation of B cells (see Fig. 17-9).

The importance of contact between cooperating cells is suggested by an **"allogeneic effect."** In this complex reaction the carrier requirement for eliciting antihapten secondary responses (Carrier effect, above) can be overcome in animals primed with hapten on protein I if, at the time they receive the hapten on a second, non-cross-reacting protein (II), they are also injected with allogeneic lymphoid cells from a donor whose incompatibility in transplantation Ags is such that the injected cells attack the host's cells (including his specifically primed, Ag-binding B cells). This "graft-vs.-host" reaction almost certainly requires cell-cell contact (see Chs. 20 and 21). The allogeneic effect is not obtained with the reverse incompatibility,[*] i.e., when the primed host's T cells attack the unprimed, allogeneic donor's cells, which argues against massive release of diffusible and stable "activating" factors as the primary basis for T-B cooperation.

Though T cells exercise an important regulatory role on responses of B cells to T-dependent immunogens it is important to note that these Ags can induce B cells, in absence of T cells, to make Abs of the IgM class, and to differentiate into memory cells, whose response to a subsequent introduction of the immunogen elicits the augmented secondary response (see below). However, the further maturation of the primary response, usually characterized by production of IgG Abs (see IgM–IgG switch and Secondary response, below), seems not to occur unless T cells are engaged (and also macrophages, below).

Macrophage Function. With Ags whose induction of Ab synthesis in primary spleen cell culture requires accessory T cells, there is a further requirement for adherent cells, prob-

---

[*] Unidirectionality in the attack of host against donor or vice versa is arranged by using animals of inbred strains and their hybrids; i.e., injection of parental lymphoid cells (AA or BB) into F1 hybrid hosts (AB) causes the graft-vs.-host reaction, and injection of lymphoid cells from hybrids into a host of parental type elicits the more commonplace host-vs.-graft response (Ch. 21). The difference comes about because T cells from one individual react against essentially all cells from genetically different (allogeneic) individuals with alien surface histocompatibility Ags (see Chs. 20 and 21, and above, discussion of transplantation as a method for studying Ab formation).

ably macrophages, suggesting that **the inductive complex has three components (ternary complex), perhaps with B and T lymphocytes binding to Ag on the sticky surface of a macrophage** (Fig. 17-9). While each of the cooperating B and T cells reacts specifically with an antigenic determinant of the immunogen, **the macrophage acts nonspecifically:** it is just as effective if drawn from a tolerant or genetically unresponsive donor as from a normal one (see below, Immunological tolerance and Genetic control of Ab formation). Macrophages and T cells are effective even when irradiated, indicating that induction does not require their proliferation, whereas multiplication of B cells is the essence of induction: their irradiation eliminates the response (Table 17-3 and Immunosuppression, below).

The B and T cells that react specifically with the immunogen must be rare, and so their simultaneous reaction in vivo with a given Ag particle would be highly improbable. However, a successive reaction would be more probable if Ag were concentrated on the nonspecifically acting macrophages, and the probability would be further increased if the macrophages were strategically stationed at critical positions along pathways followed by circulating lymphocytes (e.g., sinus spaces of lymph nodes and spleen), where large numbers of B and T cells could continuously pass over their surfaces.

For experimental analysis macrophages are often obtained from peritoneal exudates elicited by intraperitoneal injection of irritants (e.g., thioglycolic acid). However, under natural conditions in vivo it is likely that an equivalent function is also (and perhaps largely) performed by the sticky **reticular cells** that abound on the reticulum fiber meshwork permeating lymph nodes and spleen (see below).

T-independent Antigens. The focusing hypothesis is consistent with the properties of certain Ags that can induce differentiation of B cells without any assistance from T cells and macrophages. These T-independent Ags are large polymers, with many copies of the same determinant per particle (e.g., polyfructose [levan], pneumococcal polysaccharides, polyvinylpyrrolidone, some viruses, polymerized flagellin). Repetitive copies of the determinant on single Ag molecules probably facilitates formation of stable multivalent cross-links with membrane receptors on B cells, bypassing the need for ancillary binding to helper T cells and macrophages.*

Indeed, T cells may even play a **suppressive** role with T-independent Ags: their selective elimination

---

* T-independent Ags seem also to be unusually resistant to degradation by host enzymes, but it is not clear how this contributes to their independence of T cells and macrophages.

TABLE 17-3. Roles of B and T Cells and of Macrophages in Induction of Antibody Synthesis

Property	B cells	T cells	Macrophages
Role	Differentiate into Ab-secreting cells	Accessory cells	Accessory cells
Specificity*	Restricted	Restricted	Unrestricted
Memory†	Yes	Yes	No
Proliferation stimulated by Ag-binding	Yes	Yes	No
Inactive in unresponsive individuals‡	Yes (sometimes)	Yes (sometimes)	No
Helping function	No	Release stimulators for B cells§	Bind Ag on surface facilitating B-cell binding to Ag

* Variety of antigens bound per cell.

† That is, priming by an Ag increases the number of cells able to respond later to that Ag.

‡ Genetically unresponsive or made tolerant (see below).

§ See Chapter 20 for many other factors released by Ag-activated T cells.

by thymectomy or antilymphocytic serum (see below) causes an increase in the amount of Ab formed in response to pneumococcal polysaccharide and to polyvinylpyrrolidone (see Antigenic competition, below, for other evidence that Ag-activated T cells can sometimes suppress Ag-stimulation of B cells.)

ANTIGEN-BINDING RECEPTORS ON LYMPHOCYTES

These receptors have been demonstrated in various ways. For instance, in "hot suicide" experiments highly radioactive Ag (50 μCi/μg) can eliminate specifically the corresponding Ab-forming B cells and helper T cells. In another approach, red cells (used as Ags or coated with extrinsic Ags) form rosettes around the corresponding lymphocytes (Fig. 17-3). Hemolytic plaque assays show that many of the rosette-forming lymphoid cells secrete Ab and are thus of B lineage. The ability of T cells to form rosettes is disputed, perhaps because the density or affinity of their surface Ag-binding-receptors is too low to permit consistent formation of stable rosettes.

B-cell Receptors. Membrane-bound receptors are abundant on the surface of B lymphocytes (ca. 100,000/cell has been estimated with labeled ligands). Binding of Ags by B cells is blocked by antisera to Igs, but not by antisera to other surface macromolecules, such as histocompatibility Ags. Moreover, immuno-fluorescence staining of living cells with antisera to various Ig chains shows that the Ig on the surface of a given B cell is usually restricted to one class and allotype of heavy chain, and to one type and allotype of light chain (see One cell–one Ab rule, below). Hence each B cell has a particular Ig as receptor, possibly modified for purposes of attachment.

The proportion of B cells with κ or λ light chains in their surface receptors corresponds roughly to the frequency of these chains in serum Igs. However, in some species (e.g., man, mouse) the heavy chain distribution is discordant: of the approximately 15 to 30% of peripheral blood lymphocytes that have surface Igs (B cells), about 50% have μ, 35% have γ, and 10% have α chains. (The corresponding values for serum IgM, IgG, and IgA are about 5 to 10%, 80 to 90%, and

5 to 10%, respectively; see Appendix, Ch. 16.) Moreover, labeled Igs extracted from the B cell membrane are predominantly monomeric IgM$_s$ (8S), not the pentameric 19S molecules that account for most serum IgM (Ch. 16).*

IgM-IgG Switch. Indirect evidence hints that the Ig class of surface receptors on a B cell may change during an immune response. For instance, when a primary response to sheep erythrocytes is induced in cultured mouse spleen cells in the presence of anti-μ Abs during the initial 48 hours, the formation of Abs of all classes is blocked; the presence of anti-γ has little effect during the initial induction period, but if it is added 1 to 2 days later it blocks just the formation of Abs of the IgG class, suggesting that receptors on virgin B lymphocytes are IgM and that after stimulation by Ag some B cells come to have surface receptors of the IgG class. (For other evidence that individual cells can undergo the IgM-IgG switch without stimulation by Ag, see Ontogeny, below, and biclonal myeloma tumors in Ch. 16.) A switch could also account for effects in intact animals: anti-γ blocks only about 20% of the rosettes formed by spleen cells isolated 3 days after immunization with sheep red cells but about 40% of those that can form on day 8.

Cap Formation. When the living B cell reacts with fluorescein-labeled anti-Ig the cell's surface is initially stained diffusely; but after a few minutes the fluorescent material aggregates into **patches,** which then coalesce into a **polar cap** (Fig. 17-10). With further incubation the cap is shed or ingested by the cell and degraded into fragments. The cells thus lose their receptors and cannot be stained again until 6 to 8 hours later, when the surface Igs are regenerated. A similar time is required for regeneration after stripping surface Igs with trypsin; and this time is concordant with evidence for a slow, dynamic turnover of ^{125}I-labeled surface Igs.

Patch formation seems to represent a two-dimensional microprecipitin reaction, cross-linking receptor Ig molecules that are normally diffusible in the cell's fluid membrane: it does not, for instance, occur if the fluorescent reagent is prepared from the univalent Fab fragment of anti-Ig. Patches are also formed when B cells bind a multivalent Ag

---

* In some species (guinea pig) the predominant Ig on B cells seems to be IgG of the γ2 subclass (Ch. 19, Fig. 19-6).

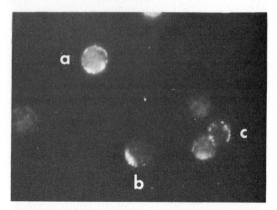

Fig. 17-10. Aggregated Igs in surface membrane of lymphocytes. Living white blood cells (of rabbit) were stained with fluorescein-labeled Abs to a rabbit Ig allotype. The speckled appearance of cells *a* and *c* represents patches of membrane Igs cross-linked by the anti-Ig; the patches are accumulated into a polar cap in cell *b*. The reaction was at 4° and the cells were examined at room temperature. At 37° most of the stained cells would have caps as in *b*. (Courtesy of Dr. Joseph M. Davie.)

and it is possible that cross-linking of surface receptor molecules (by multivalent Ag or aggregated univalent Ag and even experimentally by bivalent anti-Ig) is a crucial triggering event that sets off cell proliferation and differentiation (Blast transformation, below).

Polar caps seem to arise from patches that are swept together in the moving membrane of motile lymphocytes. Thus conditions that block motility inhibit cap formation (without blocking aggregation into patches); e.g., lowering temperature to 4°, blocking ATP generation (with azide or cyanide), or adding colcemid, an agent that disaggregates cytoplasmic microtubules and disorganizes the cell's locomotory system. Patches can also be formed on the surface of various nonlymphoid cells by fluorescein-labeled Abs to their surface histocompatibility Ags; coalescence of patches into a polar cap occurs in motile fibroblasts but not in nonmotile epithelial cells.

T-cell Receptors. The nature of Ag-binding receptors on T cells is uncertain. The immunological activities of these cells (e.g., in graft-vs.-host reactions, see Ch. 21) are not consistently blocked by antisera to Igs; and these cells have virtually no surface Ig detectable by immunofluorescence ($< 1\%$ of the cells are stained).

Quantitative adsorption of trace amounts of radio-iodine-labeled anti-Igs suggests that the average T cell has on its surface the equivalent of about 100 molecules of Ig per cell, or about 0.1% of the amount present on the average B lymphocyte. Whether this small amount is functionally significant is not known. Some of the difficulties in evaluating surface Igs of T cells could derive from the use of antisera to class-specific (isotypic) determinants (Ch. 16), which could be buried in the T cell membrane or sterically hindered by other surface macromolecules; and since Ag binding seems perhaps to be blocked more by antisera to light chains than by those to the known heavy chains (including μ) the T-cell receptors might belong to an as yet uncharacterized class (IgT). The receptors could also lack domains with isotypic determinants and consist of just the V_H plus V_L regions required to constitute the Ag-binding site of an Ig (Ch. 16). The most intriguing possibility is that a novel family of diversified proteins, not Igs at all, makes up the Ag-binding receptors on T cells (see discussion of Ir genes below under Genetic control of antibody formation).

BLAST TRANSFORMATION

Incubation with Ag causes small lymphocytes with the corresponding surface receptors to undergo "blast transformation": the cells enlarge; the nucleolus swells; polysomes, rough endoplasmic reticulum, and microtubules develop; and rates of macromolecule synthesis increase markedly (Ch. 20, Fig. 20-9). Similar changes are initiated by the binding of anti-Ig Abs to surface receptors of B cells, and of certain mitogenic plant proteins to the surface of B and T cells. The changes suggest that a membrane perturbation brought about by cross-linking appropriate surface macromolecules stimulates lymphocytes to divide.

The **plant mitogens** are specific for various sugars of different surface glycoproteins (not Igs), which seem to be approximately equally represented in B and T lymphocytes. However, the two cell types respond differently; soluble **phytohemagglutinin (PHA)** and **concanavalin A** stimulate transformation in T cells only, but when these proteins are insolubilized by attachment to large particles (Sephadex beads) they also stimulate B cells, which can even start secreting Igs. Another protein, **pokeweed mitogen,** stimulates transformation of B and T cells. The lack of a response of blood lymphocytes to soluble

PHA is used clinically to reveal T-cell deficiencies in rare developmental anomalies (see below, Immunodeficiency diseases) and in certain neoplastic diseases (e.g., Hodgkin's disease).

Lipopolysaccharides (endotoxin) of gram-negative bacteria are mitogenic for B cells. Unlike the plant mitogens, which react with cell surface glycoproteins, the lipid moiety of endotoxin **(lipid A,** see Chs. 6, 29) probably reacts with lipids of the lymphocyte membrane.

PLASMA CELLS

Attention focused on plasma cells as the principal Ab-producing cells because their frequency in a tissue reflects the level of Ab synthesis:

1) As lymphoid tissues become hyperplastic in response to immunogenic stimulation, plasma cells become conspicuous. They are especially numerous when Ab production is at its height.

2) In intensively immunized animals the amount of Ab extractable from various tissues correlates roughly with plasma cell content.

3) Plasma cells in tissues are unusually prominent in those diseases in which serum Igs are markedly elevated: e.g., in multiple myeloma (which is a plasma cell tumor), various chronic infectious diseases, cirrhosis of liver, and certain diseases of unknown origin, such as Boeck's sarcoid.

Ag-stimulated small B lymphocytes differentiate into plasma cells, which synthesize and secrete Abs more actively than any other cell type (Fig. 17-11). "Immature plasma cells"

Fig. 17-11. Electron micrographs of representative Ab-secreting cells (hemolytic plaque-forming cells, PFC, as in Fig. 17-4). Cells in **A,B,C** are from lymph nodes and spleen; the one in **D** is characteristic of PFC in efferent lymph emerging from an antigenically stimulated lymph node. Most PFC from within lymph nodes and spleen are plasma cells **(C),** except during the first few days after immunization when lymphocytes **(A)** and transitional cells **(B)** constitute the majority. [From F. G. Gudat, T. N. Harris, S. Harris, and K. Hummeler, *J Exp Med 134:*1155 (1971) **[A,B]** *J Exp Med 132:*448 (1970) **[C];** K. Hummeler, T. N. Harris, S. Harris, and M. B. Farber, *J Exp Med 135:*491 (1972) **[D].**]

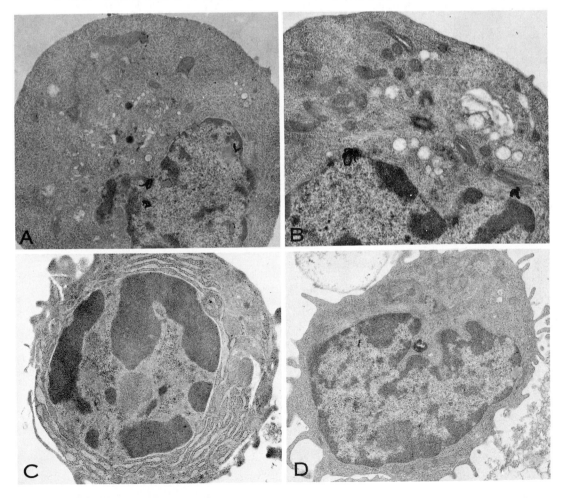

and "large lymphocytes" are arbitrary designations for transitional stages between the small B lymphocyte and the fully differentiated plasma cell. In its fully differentiated form the plasma cell is anatomically distinctive: the nucleus is eccentric and contains coarse, radially arranged chromatin (cartwheel), the cytoplasm has a conspicuous Golgi apparatus, and abundant rough and smooth endoplasmic reticulum is usually packed into thin onionskin-like lamellae or sometimes distended with Igs (as shown by immunofluorescence; Figs. 17-6 and 11).

The mature plasma cell is believed to survive only a few weeks and to die after a few (or no) cell divisions; in contrast, neoplastic plasma cells (myeloma cells), like other neoplastic differentiated cells, are capable of an indefinite number of cell divisions. Synthesis of Igs decreases during the mitotic stage of the cell cycle in myeloma cells.

ONE CELL–ONE ANTIBODY RULE

The Igs in individual plasma cells appear to be uniform in staining reactions with fluorescent Abs to diverse Ig chains: a given cell has only one class and one allotype of heavy chain and one type and allotype of light chain. The Abs used as reagents in establishing this one cell–one Ig rule are usually specific for the invariant parts of Ig chains, but the rule also applies to the variable regions, which determine the Ig's ligand-binding site: in animals immunized with two Ags or one Ag with two distinguishable determinants (e.g., arsanilate and polyalanyl groups) some plasma cells make Abs to one, others make Abs to the second, and none make Abs to both.* Hence the rule is one plasma cell–one Ab. The uniformity of the heavy chains and of the light chains produced in each Ig-synthe-

sizing cell accounts for the **homospecific symmetry** of the Ab molecule (i.e., the same specificity at each of its combining sites), and it explains the absence of natural "hybrids," with different heavy or different light chains in the same molecule.

Cross-reactions show that different cells producing Abs to the same immunogen can differ in their respective Abs' active sites: by testing individual cells in microdrops with different phages (T2 and T4) labeled with cross-reacting haptens (mono- or dinitroiodophenyl, NIP or NNP), some cells from an animal immunized with NIP-BγG were found to neutralize NIP-phage but not NNP-phage, and other cells neutralized both. In addition, individual cells from an animal immunized with a Dnp-protein differ in the concentration of Dnp-hapten required to block their formation of hemolytic plaques in vitro, showing that the Abs secreted by different cells can differ in affinity for the hapten. **Thus the great diversity of Igs in an individual, and the often immense heterogeneity of the Abs he forms against a given Ag, arise from corresponding diversity among Ab-producing plasma cells.**

Small B cells also conform to the one cell–one Ab rule. As noted above, immunofluorescence shows that the surface Igs on a given cell have one isotypic and allotypic form of heavy chain and of light chain (B-cell receptors, above), and reactions with antiidiotypic antisera suggest that there is also one idiotype per cell (see Idiotype suppression, below). Thus the Ig molecules produced by an individual cell of B type (small lymphocyte or plasma cell) are probably as uniform in primary structure as the myeloma protein produced by a myeloma tumor (each of which is a clone of neoplastic plasma cells).

All these findings emphasize that synthesis of Ig molecules in cells of B lineage is subject to the principle of **allelic exclusion:** the cell expresses only one of its several alleles for light chains and only one of its many alleles for heavy chains† (for possible exceptions see

---

* One search for double-producing plasma cells was carried out by an interesting modification of the hemolytic plaque assay with a mixture of rabbit and camel red cells, each coated with a different Ag: a clear plaque meant that the central Ab-forming cell secreted Abs to both Ags, while turbid plaques meant Ab to only one of the two Ags. Over 40,000 plaques were examined from animals immunized with two different Ags or one Ag with two determinants: no clear plaques were found above the low number observed as background with cells from unimmunized animals.

---

† A somewhat similar situation occurs in mammalian females, where random inactivation of one of the two X-chromosomes per cell during embryogenesis causes **mosaicism:** one X is active in some cells and the other X in other cells (the Lyon effect). But structural genes for Igs are not X-linked, and allelic exclusion among autosomal genes appears to be unique for Igs. It does not, for instance, occur

IgM-IgG shift, below). It also secretes Ig molecules or produces Ig membrane receptors that in each cell are restricted to a particular Ag-binding specificity and idiotype. Though all cells express only a small portion of their genes, the degree of restriction seems to be extreme in regard to Ig genes; but it is not clear just how or when the selective expression of particular Ig alleles is initiated in differentiation of stem cells into B cells. Nevertheless, **the restricted specificity of single lymphocytes and the resulting diversity of the mass of lymphocytes in a given individual strongly support the clonal selection hypothesis.**

The **frequency** of a given Ig-producing plasma cell in lymphoid tissues is roughly proportional to the level of the corresponding protein in serum. For instance, there are about 3 to 6 plasma cells that produce δ chains per 1000 that produce γ chains, in accord with the much lower level of IgD than of IgG in serum. And cells that form α chains constitute the vast majority of Ig-forming cells in intestinal and respiratory tracts, and in a number of secretory glands, in accord with the preponderance of IgA over other Igs in mucinous secretions.

In contrast to fully differentiated plasma cells, most of the small Ag-sensitive B lymphocytes that represent the beginning of the differentiation pathway seem to produce only IgMs (see B cell receptors, above). The difference suggests that during the differentiation triggered by Ag some cells switch from production of IgM to IgG or IgA or another class (see below).

IgM-IgG Shift. Rare individual cells in microdrops seem to secrete anti-*Salmonella* Abs of both IgM and IgG classes; and immunofluorescence reveals rare lymphocytes with IgM on the surface and IgG internally. These "double-producers" could correspond to cells in the process of shifting from synthesis of IgM to IgG Abs.* This shift, if it occurs consistently following immunization, could contribute to the shift in preponderance of serum Abs from IgM to IgG that occurs early in most immune responses (see discussion of Change with time after immunization, below). A shift from IgM to IgG production can apparently occur independently of Ag stimulation during embryogenesis of B cells (see Ontogeny, below).

Two considerations can reconcile the double-producers with the one cell–one Ab rule: 1) The rule refers to the activity of cells at a given time: if a cell stops making IgM molecules and starts making IgG molecules, it could for some hours contain and possibly even secrete both Igs without actually synthesizing both of them at the same time. 2) The two Igs of double-producers probably have the same idiotype and presumably therefore the same Ag-binding specificity; i.e., they are likely to differ in just the isotype of the heavy chain.

The two genes–one chain hypothesis (Ch. 16) suggests how the shift could occur with minimal perturbation: in making an IgM Ab the cell expresses genes for V_L, C_L, V_H, and $C\mu$ domains, and in shifting to production of IgG only the gene for $C\mu$ would have to be shut off and the one for $C\gamma$ turned on. Both the IgM and the IgG molecules would thus have the same V_L and V_H and, therefore, the same idiotype and same combining-site specificity. The plausibility of this sequence is supported by several observations. For instance, the IgM and the IgG myeloma proteins made by one **biclonal human myeloma tumor** seem to be identical (by peptide map, idiotypic determinants, partial amino acid sequences) except for C_H, which was μ in one protein and γ in the other (Ch. 16).

As noted above, in the absence of T cells the T-dependent Ags can stimulate B cells to make Abs of the IgM class, but the copious production of IgG molecules to these Ags requires the assistance of T cells and macrophages. The IgG response could either reflect a shift within individual cells (from IgM to IgG production) or a requirement by B cells of the IgG class for some product of stimulated T cells.

---

with hemoglobin (Hgb): in a heterozygote with normal and sickle cell alleles each red cell has both normal and abnormal Hgb molecules.

* Some cultures of permanent lymphoid cell lines consistently produce two kinds of Igs (IgM and IgG, or IgG and IgA). However, these cells are usually aneuploid (abnormal number of chromosomes) and may have many anomalous regulatory mechanisms; it is possible, nevertheless, that a very small proportion of normal lymphoid cells also can simultaneously secrete Igs of two classes.

SYNTHESIS, ASSEMBLY, AND SECRETION OF IMMUNOGLOBULINS

In plasma cells pulse-labeled with radioactive amino acids it appears that Igs, like secreted proteins in general, are synthesized on polyribosomes attached to the rough endoplasmic reticulum, rather than on unbound polyribosomes. Though the cells promptly incorporate radioactive amino acids, the newly synthesized Ig molecules are secreted only after a

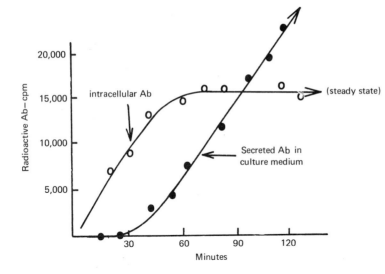

Fig. 17-12. Lag in secretion of antibodies. Labeled amino acid was added at zero time to a suspension of lymph node cells from an immunized rabbit, and cells and supernatant were then assayed at intervals for newly synthesized Abs. [Based on Helmreich, E., Kern, M., and Eisen, H. N. *J Biol Chem 236*:464 (1961).]

20 to 30 minute lag (Fig. 17-12), during which they presumably enter and pass through cisternae of endoplasmic reticulum, traverse the Golgi apparatus, and then move through secretory vesicles toward the cell surface, from which Ig molecules are shed as the vesicles fuse with the surface membrane. During this migration the completed chains are assembled into molecules, the interchain S-S bonds are formed, and sugars are added successively by hexosetransferases to form the oligosaccharide groups of complete Ig molecules (Fig. 17-13).

The order of assembly of chains has been studied primarily in myeloma tumors, in which various patterns have been deduced from the variety of in-

complete molecules found intracellularly and from pulse-chase experiments. Thus, when cells are harvested at various times after a 30-second pulse of radioactive amino acid the labeled nascent light (L) or heavy (H) chain can be followed as it joins with other chains to establish complete four-chain Ig molecules ($H_2 \cdot L_2$). In some tumors complete molecules are made by joining two $H \cdot L$ half-molecules; in others, H-chain dimers (H_2) add one L chain at a time; in still other tumors both patterns are observed. Regardless of the particular pattern, assembly and secretion are orderly: interchain S-S bonds form slowly (2 to 20 minutes after the constituent chains are completed); the rate of secretion equals the rate of synthesis and, accordingly, the intracellular level of Ig molecules is constant; the more recently synthesized molecules leave the cell only after pre-

Fig. 17-13. Scheme for assembly, intracellular transport and secretion of Igs. RER = rough endoplasmic reticulum, i.e., with bound polyribosomes. [Based on Uhr, J. W. *Cellular Immunol 1*:228 (1970).]

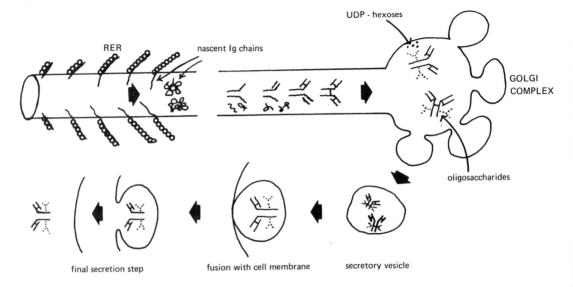

viously synthesized ones have been secreted (Fig. 17-12).

In myloma cells that make IgA or IgM molecules the intracellular Ig seems not to progress beyond the four-chain monomer, though polymers are found in the culture medium. The monomers probably associate with each other and with J chains (which are made in the same cells) as Ig molecules are secreted (for J chains, see Ch. 16).

The order of incorporation of radioactive sugar precursors (hexoses and hexosamines) is in accord with the sequence of sugar residues in Ig oligosaccharides (Ch. 16). Glucosamine, which links oligosaccharides to Ig chains, is incorporated first, and followed by mannose, galactose, and later by sialic acid groups. Fucose appears to become attached last, as Ig molecules exit from the cell.

The addition of sugars may not be necessary for secretion, as has been suggested, because some myelomas secrete only light chains (Bence Jones protein), many of which lack carbohydrate.

LYMPHATIC ORGANS

Besides circulating through blood, lymph, and tissue spaces, lymphocytes are aggregated into primary and secondary lymphatic structures, where different stages in their differentiation are carried out. In the primary organs (thymus, bursa of Fabricius or its analog in nonavian species) lymphocytes become committed to react specifically with particular Ags, and in secondary lymphatic organs the committed cells react with Ags, which stimulate their terminal differentiation: B cells into Ab-secreting plasma cells, T cells into effectors of cell-mediated immunity (Ch. 20), and both into their respective memory cells, which probably also look like small lymphocytes.

PRIMARY LYMPHATIC ORGANS

Thymus. A role for the thymus in the immune response was long suspected (because it is essentially a mass of lymphocytes) but largely discounted, because decades of study showed that this organ did not form Abs, trap Ags, or contain more than a rare plasma cell. Beginning, however, in 1960 with Jacques Miller's observations in England, mice that were thymectomized **at birth** were found to develop a coherent variety of defects, which

illuminate the contribution of the thymus and define properties of T cells.

Neonatally thymectomized mice have a drastically reduced number of blood lymphocytes, depleted T-cell areas in lymph nodes and spleen (Fig. 17-8), and reduced ability to reject allografts (Chs. 20 and 21); moreover, in response to many Ags they produce few if any Abs, and what is produced seems to be largely limited to the IgM class. They can, however, form Abs normally in response to other, T-independent Ags (e.g., highly polymerized proteins, viruses, polysaccharides; Table 17-4).

The effects of thymectomy are confirmed in mice born without a thymus. The defect is inherited as a recessive autosomal trait linked to hairlessness: the resulting **nude, thymus-less** mutants do not usually survive more than a few months, probably because of extreme susceptibility to infections.* Practically all their lymphocytes have readily demonstrable surface Igs (i.e., they are B cells). Their serum IgM levels are normal but Igs of other classes are depressed, and most of the Abs they make in response to experimental immunization are IgM, suggesting that the switch from IgM to IgG production is largely blocked. Perhaps because some T cells migrate out of the thymus before birth, neonatally thymectomized normal mice seem not to be as deficient in T cells or in T cell functions as the nude mutants.

The thymus is a "lymphoepithelial" mixture of lymphoid and epithelial cells. It develops in the embryo from branchial pouches of the pharynx: epithelial buds grow out, pinch off, and migrate (in higher vertebrates) to the midline of the upper thorax where they become infiltrated with lymphocytes. The transfer of cells from diverse tissues in mice with the T6 chromosomal marker to syngeneic mice lacking the marker has shown that thymus lymphocytes derive from migratory blood-forming (hematopoietic) stem cells (originating in yolk sac or liver of the fetus and in bone marrow of the adult). A high incidence of mitotic figures in the thymus, and rapid incorporation of radioactive thymidine into DNA, show that the immigrant cells divide rapidly; but only a small proportion of their progeny survive and be-

---

* These mice are, accordingly, produced in special colonies maintained for high frequency of the defective chromosome.

TABLE 17-4. Effects of Extirpation of Thymus or Bursa of Fabricius*

Property	Thymectomy	Bursectomy
Cellular changes		
Circulating lymphocytes	↓↓	0
Spleen		
Germinal centers	0(↓)	↓↓
B zones†	0	↓↓
T zones†	↓↓	0
Plasma cells	0(↓)	↓↓
Functional changes		
Serum Ig level	0(↓)	↓↓
Antibody formation	0(↓)	↓↓
Cell-mediated immunity		
(e.g., rejection of skin		
allografts)	↓↓	0

* Composite effects of bursectomy and thymectomy in chicks at hatching and of thymectomy in newborn mice.

† Lymph nodes in birds are poorly organized clusters of lymphocytes alongside lymphatic channels; their B and T zones are readily discernible in the spleen.

0 = No change; ↓↓ = marked decrease; ↓ = modest decrease; 0(↓) = variable decrease, probably secondary to role of T cells as helpers in induction of Ab synthesis.

come mature T cells. About 90% of thymus lymphocytes are readily destroyed by corticosteroids. The resistant 10%, located mostly in the medulla (Fig. 17-14), have the characteristic surface Ags of mature T cells (Table 17-2), which they also resemble in having marked reactivity with foreign (allogeneic) cells (Ch. 21, Graft-vs.-host reaction).

In most species the thymus is fully developed at birth. It atrophies gradually with time ("age involution"), or in occasional rapid bursts after severe stress ("accidental involution" after severe infection, starvation, trauma), probably in response to high levels of adrenal corticosteroids (Immunosuppressive agents, below). Removal of the thymus from an adult usually has no obvious effects, because peripheral tissues are already fully populated with a great many diversified T cells. However, the adult thymus is functional: its cells serve as competent T cells and T-cell precursors in adoptive transfer, and thymectomy delays recovery of immunological activity after whole-body X-irradiation (see Fig. 17-29).

Thymic Hormone. It is possible that a hormone elaborated by thymus epithelial cells promotes differentiation of precursor lymphocytes into T cells.

Thus the cellular and functional deficiencies of neonatally thymectomized mice can be largely corrected with thymic grafts enclosed in chambers whose porous membrane passes macromolecules but not cells. Moreover, a glycoprotein ("thymosin") in calf thymus extracts seems to repair some defects in thymectomized mice (e.g., the ability to reject allografts).

Bursa of Fabricius. One of the earliest clues to the distinction between B and T cells derived from Glick's serendipitous discovery that chicks deprived at birth of the bursa of Fabricius are unable to produce Abs. Resembling the thymus anatomically, the bursa also develops by lymphocytic infiltration of an epithelial outpouching from the intestine, but in the hind gut (cloaca) instead of the foregut. Lymph follicles of the bursa, unlike those of thymus, are packed with plasma cells. The bursa also undergoes atrophy at puberty (4 months of age in chickens), probably as a result of rising levels of steroid sex hormones. In fact, the bursa can be eliminated ("hormonally extirpated") by simply dipping embryonated eggs for a few minutes in a solution of testosterone.

Extirpation has shown that the bursa and thymus regulate complementary functions

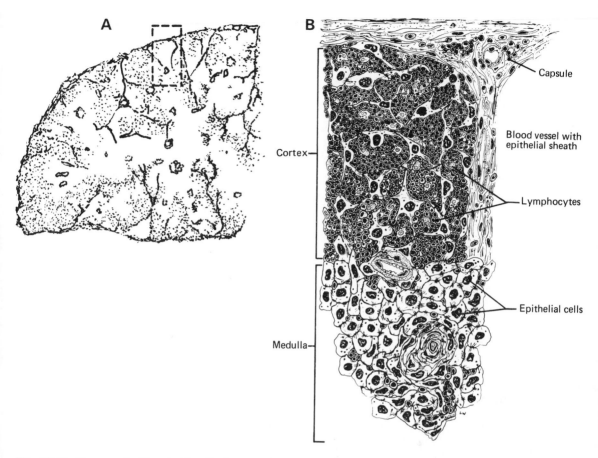

Labels on figure: Cortex, Medulla, Capsule, Blood vessel with epithelial sheath, Lymphocytes, Epithelial cells

A   B

Fig. 17-14. Thymus. **A.** The darkly stippled cortex consists of a dense mantle of T lymphocytes surrounding the lightly stippled medulla, which is made up of epithelial cells plus some lymphocytes (more mature T cells). **B.** Portion of thymus lobule (area enclosed in **A**) in some detail. (Based on Weiss, L. *The Cells and Tissues of the Immune System.* Prentice-Hall, Englewood Cliffs, N.J., 1972.)

(Table 17-4). In contrast to thymus-less animals, neonatally bursectomized chicks have normal cell-mediated immune responses (e.g., they reject skin allografts, Ch. 21) and they have normal levels of lymphocytes in blood and also in T zones of lymph nodes and spleen. However, they are devoid of plasma cells, and their severe deficit in serum Ig levels and in Ab-forming ability is greater the earlier in life the bursa is removed (Ontogeny, below).

Mammals lack a bursa of Fabricius and their structure with equivalent function has not been identified. Possibilities include the bone marrow itself, lymph nodes (which are rudimentary in chickens), various gut-asso-ciated lymphoepithelial structures (appendix, tonsils), and the lymphocyte-infiltrated villous epithelium that stretches the length of the intestinal tract.

SECONDARY LYMPHATIC STRUCTURES

The spleen, many lymph nodes, and smaller, less organized clusters of lymphoid cells in many tissues and organs constitute the secondary structures in which committed lymphocytes undergo terminal differentiation in response to Ag stimulation. These structures are highly effective Ag-trapping filters in which lymphocytes pack the interstices of a dense three-dimensional fibrous network, with many sticky reticular cells attached to reticulum fibers. Injected lymphocytes accumulate in spleen and lymph nodes, as though expressing the **homing** instinct that normally causes circulating lymphocytes to leave blood vessels in these structures (via postcapillary venules or sinusoids), and to reside for a time in appropriate areas (B and T zones, Fig. 17-8) before recirculating.

Lymph Nodes. These ovoid structures are widely distributed in extremities, trunk, mediastinum, omentum, etc., where they generally are situated at major junctions of the network of lymphatic channels, which pass tree-like from twigs in the more superficial tissues to a large central collecting trunk, **the thoracic duct;** this vessel pours lymph and lymphocytes into the great vein that returns blood to the heart. Ags deposited in tissues are carried via lymphatic channels through successive lymph nodes, in which they are likely to be trapped by reticular cells and macrophages. (Brain, spinal cord, and eye lack lymphatic drainage, and Ags carried away in blood from these areas are likely to be trapped in the spleen or distant lymph nodes.)

At the center of the subcapsular B-cell nodules the **germinal center** is made up of a mass of rapidly dividing large B lymphocytes (generation time ca.

6 hours; Fig. 17-15). Macrophages with ingested pyknotic nuclei and DNA debris are also abundant, as in many other areas with rapidly dividing cells (as though many of the rapidly formed progeny are defective and are disposed of by phagocytosis). **The size of germinal centers is proportional to the intensity of antigenic stimulation:** they are greatly enlarged in secondary responses (below) and are essentially absent in germ-free mice. These centers become similarly hyperplastic in other secondary lymphatic structures when intensely engaged in producing Abs.

Spleen. This large encapsulated vascular organ (about 200 gm in adult man) traps Ags carried in blood. Like other lymphatic organs, its cortex has densely packed lymphocytes (with germinal centers), and its loose medulla has wide vascular spaces with a variety of lymphoid and other cells (Fig. 17-16). In the spleen, however, the medulla (called "red pulp") encloses cortical areas (called "white pulp"), rather than the reverse, as in other lymphatic structures. Cortical areas surround small central arteries with leaky walls, through which Ags are probably driven by the arterial blood pressure. Separate T and B zones are also discernible in the white pulp (Fig. 17-8); the T area is relatively smaller in spleen than in lymph nodes,

Fig. 17-15. Mammalian lymph node. **A.** Schematic view showing afferent (AL) and efferent (EL) lymph channels and the subcapsular sinus (SS) with criss-crossing reticulum fibers that extend throughout the node. Reticular macrophages, attached to the fibers, trap Ags, especially when in the form of Ab-Ag complexes. GC = germinal center; MS = medullary sinus. **B.** Human lymph node (×45). The "secondary nodule" points to a germinal center with its surrounding mantle of B lymphocytes. The "tertiary cortex" is a mass of T cells. (**A** courtesy of Dr. S. Clark, Jr. **B** from Weiss, L. *The Cells and Tissues of the Immune System.* Prentice-Hall, Englewood Cliffs, N.J., 1972.)

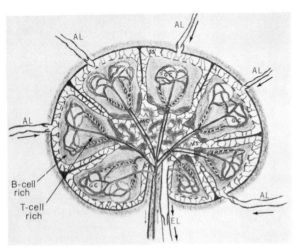

A

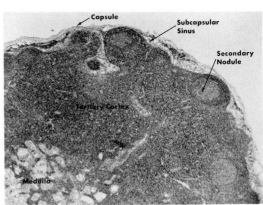

B

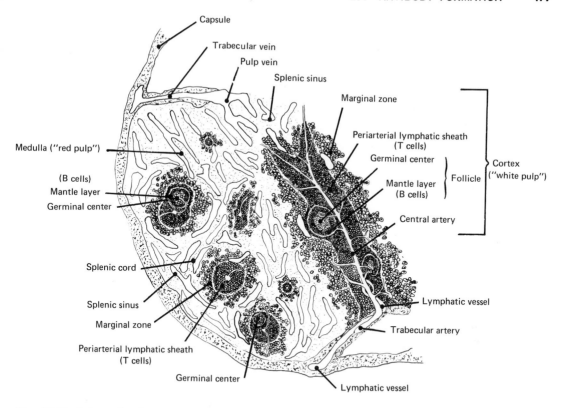

Capsule
Trabecular vein
Pulp vein
Splenic sinus
Marginal zone
Periarterial lymphatic sheath
(T cells)
Germinal center
Medulla ("red pulp")
Mantle layer
(B cells)
Follicle
Cortex
("white pulp")
(B cells)
Mantle layer
Germinal center
Central artery
Splenic cord
Splenic sinus
Marginal zone
Lymphatic vessel
Trabecular artery
Periarterial lymphatic sheath
(T cells)
Germinal center
Lymphatic vessel

Fig. 17-16. Schematic view of a representative area of the spleen showing masses of lymphoid cells (white pulp) distributed around the central arteries. T cells make up the periarterial lymphatic sheath; B cells form the mantle layer around germinal centers. See also Figure 17-8. (From Weiss, L. *The Cells and Tissues of the Immune System.* Prentice-Hall, Englewood Cliffs, N.J., 1972.)

and after intense antigenic stimulation T cells are virtually replaced by sheets of plasma cells (in contrast to lymph node T areas, where plasma cells are almost never seen).

Gut-associated Lymphoid Cells. Lymphocytes and plasma cells (predominantly with IgA) are spread throughout the inner layers of the intestinal wall as isolated cells or as small cell clusters. Larger clusters form distinct follicles with germinal centers; some follicles become confluent and interdigitated with overlying epithelium, forming small **lymphoepithelial** structures which (unlike thymus and bursa) remain associated with the intestinal wall throughout life. The main ones in man are 1) tonsils (in the pharyngeal wall), 2) appendix (at junction of small and large intestine), and 3) Peyer's patches (oblong lymphoid aggregates found mostly in the wall of the terminal part of the small intestine). As in other secondary lymphatic structures, follicular (B) areas around germinal centers are well developed and interfollicular (T) areas are atrophic in thymus-less individuals.

GENETIC CONTROL OF ANTIBODY FORMATION

Selective breeding can generate strains of animals able to make high or low titers of Abs to complex Ags (foreign red cells, salmonellae, etc.). However, insight into genetic control began to accumulate rapidly only after systematic use was made of 1) inbred mice and guinea pigs, and 2) Ags of limited immunogenicity, such as synthetic polypeptides, unusually small doses of conventional proteins, and alloantigens.

Ability of mice to make high Ab titers to many of these Ags is determined by a dominant, autosomal (not sex-linked) locus, Ir-1: e.g., mice of the C57Bl strain make about 10 times higher titers than CBA mice to the tyrosine-glutamate (T,G) determinant of (T,G)–A—L (Fig. 17-17); and all F_1 hybrids

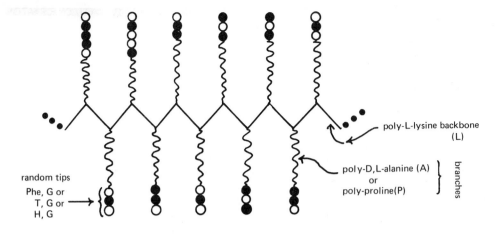

Immunogen:	Phe, G-Pro--L		T, G-Pro--L	T, G-A--L	Phe, G-A--L	H, G-A--L
Abs specific for:	Phe, G	Pro, L	Pro, L	T, G	Phe, G	H, G
Mouse strains						
High responders	DBA	SJL	SJL	C57B1	DBA	C3H, CBA
Low responders	SJL	DBA	DBA	SJL, C3H, CBA	SJL	C57B1, SJL
Ir gene linked to:	H-2	not H-2	not H-2	H-2	H-2	H-2

Fig. 17-17. Genetic control of Ab formation to synthetic branched polypeptides. The most useful ones have a poly-L-lysine (L) backbone and poly-D,L-alanine (A) or polyproline (P) branches, with tips carrying short random amino acid sequences of tyrosine and glutamate (T,G) or histidine and glutamate (H,G) or phenlyalanine and glutamate (Phe,G). The corresponding polymers are designated (T,G)-A—L, (H,G)-A—L, and (Phe,G)-A—L. The antigenic determinants are usually the short terminal sequences (Phe,G or T,G or H,G); but in a few mouse strains the branched backbone (poly-pro-poly-lysine) is immunogenic. [Based on Sela, M. *Harvey Lect* 67:213 (1973).]

(i.e., C57 × CBA) are high responders, as are ca. 50% of the progeny of the back-cross between hybrids and the low-responding homozygous parental strain (F_1 × CBA). Parallel effects have been obtained in other strains with this and other Ags: for instance, with another branched polypeptide, (H,G)–A—L, the high responders are CBA and the low responders are C57B1 mice (Fig. 17-17).

The ability of a mouse strain to respond to certain Ags was found by McDevitt to be associated with the strain's major histocompatibility Ags, which are located on cell surface membranes: both phenotypes are consistently carried together in the progeny of diverse matings, establishing genetic linkage of Ir-1 with the H-2 locus, which specifies the most potent histocompatibility Ags in mice (Ch. 21). This unexpected association turned out to be remarkably useful, because independent genetic analyses provided rare mice that represented recombinants between the two ends of the H-2 locus: and by selective breeding the recombinant chromosome could be introduced in homozygous form into mice whose immune responses to branched polypeptides then made it possible to map the Ir-1 locus close to the center of the H-2 locus (Fig. 17-18). A few other Ir genes, segregating from Ir-1, specify ability to make high Ab titers to different Ags; some are linked to other loci (not H-2) (Fig. 17-17).

Similar relations were found independently by Benacerraf *et al.* in inbred guinea pigs, in whom the additional ability to exhibit delayed-type hypersensitivity skin responses provided

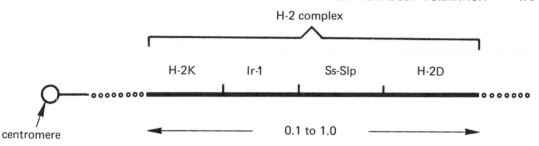

Fig. 17-18. Map of a mouse chromosome (IXᵗʰ linkage group) showing the immune response-1 (Ir-1) locus and the complex locus for the most potent histocompatibility Ags (H-2). *Ir-1* falls between *H-2K* and *H-2D*, the two genes that define the limits of the *H-2* complex (Ch. 21). *Ss-Slp* governs the quantitative level of a serum protein, Ss, and a cross-reacting protein whose production is limited to males (Slp, sex-limited protein). Products of H-2 and of Ss-Slp are probably entirely unrelated in function. The recombination frequency between the ends of *H-2D* and *H-2K* is between 0.1 and 1.0%, which means that the *H-2* complex might include ca. 1000 genes. By convention, the markers are aligned from left to right starting with the centromere. [From Klein, J. and Shreffler, D. C. *Transplant Rev 6*:3 (1971).]

additional information about genetic control of cell-mediated immunity (Ch. 20). Guinea pigs of one inbred strain (2) are high responders to poly-L-lysine (PLL) carrying Dnp or other haptenic groups: they develop cell-mediated hypersensitivity to the immunogen (Ch. 20) and high Ab titers to the haptenic group. Those of another strain (13) are low responders: they develop no hypersensitivity to the immunogen and little if any antihapten Ab. As with purebred strain 2, all F₁ hybrids (2 × 13) are high responders, and so also are ca. 50% of the progeny of the back-cross of hybrids to the low-responder strain (F₁ × 13). Hence the response to hapten-PLL also depends on a dominant autosomal locus, the PLL gene, which, like Ir-1 of mice, has also turned out to be closely linked to the main locus for guinea pig histocompatibility Ags.

Guinea pigs that lack the PLL⁺ gene can, nevertheless, make the same anti-hapten Abs as responders if the hapten-PLL Ag (Dnp-PLL) is administered as a complex with an immunogenic carrier, such as bovine serum albumin (BSA). Similarly, mice that ordinarily make little response to (T,G)–A—L can make a high Ab response if this Ag is administered as a complex with an immunogenic carrier (e.g., methylated BSA). Hence the Ir genes do not specify the V-region amino acid sequences that determine Ab specificity (Ch. 16), but rather some element that seems to be concerned with recognition of the carrier moiety of the immunogen (e.g., PLL). From what is known about carrier recognition (see

above), products of the Ir-1 gene should be expressed on T cells.

The following circumstantial evidence supports this view.

1) T lymphocytes are the effector cells for cell-mediated immunity (such as delayed-type skin reactions, Ch. 20), and this type of reaction to Dnp-PLL is entirely lacking in PLL⁻ guinea pigs, even when they are induced to make anti-Dnp Abs in response to Dnp-PLL in complex with an immunogenic carrier.

2) T cells seem to regulate the production of the 7S, rather tnan the 19S, Abs made in response to T-dependent Ags; correspondingly, mice that are genetic nonresponders to a given Ag are blocked in the formation of the appropriate 7S Abs, but not in the production of the 19S Abs.

Adoptive transfers suggest, however, that while some Ir genes are expressed on T cells, others seem to be manifested on B cells. Thus titrations of cells from donors carrying Ir⁺ or Ir⁻ genes have been carried out in irradiated, syngeneic recipients by transfer of an excess number of T cells plus varying numbers of B cells, or the reverse (excess B and varying number of T cells): the proportion of recipients making Abs to the subsequently injected Ag indicates the frequency of Ag-sensitive cells in the transferred thymus and bone marrow populations.* With some Ags the responder and nonresponder strains differ in the frequency of Ag-sensitive cells

---

* By application of the Poisson distribution: the frequency of Ag-sensitive cells in a given number of T or B cells (the complementary cell population being given in excess) is based on the proportion of recipients who make no Ab response to an optimal dose of Ag (see Ch. 18, One-hit theory in complement lysis).

in the thymus, not in the bone marrow, while with other Ags the strains differ in marrow cells, not in thymus. While the Ir-1 genes of the H-2 locus seem to be expressed on T cells, it is also possible that they and other Ir genes are expressed on B cells.

The Ir genes seem also to control immune responses to many complex Ags, such as red cells, serum proteins (including Igs). With serum proteins as Ags, very small doses elicit responses in certain inbred mouse strains, but not in others, and the response is again genetically controlled by single autosomal dominant loci, which in a number of instances have been linked to the H-2 locus. Evidently with sufficiently low doses of immunogen only the dominant determinant is effective, and complex Ags can approach the simplicity of single haptenic groups.

The linkage of Ir-1 to the H-2 locus suggests that the product of the Ir-1 gene might be simply another histocompatibility Ag that happens, perhaps because of proximity, to modify the specificity or affinity of the cell-bound Ig that serves as Ag-binding receptor. If so, various Ir-1 genes would be expected to be scattered throughout the H-2 locus. However, the recombinant chromosomes so far analyzed show the Ir-1 gene(s) to be consistently clustered in a discrete region next to but distinct from the left-hand end of the H-2 locus (Fig. 17-18). It seems possible, therefore, that the product of Ir-1 genes are the T-cell Ag-binding receptors themselves (or an essential part of them): if so, the receptors would have to be something other than Igs, for Ir-1 is not a structural Ig gene: it is not linked to the locus for heavy Ig chains and responder and nonresponder strains form indistinguishable Abs when the discriminating Ag is attached to a suitable carrier (see above).

The products of the Ir-1 locus could be sufficiently diversified to account for the great range of specificities of T-cell receptors. The recombination frequency between the two ends of the H-2 locus suggests that the area in between, including Ir-1, could accommodate perhaps 1000 genes; moreover, diversity could be amplified by the mechanisms envisioned to help account for Ig diversification—e.g., mutations in dividing stem cells or assembly of various combinations of subunits (Ch. 16, Origin of Ig diversity).

Whatever their product turns out to be, the Ir genes probably have an important role in many diseases. Susceptibility to various leukemogenic viruses, to lymphocytic choriomeningitis virus, to mouse smallpox infection, and perhaps even to some autoimmune diseases in certain hybrid mice seems to be linked to the H-2 locus and many of these phenotypes could be under control of immune responses and thereby of Ir genes.

ANTIBODY FORMATION IN THE WHOLE ANIMAL

The rates of formation, steady-state levels, and types of Abs formed vary widely with conditions of immunization, which are reviewed in this section.

ADMINISTRATION OF ANTIGEN

ROUTE

Natural Immunization. Lymphatic tissues are probably bombarded almost constantly with Ags from transiently invasive or indigenous microbes (normal flora of skin, intestines, etc.). The resulting stimulation is probably responsible for the familiar histological appearance of lymph nodes and spleen, the normal concentration of Igs in serum (ca. 15 mg/ml), and **natural antibodies**—those Igs that react or cross-react (one cannot be sure which) with Ags that have not been known to serve as immunogens in the individual under test. Animals reared under germ-free conditions synthesize Igs at ca. 1/500 the normal rate, have exceedingy low serum levels (especially IgG), and have markedly hypoplastic secondary lymphatic tissues. Nonmicrobial immunogens can also enter the body naturally by inhalation (e.g., plant pollens), ingestion (e.g., foods, drugs), and penetration of skin (e.g., catechols of poison ivy plants).

Deliberate Immunization. For this purpose immunogens are usually injected into skin (intradermally or subcutaneously) or muscle, depending upon the volume injected and the irritancy of the immunogen. Intraperitoneal and intravenous injections are also used in experimental work, especially with particulate Ags. Usually, regardless of route, the Ag eventually becomes distributed widely throughout the body via lymphatic and vascular channels.

Because most Ags are degraded in the intestines, **feeding** is effective only under special circumstances; e.g., with attenuated poliomyelitis vaccine (Ch. 55), which can invade the intestinal wall, and allergic responses to food are often due to earlier antigenic stimulation by ingestion of the same substances. **Inhalation** can also be used: e.g., aerosol administration of attenuated strains of *Pasteurella tularensis*. Preferential synthesis of IgA Abs can occur when immunogens are introduced into the respiratory and intestinal tracts, many of whose abundant plasma cells are committed to produce Igs of this class. Direct **application to the skin** is effective with certain penetrating substances of low molecular weight, which tend especially to induce cell-mediated immune responses (Ch. 20, Contact skin sensitivity).

ADJUVANTS

The immunogenic potency of soluble proteins is enhanced if they persist in tissues; for example, repeated small injections of diphtheria toxoid evoke a greater Ab response than the same total amount of toxoid given as a single injection. Accordingly, a widely used procedure involves administration of inorganic gels (e.g., alum, aluminum hydroxide, or aluminum phosphate) with adsorbed immunogens that are released slowly for a prolonged period. These gels are called **adjuvants,** a term which applies broadly to any substance that increases the response to the immunogen with which it is injected.

The most effective adjuvants are the water-in-oil emulsions developed by Freund, particularly those in which living or dead mycobacteria are suspended. After a single subcutaneous or intramuscular injection (e.g., 0.5 ml in a rabbit) droplets of emulsion metastasize widely from the site of injection; Ab formation can be detected as early as 4 or 5 days later, and it may continue for 8 or 9 months or longer (Fig. 17-19). The intense, chronic inflammation around the deposits of emulsion precludes their use in man. However, emulsions without mycobacteria ("incomplete" Freund's adjuvant) are less irritating and have been used clinically; their enhancing effect is less than that of "complete" Freund's adjuvant. Some other adjuvants are bacterial endotoxin; large

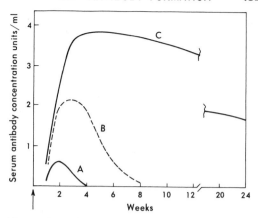

Fig. 17-19. Influence of adjuvants. Schematic view of amounts of Ab produced by rabbits in response to one injection (arrow) of a soluble protein, such as Bovine γ-globulin in dilute salt solution (A), adsorbed on precipitated alum (B), or incorporated in a water-in-oil emulsion containing mycobacteria (Freund's complete adjuvant, C).

polymeric anions (certain synthetic polyribonucleotides [poly AU], dextran sulfate, but not dextran itself); and *Bordetella pertussis*.

Most adjuvants promote the maintenance of low, effective Ag levels in tissues and provoke inflammation, in which accumulated macrophages could bind Ag for reaction with B and T cells. Some adjuvants (e.g., mycobacteria) aid responses only to T-dependent Ags: perhaps by acting as independent immunogens or as carriers for Ags that they adsorb, these adjuvants cause proliferation of T cells (evident as hyperplasia in T zones of regional lymph nodes) and might also increase their output of B-cell-stimulating factors (Antigenic promotion, see below).

DOSE

The smallest effective dose of an immunogen depends on the method of administration. Thus 100 μg of the human serum albumin will usually not evoke detectable Ab formation when injected intravenously in a rabbit, whereas the same dose is highly effective if injected subcutaneously in Freund's adjuvant. With the adjuvant as little as 1 to 10 μg might represent the threshold, which is usually much lower in animals that have been previously stimulated by the same immunogen (Secondary response, below). Moreover, a subthreshold dose can sometimes "prime" animals for a subsequent, augmented secondary response (below) without actually eliciting the formation of detectable Ab.

Once the threshold is exceeded, increasing doses lead to increasing, but generally less than proportionate, responses (which can be measured over an approximately 10 million-fold range: from ca. 0.001 μg Ab/ml, about the lowest measurable concentration, to ca. 50 mg/ml in animals intensively immunized with the most potent immunogens).

Doses that are excessive (or, with certain Ags, that are just below the threshold) not only fail to stimulate Ab synthesis, but can establish a state of specific unresponsiveness (Immunological tolerance, below).

THE PRIMARY RESPONSE

The initial exposure to most Ags evokes a smaller and somewhat different Ab response than subsequent exposures. The differences are of cardinal importance in resistance to microbial infections.

The first introduction of immunogen, the **primary stimulus,** evokes the **primary response** in which Abs are first detectable after 1 to 30 days or more (Fig. 17-20). The lag varies with dose, route of injection, the particulate or soluble nature of the immunogen, the type of adjuvant used, and with the sensitivity of the assay. It is common for Abs to be detected 3 to 4 days after injection of foreign erythrocytes, 5 to 7 days after soluble proteins, and 10 to 14 days after bacterial cells.

Special immunogens are needed to follow early rates of Ab formation. Bacteriophages are particularly useful: exceedingly small quantities are immunogenic, avoiding significant masking of newly formed Ab by persistent Ag. In addition, neutralization of phage infectivity (for *E. coli*) can measure extremely low concentrations of Ab, including molecules of low affinity (see Ch. 15, Rates of reaction and Table 15-5). As is shown in Figure 17-21, the phage evokes detectable Abs as early as 1 day after an intravenous injection. The activity in serum increases thereafter for the next 4 to 5 days at an exponential rate (i.e., the rate of increase at any time is proportional to the level of activity at that time), and the doubling time for serum Ab is as short as 6 hours.

The time required to attain maximal Ab levels, and the duration of the peak titer, vary with different immunogens and methods of immunization. The peak is often reached 4 to 5 days after an injection of red cells, and 9 to 10 days after soluble protein is common;

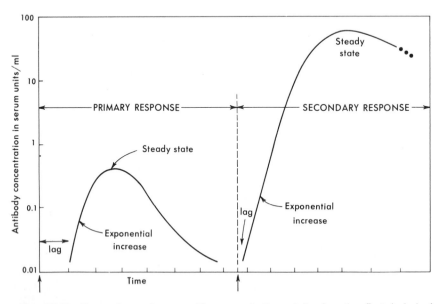

Fig. 17-20. Comparison of serum Ab concentrations following the first (priming) and second injections of the immunogen (arrows). Note the logarithmic scale for Ab concentration. Time units are left unspecified to indicate the great variability encountered with different immunogens under different conditions.

diphtheria toxoid in man may require as long as 3 months. The serum concentration of Abs to soluble proteins may begin to decline within 1 or 2 days after reaching the maximum, but after the same immunogen is given in Freund's adjuvant it may remain elevated for many months (Fig. 17-19).

Antibody Turnover and Distribution. The level of Ab in serum reflects the balance between rates of synthesis and degradation. When the rates are equal, the serum Ab concentration is constant (steady state). The rate of synthesis depends upon the number of Ab-producing cells, which varies enormously with conditions of immunization. However, Ab is degraded at a rate (expressed as half life or $t_{\frac{1}{2}}$) which is determined by its Ig class (Table 17-5): **IgM and IgA are normally broken down much more rapidly than IgG molecules.**

However, infusions of trace amounts of ^{125}I-labeled IgG into individuals with widely varying IgG levels (agammaglobulinemia or multiple myeloma) revealed an inverse relation between the half-time for IgG degradation and the total concentration of this Ig class: at high and low levels of IgG the $t_{\frac{1}{2}}$ was about 11 and 70 days, respectively, as compared with 23 days at normal levels. Injected Fab fragments and light chains disappear rapidly ($t_{\frac{1}{2}} < 1$ day), but the Fc fragment has the same half life as intact IgG. By analogy with some other serum pro-

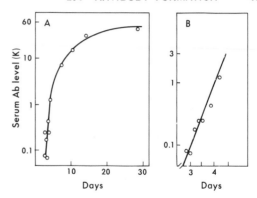

Fig. 17-21. A. The primary response in a guinea pig injected at zero time with 6×10^8 bacteriophage ϕX174 (about 0.01 μg protein). **B.** The first 4.5 days in **A** is repeated with an expanded scale to demonstrate that the increase is exponential. [From Uhr, J. W., Finkelstein, M. S., and Baumann, J. W. *J Exp Med* 115:655 (1962).]

teins, it is possible that shortening of oligosaccharide branches, by random removal of terminal sialic acid or other residues by blood glycosidases, makes Ig molecules susceptible to uptake and degradation in the liver.

The actual serum concentration of Ig depends also upon the volume in which the molecules are distributed. The total mass of IgG is about the same in blood and in extravascular fluids. About 25% of the plasma IgG diffuses out of the vascular compartment each day, and an equal amount is returned via lymphatic channels.

TABLE 17-5. Degradation Rates and Some Other Metabolic Properties of Human Immunoglobulins

Properties	IgG*	IgA	IgM	IgD	IgE
Serum concentration (mg/ml) (average, normal individuals)	12.1	2.5	0.93	0.023	0.0003
Half life (days)†	23	5.8	5.1	2.8	2.5
Rate of synthesis (mg/kg body weight per day)	33	24	6.7	0.4	0.016
Catabolic rate (% of intravascular pool broken down per day)	6.7	25	18	37	89

* IgG-1, IgG-2, and IgG-4 have the same half life (ca. 23 days), but that of IgG-3 is shorter ($t_{\frac{1}{2}} = 8$ to 9 days). The half life of IgG in some other species is (in days): rabbit (6), rat (7), guinea pig (7 to 9).

† Half life ($t_{\frac{1}{2}}$) is the time required for the concentration (at any particular moment) to drop to $\frac{1}{2}$ the value; it is related to the first-order rate constant for degradation, k (in days^{-1}), by: $t_{\frac{1}{2}}$ (in days) $= 0.693/k$.

Based on Waldmann, T. A., Strober, W., and Blaese, R. M. in *Immunoglobulins* (E. Merler, ed.). National Academy of Sciences, Washington, D.C., 1970.

CHANGES WITH TIME

The Abs made at various times after immunization differ in type of Ig chain and in affinity for Ag.

Changes in Ig Class. Most immunogens elicit detectable Abs of the IgM class before those of the IgG class (Fig. 17-22).*

---

* Human IgM and IgG Abs can usually be distinguished by treating dilute serum with a reducing agent, such as mercaptoethanol: IgM molecules dissociate into 7S subunits, which lose ability to cross-link Ag particles (as in hemagglutination), though the subunits still bind Ags. IgG molecules, in contrast, retain full activity even when all of their interchain S-S bonds are cleaved (Chs. 15 and 16). The inability of reduced IgM molecules to cross-link Ags may reflect the low intrinsic affinities of most IgM Abs and a correspondingly great need for cooperative multivalent binding (Ch. 15, Monogamous binding; Avidity; Appendix).

It is possible that this sequence is related to the IgM-IgG switch that appears to take place in some B cells following Ag stimulation (see above). Nevertheless, it is not clear whether IgM Abs are always produced in significantly greater bulk before the corresponding IgG molecules, or whether IgM Abs are simply more readily detected because of the greater sensitivity of conventional assays for more avid Abs: with 10 combining sites per IgM molecule, and 2 per IgG, the IgM Abs tend to be more avid (Ch. 15, Avidity; Appendix). Indeed, special analyses suggest that low-avidity IgG (see below) can be produced as early as the more readily detectable IgM molecules.

If the immunogen is administered in complete Freund's adjuvant both IgM and IgG Abs can continue to be synthesized for many months. Otherwise, synthesis of IgM usually ceases to be easily detectable after 1 to 2 weeks, while IgG titers continue to rise (Fig. 17-22). The synthesis of IgM Abs can be arrested by passive transfer of IgG molecules of the same specificity **(feedback inhibition)**; this lowers the level of residual immunogen and suggests that Ag levels have to be relatively high to elicit synthesis of IgM Abs, which would be in ac-

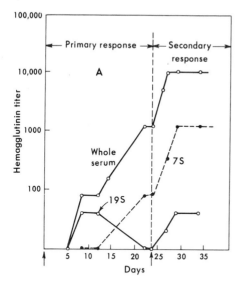

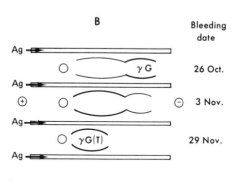

Fig. 17-22. Sequential changes in class of Ab made after immunization. **A.** A rabbit was immunized with diphtheria toxoid as shown (arrows). Antitoxin was measured by passive hemagglutination, using sucrose density gradient centrifugation to separate IgM (19S) and IgG (7S) Abs. **B.** A horse was immunized with tetanus toxoid. Antisera were subjected to electrophoresis, then Ag (toxoid) was added to the long troughs to precipitate antitoxin (Fig. 15-29, Ch. 15). The earliest precipitating antitoxin belonged to one IgG subclass; the more anionic antitoxin that appeared later, IgG (T), belonged to another. [**A** from Bauer, D. C., Mathies, M. J., and Stavitsky, A. B. *J Exp Med 117*:889 (1963). **B** from Raynaud, M. in *Mechanisms of Hypersensitivity*, Shaffer, J. H., LiGrippo, G. A., and Chase, M. W., eds. Little, Brown, Boston, 1959.]

cord with the generally low intrinsic affinities of these molecules for their ligands (see discussion of Changes in affinity, below).

Some thymus-independent Ags seem to elicit the formation of IgM Abs almost exclusively. For instance, the Abs made in horses to pneumococcal capsular polysaccharides, and in rabbits to the Forssman antigen of red cell stroma (Ch. 18) and to *Salmonella* lipopolysaccharide (endotoxin), are predominantly and persistently IgM molecules.

Other Ig chains are also occasionally used preferentially in the formation of Abs to certain other Ags. For instance, in human Abs ("cold agglutinins") to certain red cell Ags and in high-affinity guinea pig Abs to the Dnp group, the light chains seem always to be of κ type; and in horse antitoxin formed late in immunization (Fig. 17-22) and in human Abs to teichoic acid, the heavy chains are of a particular γ subclass. The basis for these restrictions is obscure.

Increase in Affinity. The antihapten Abs formed initially after injection of a hapten-protein immunogen usually have low affinity for the hapten, while the average affinity of the Abs formed later is much higher. These changes are especially pronounced with IgG molecules, and they take place more rapidly after a small than after a large dose of immunogen (Table 17-6). They probably derive from the following: 1) the level of immunogen decreases with time, and 2) the Ag-binding sites of receptor-Igs on an Ag-sensitive B cell are probably the same as on the Ab molecules secreted by the stimulated cell's differentiated progeny (plasma cells). Hence the concentration of Ag required to stimulate a B cell should be inversely related to the affinity of the Ab molecules secreted by the resulting clone: e.g., high Ag levels generally elicit production of low-affinity Abs.

In previously unimmunized animals most of the B cells that bind a given immunogen are likely to have low affinity for it. The relatively high level of Ag prevailing soon after the immunogen is injected can stimulate many of these cells, leading to the initial production of low affinity Abs. As the Ag level declines, increasingly selective stimulation and expansion of high-affinity Ab-producing clones probably occurs, leading to a rise in average intrinsic affinity of serum Abs. Thus with time after immunization the formation of hemolytic plaques by isolated Ab-secreting cells can be specifically inhibited by increasingly low concentrations of haptens. As expected, prolonged high levels of Ag delay the onset of selective production of high-affinity Abs (Table 17-6).

An immunogen generally has diverse antigenic determinants, and the corresponding Ab molecules can appear after different lag periods: hence the variety of Ab specificities tends to increase with time. This increase and the late appearance of high-affinity Ab molecules may explain why a given Ag behaves as though it has more binding sites per molecule when it reacts with a late antiserum than with an early one (Fig. 17-23). The Ab-Ag complexes formed in late antisera are correspondingly less dissociable: **avidity of antisera increases with time.**

TABLE 17-6. Sequential Changes in Affinity of the Anti-Dnp Antibodies (IgG Immunoglobulins) Made with Increasing Time After Immunization*

Group	Ag injected per rabbit (mg)	Average intrinsic association constants for binding ε-Dnp-L-lysine at		
		2 weeks	5 weeks	8 weeks
I	5	0.86	14	120
II	250	0.18	0.13	0.15

* Immunogen was 2,4-dinitrophenyl bovine γ-globulin. Values are averages for five animals per group, and are given in liters mole^{-1} $\times$ 10^{-6} (30°).

From Eisen, H. N., and Siskind, G. W. *Biochemistry* 3:996 (1964).

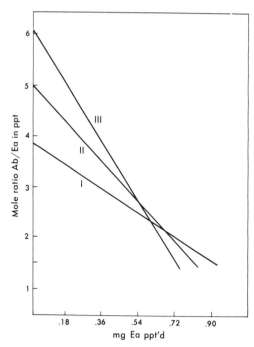

Fig. 17-23. Sequential changes in antisera reflected in the increasing number of functional groups detected per molecule of Ag. Rabbits were immunized with several courses of injections of hen's ovalbumin (Ea). Precipitin reactions with sera obtained after courses I, II, and III show, from the limiting mole ratio in extreme Ab excess (intercept on ordinate), that with time the serum Abs react with an increasing number of sites per Ea molecule (see Ch. 15., Avidity). [Based on Heidelberger, M. and Kendall, F. *J Exp Med 62*:697 (1935).]

Cross-reactivity also increases with time, because Abs with high affinity for the immunogen usually cross-react with related ligands more extensively than low-affinity Abs (Ch. 15), and perhaps also because a greater variety of Ab populations appear.

THE SECONDARY RESPONSE

After Ab levels in the primary response have declined, even to the point of being no longer detectable, a subsequent encounter with the same Ag usually evokes an enhanced **secondary (anamnestic, memory) response** (Gr. *anamnesis* = recall). By comparison with the primary response it is characterized by 1) a lower threshold dose of immunogen,* 2) a shorter lag phase, 3) a higher rate and longer persistence of Ab synthesis, and 4) higher titers (Fig. 17-24A). In addition, the Abs formed in the secondary response are overwhelmingly of the IgG class, and they have from the outset about the same high affinity for the immunogen as those synthesized at the end of the response to the primary stimulus (Table 17-7). **The capacity for a secondary response can persist for many years and provide long-lasting immunity against infection: long after Abs cease to be detectable, the immunogen can evoke unusually prompt synthesis of relatively large amounts of highly efficient Abs.** The primary response is less protective, because Abs appear more slowly and their combining power is relatively poor, at least initially.

The doubling time of serum Abs in the secondary response appears to be about the same as in the primary response, but the rate of Ab production is much greater (Figs. 17-21 and 17-24A); the difference evidently depends upon the increased number of Ag-sensitive ("memory") cells at the time of the secondary stimulus (Fig. 17-24B). If administered 2 to 3 days after the primary stimulus, agents that prevent cell proliferation (X-rays, 6-mercaptopurine) can block development of the capacity to give a secondary response, showing that cell division is necessary for production of memory cells.

Memory resides in B and in T cells. The carrier effect is not always evident in secondary antihapten responses. Thus, 1 and 2 years after rabbits are primed with Dnp on BγG a vigorous secondary response with prompt production of high-affinity anti-Dnp molecules can be elicited with Dnp conjugated onto hemocyanin (which does not cross-react with BγG): memory is evidently represented in the B cells that promptly produce high-affinity antihapten Abs (see Table 17-7). However, other secondary responses, elicited with primed, cultured spleen cells (B plus T cells) can be blocked with anti-θ sera, indicating a need for T cells; and the greater helping effect of T cells from primed than from unprimed donors in adoptive secondary responses shows that

---

* For instance, the minute amount of diphtheria toxoid injected intradermally in a man in the Schick test (0.003 μg) is usually enough to cause a secondary response in the production of antitoxin, though it is far too little to cause a primary response.

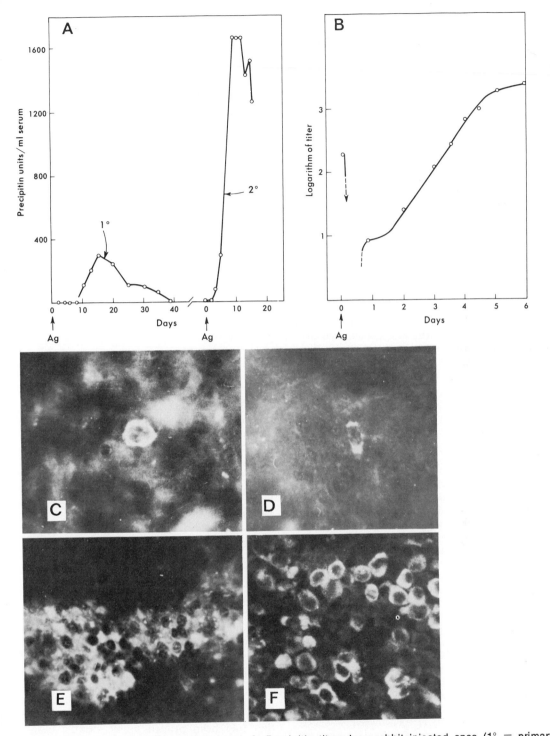

Fig. 17-24. Secondary response in rabbits. **A.** Precipitin titers in a rabbit injected once (1° = primary response), and in another rabbit injected with the same Ag about 4 weeks after a series of priming injections (2° = secondary response). **B.** A rabbit previously immunized with staphylococcal toxoid was given a second large dose intravenously. Note the initial drop in titer (negative phase) followed by the exponential increase; the doubling time is ca. 9 hrs, about the same as in the primary (and secondary) responses to bacteriophage φ✕174 (see Fig. 17-21). [**A** based on Dean, H. R., and Webb, R. A. *J Path Bact* *31*:89 (1928). **B** based on Burnet, F. M. Monograph No. 1, Walter and Eliza Hall Institute, 1941.] Greater proliferation of B cells in secondary than in primary response. Following footpad injections with diphtheria toxoid or bovine serum albumin sections of regional lymph nodes were treated with the Ag and then with the corresponding fluorescein-labeled Abs. **C** and **D** show rare Ab-producing cells 4 days after the first injection; **E** and **F** show clusters of Ab-producing cells 4 days after the second injection (see Fig. 17-2). [From Leduc, E. H., Coons, A. H. and Connolly, J. M. *J Exp Med 102*:61 (1955).]

TABLE 17-7. Increased Affinity of the Anti-Dnp Antibodies Formed in the Secondary Response

Group	Rabbit No.	Average intrinsic association constant for binding 2,4-dinitrotoluene (liter mole$^{-1} \times 10^{-6}$)
I. Bled 14 days after primary stimulus	1	0.14
	2	.03
	3	.20
	4	.15
II. Bled 8 days after secondary stimulus	5	34.
	6	84.
	7	>500.

Rabbits were injected with 1 mg Dnp-hemocyanin in Freund's adjuvant and anti-Dnp Abs were isolated 14 days later (group I, primary stimulus). Seven months later animals with less than 100 μg anti-Dnp Ab per milliliter of serum were reinjected with 1 mg of the same immunogen: 7 to 8 days later the level of anti-Dnp Abs had increased to 2 to 6 mg/ml, and affinity for ε-Dnp-L-lysine, the haptenic group of the immunogen, was too high to measure. Hence affinities were all measured with 2,4-dinitrotoluene, a less strongly bound analog. A secondary response to the Dnp group has been elicited in rabbits as long as 2 years after the primary injection.

From Eisen, H. N. *Cancer Res 22*:2005 (1966).

memory can also reside in "educated" T cells (Carrier effect, above).

Indeed, memory T cells are probably more important for most secondary responses than memory B cells. This would account for the lack of secondary responses to T-independent Ags, such as pneumococcal polysaccharides, and the strong secondary responses elicited by most proteins, which are usually T-dependent: tetanus toxoid, for instance, can evoke a powerful secondary response in man 10 to 20 years after primary immunization.

The magnitude of secondary responses also depends on other variables, such as the interval between injections. If it is too short, a substantial level of Ab is likely to be still present from the primary injection: hence immune complexes can form, leading to accelerated degradation of Ag, less stimulation of new Ab production, and even a transient decrease in the serum concentration of free Ab (so-called "negative phase," Fig. 17-24A). With too long an interval the secondary response can also be reduced, probably because Ag-sensitive cells are not infinitely durable. Indeed, it has been estimated from successive transfers of Ag-activated Ab-secreting cells through a series of X-irradiated, syngeneic recipients that a clone of B cells undergoes "senescence" (i.e., stops responding to Ag) after about 80 cell divisions. However, with an interval of many months or even years between mitoses of nonactivated lymphocytes, immunological memory can persist for practically a lifetime after the primary

stimulus with some Ags (see Appearance and generation times of lymphocytes, above).

Enhanced synthesis of Abs of the IgM class is normally inconspicuous in the secondary response, but it can become evident when IgG molecules are absent, as in certain severe immunodeficiency states. Increased affinity of IgM Abs in the secondary response is slight and difficult to demonstrate.

CROSS-STIMULATION

A secondary response can sometimes be elicited with an immunogen that is not quite identical to the primary Ag. Most of the Abs made will then react more strongly with the first than with the second immunogen. This phenomenon, called **"original antigenic sin,"** was initially recognized in epidemiological studies with cross-reacting strains of influenza virus. An example is shown in Table 17-8, where the secondary response evoked with 2,4,6-trinitrophenyl (Tnp)-proteins in rabbits that had been primed many months before with 2,4-dinitrophenyl (Dnp)-proteins consisted primarily of Abs with the physicochemical and ligand-binding properties of anti-Dnp, rather than of anti-Tnp, molecules: the effect is probably due to specific cross-stimulation by Tnp-proteins of an en-

TABLE 17-8. Cross-Stimulation (Original Antigenic Sin) Illustrated in the Secondary Response to 2,4-dinitrophenyl (Dnp)-protein and to 2,4,6-trinitrophenyl (Tnp)-protein

Rabbit No.	Primary stimulus	Secondary stimulus	Affinity of antibodies formed 7–8 days after secondary stimulus		Ratio of affinities DNT/TNT
			For 2,4-dinitrotoluene (DNT) (liters mole$^{-1} \times 10^{-7}$)	For 2,4,6-trinitrotoluene (TNT) (liters mole$^{-1} \times 10^{-7}$)	
1	Dnp-BγG	Tnp-BγG	25.	0.49	50.
2	Dnp-BγG	Tnp-BγG	17.	.85	20.
3	Dnp-BγG	Tnp-BγG	34.	.84	40.
4	Tnp-BγG	Dnp-BγG	0.20	0.30	0.7
5	Tnp-BγG	Dnp-BγG	0.62	1.0	0.6

The primary stimulus was 1 mg Dnp-bovine γ-globulin Dnp-BγG or 1 mg Tnp-BγG; 8 months later animals with no detectable Ab in serum were reinjected with the immunogen shown, and they produced Abs in abundance. In control rabbits given Dnp-BγG in both injections the ratio of affinities for DNT/TNT ranged from 2 to 100 (i.e., they formed anti-Dnp Abs). In other controls given Tnp-BγG in both injections this ratio ranged from 0.2 to 0.9 (i.e., they made anti-Tnp molecules). Most of the Abs produced within 1 week of the second stimulus had binding properties that corresponded to the primary rather than the secondary immunogen.

Based on Eisen, H. N., Little, J. R., Steiner, L. A., and Simms, E. S. *Isr J Med Sci 5*:338 (1969).

larged population of anti-Dnp memory B cells remaining after the primary response to the Dnp immunogen.

This principle has been exploited in "serological archaeology," testing human sera during an influenza epidemic with diverse strains of the virus. A given patient's serum tends to react less strongly with the strain that causes his current illness than with a strain that caused his first attack of influenza in some previous epidemic. From the study of sera from very elderly patients it has thus been possible to identify strains that probably caused major epidemics in the past, e.g., in 1918, long before the influenza virus was discovered.

Nonspecific Anamnestic Response. Secondary responses can sometimes be triggered by stimuli that appear to be unrelated to the priming immunogen. For instance, patients with typhus fever, due to *Rickettsia*, sometimes exhibit a rise in Ab titer to unrelated bacteria against which they were previously immunized. These nonspecific responses are probably due to stimulation of one Ag's memory B cells by diffusible factors released by nearby T cells that are activated by the unrelated immunogen (see Cell cooperation, above, and Antigenic promotion, below). A plant (pokeweed) mitogen that causes blast transformation of B cells can also cause a slight secondary response in antihapten Abs in animals previously primed against the hapten (see also Antigenic promotion, below).

FATE OF INJECTED ANTIGEN

Following intravenous injection of a soluble Ag the decline in its concentration in serum exhibits three sharply distinguishable phases (Fig. 17-25): 1) a brief **equilibration phase** due to rapid diffusion into extravascular space, 2) slow **metabolic decay** during which the Ag is degraded, 3) rapid **immune elimination,** which identifies the onset of Ab formation; during this phase the Ag exists as soluble Ab-Ag complexes, which are taken up and degraded by macrophages. Free Ab appears at the end of the immune elimination stage (Fig. 17-25).

Extensively phagocytized particulate Ags, such as bacteria and red cells, do not diffuse into extravascular spaces, and hence do not exhibit the initial equilibrium phase of rapid decrease in serum concentration after intravenous injection. Trace antigenic fragments can persist in lymphoid tissues, long after the Ag is no longer detectable in blood. Ags that readily establish tolerance (below) tend to be unusually persistent (e.g., pneumococcal poly-

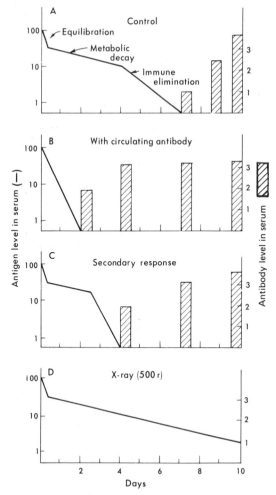

Fig. 17-25. Accelerated elimination of Ag as an index of Ab formation in rabbits injected intravenously at zero time with 75 mg ^{131}I-labeled BγG. The vertical bars represent serum Ab levels. **A.** Control animals, not previously immunized with BγG. **B.** Accelerated elimination begins at time zero when BγG is injected into animals that still have circulating anti-BγG from an earlier immunization; and it begins after an abbreviated lag in previously immunized rabbits (without residual Abs) that make a secondary response **C.** X-irradiation (500 r) before administration of BγG blocks Ab formation and accelerated elimination **D.** [Based on Talmage, D. W., Dixon, F. J., Bukantz, S. C. and Dammin, G. J. *J Immunol* 67:243 (1951).]

saccharides can be detected for about a year after their injection in mice).

EFFECT OF ANTIBODIES

High levels of Ab, whether due to active immunization or to injected antisera, can intercept Ags and block their immunogenicity (Suppression by Ab as antiimmunogen below). However, small quantities of Abs are actually enhancing, as though small Ab-Ag complexes can be more immunogenic than free Ag, perhaps because some complexes (such as bimolecular Ab · Ag) stick more readily on macrophages. For instance, newborn piglets, who have no Igs, form Abs in high titer in response to an Ag administered with small amounts of the corresponding Abs, but not to the Ag alone. In fact before diphtheria toxoid was available humans were immunized against diphtheria with nontoxic mixtures of toxin and antitoxin. But unless very carefully selected doses are given the simultaneous administration of Ab is more likely to block than to enhance immunogenicity (Antibodies as immunosuppressive agents, below).

ANTIGENIC PROMOTION AND COMPETITION

The response to immunogen X can sometimes be enhanced by simultaneous administration of immunogen Y, especially if the responding cell population has been previously primed with Y. This **antigenic promotion** of the response to X could be due to interaction of Y with the corresponding T cells, which release factors that stimulate neighboring B cells with specifically bound X.

Antigenic competition can also occur: the response to one Ag may be reduced if an unrelated, non-cross-reacting Ag is injected at the same time. For instance, poly-L-alanyl-protein readily elicits Abs to the L-polypeptide, but on coimmunization with poly-D-alanyl-protein only the latter elicits Abs to its polypeptide **intermolecular competition).** Moreover, different determinants on the same molecule can also compete **(intramolecular competition):** thus a protein with both D- and L-polyalanyl peptides substituted on the same molecule evokes synthesis only of Abs to the D-polyalanyl groups. Presumably the available receptors for the two determinants differ in affinity, and one determinant becomes dominant because the corresponding cells bind the limited supply of Ag. Intermolecular competition is more obscure: it could involve a suppressive effect of T cells on B cells, rather than the usual augmentation (see, for instance, Allotype suppression, below). Thus the phenomenon was not obtained in thymus-deprived mice unless they were given thymus cells, and the extent to which competition was restored was proportional to the number of injected T cells.

VACCINATION AGAINST MICROBIAL ANTIGENS

The list of procedures that increase resistance to infectious agents (Table 17-9)

TABLE 17-9. Vaccines Preventing Infectious Disease in Man

Disease	Immunogen
Diphtheria	Purified diphtheria toxoid
Tetanus	Purified tetanus toxoid
Smallpox	Infectious (attenuated) virus
Yellow fever	Infectious (attenuated) virus
Measles	Infectious (attenuated) virus
Mumps	Infectious (attenuated) virus
Rubella	Infectious (attenuated) virus
Polio	Infectious (attenuated) virus or inactivated virus
Influenza	Inactivated virus
Rabies	Inactivated virus
Typhus fever	Killed rickettsiae (*Rickettsia prowazeki*)
Typhoid and paratyphoid fever	Killed bacteria (*Salmonella typhi, S. schottmülleri,* and *S. paratyphi*)
Pertussis	Killed bacteria (*Bordetella pertussis*)
Cholera	Crude fraction of cholera vibrios
Plague	Crude fraction of plague bacilli
Tuberculosis	Infectious (attenuated) mycobacteria (bacille Calmette Guérin or BCG)
Meningitis	Purified polysaccharide from *Neisseria meningitidis*
Pneumonia	Purified polysaccharide from *Diplococcus pneumoniae*

justifies Edsall's statement: "Never in the history of human progress has a better and cheaper method of preventing illness been developed than immunization at its best." Unfortunately, the development of the best procedure for a given microbe is a laborious and almost entirely empirical process. Useful generalizations are meager; some of them follow.

Number of Injections. Multiple injections of immunogen (commonly at 1- to 6-month intervals) are usually necessary to establish long-lasting ability to give an effective secondary response, either to natural infection or to a prophylactic ("booster") injection.

Soluble vs. Insoluble Antigens. Immunogens that are aggregated, or are adsorbed on alum or other gels, are usually more effective than soluble immunogens. The increased multivalency of aggregated Ags probably enhances ability to cross-link receptors on B cells; and the slow desorption of Ags from gels maintains low concentration of Ag in tissues for long periods. Freund's complete adjuvant is too irritating for use in man, and the clinical safety of the incomplete adjuvant (without mycobacteria) is still under consideration.

Systemic vs. Local Immunization. The choice of site for injection of Ag is usually determined by convenience, because the ensuing immunity is generally due to systemically disseminated Ig molecules (or to T lymphocytes in cell-mediated immunity, Ch. 20). However, preferential activation of local groups of Ag-sensitive cells can sometimes be valuable, by concentrating the immune response at sites where target microbes invade; e.g., by achieving high IgA Ab levels in secretions of respiratory or intestinal tracts for agents that primarily infect these regions. This may, in part, account for the effectiveness of the attenuated polio vaccine (below), which is administered orally, and for the contention that influenza vaccine elicits more protection when given by aerosol inhalation than by injection into skin or muscle. Trachoma vaccines instilled in the conjunctival sac may similarly generate more protection against trachoma eye infections than injected vaccine.

Though current immunization practices stimulate immune responses effectively, it is still not possible to stimulate them selectively: e.g., to elicit Ab formation without cell-mediated immunity (Ch. 20) or vice versa, or to avoid producing certain types of Abs, such as those of the IgE class that can cause serious allergic reactions (Ch. 19).

INTERFERENCE WITH ANTIBODY FORMATION

IMMUNOLOGICAL TOLERANCE

The ability of an individual's immune response to distinguish between his own and foreign Ags has been recognized at least since 1900, when Ehrlich's doctrine of *horror autotoxicus* maintained that one can form Abs to almost anything except components of his own tissues. The medical importance of this principle, now called "self-tolerance," is apparent from the serious consequences of its occasional breakdown, which can result in autoimmune diseases (Ch. 20). Its key role in the biology of immune responses is also evident, for central to these processes are the regulatory mechanisms that prevent formation of Abs to self-Ags while permitting it to an almost unlimited range of foreign Ags.

Analysis of mechanisms responsible for self-tolerance became possible with the finding that under certain experimental conditions a foreign Ag may be treated in the same way as a self-Ag: i.e., it not only fails to act as immunogen but acts as **tolerogen,** establishing a

specific **unresponsive state.** In this state the animal fails to form Abs (or to develop cell-mediated immunity) even when the Ag is given under what would otherwise be immunogenic conditions. The alternative responses suggest that the tolerogen somehow causes the Ag-sensitive lymphocytes, or their receptors, to be physically eliminated or functionally blocked: the immunogen can then no longer stimulate cell proliferation and differentiation.

Pseudotolerance. When Ags are present at moderately high levels they can both stimulate Ab production and thoroughly neutralize or mask the Ab molecules that are formed (for example, see 10 μg Ag in Fig. 17-26). If tolerance were generally due to this "treadmill" mechanism, the continuing synthesis and elimination of Ab should be accompanied by accelerated elimination of labeled Ag. However, this is not ordinarily observed. Instead, truly tolerant animals not only lack circulating Abs but also lack the cells that synthesize Abs,

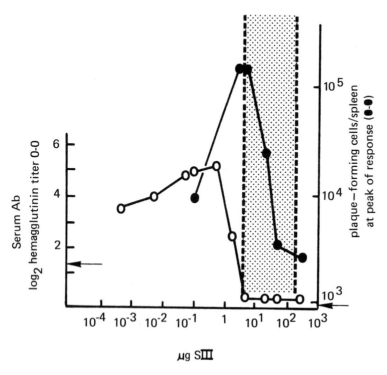

Fig. 17-26. Pseudotolerance; discordance between serum Ab titers and Ab-producing cells in tissues. Mice were injected with various doses of pneumococcal polysaccharide type 3 (SIII) and tested 10 days later for serum Ab titers and for the frequency of Ab-secreting (plaque-forming) cells in the spleen (see Fig. 17-4 for assay). At doses between 10 and 100 μg of SIII per mouse the absence of serum anti-SIII is not due to true tolerance: the Ab produced was neutralized by persistent nondegradable polysaccharide (cross-hatched area). At 250 mg per mouse (not shown) true tolerance was approached: the incidence of plaque-forming spleen cells fell below even the low background level in unimmunized controls (←). [Based on Howard, J. G., Christie, G. H., and Courtenay, B. M. *Proc R Soc Lond, Biol* 178:417 (1971).]

as shown by the hemolytic plaque assay with isolated cells or by immunofluorescence staining for intracellular Ab. **Hence tolerance of an immunogen signifies the absence of synthesis of the corresponding Abs.**

CONDITIONS PROMOTING TOLERANCE

The alternative effects of **dosage** were clearly demonstrated in the 1940s by Felton *et al.*: mice injected with 0.01 to 1.0 μg of a pneumococcal polysaccharide, say of type 2, became resistant to infection with type 2 pneumococci and produced Ab to its polysaccharide; but if given 1000 μg of the same substance they failed to become resistant or to form detectable Abs. This **immune paralysis or unresponsiveness** was persistent and specific: though no response to type 2 could be elicited, the mice reacted normally to immunogenic doses of other Ags including other capsular polysaccharides.

Route of administration is another determinant: soluble Ags tend to be immunogenic when injected with adjuvants into the tissues, but to be tolerogenic when given alone intravenously (perhaps because, like a large dose in tissues, this creates a higher circulating concentration).

Another factor with many Ags is their **physical** state: with BγG, for instance, **aggregated molecules tend to be immunogenic and monomers to be tolerogenic.** Specific unresponsiveness to BγG is induced not only by doses that exceed the immunogenic level **(high-zone tolerance),** as is true with virtually all Ags,* but also by doses just below the threshold for initiating Ab formation **(low-zone tolerance; Fig. 17-27).** Since many Ag preparations contain both immunogenic aggregates and tolerogenic monomers, which probably compete for the same cell receptors, low-zone tolerance would be produced if the tolerogen were effective at lower concentrations than the immunogen.

Diversity and Specificity. Tolerance can be established for any of the substances that induce Ab formation: proteins, polysaccharides, synthetic polypeptides, haptenic groups, etc. Because of their greater immunogenicity, it is more difficult to establish tolerance with particulate Ags (viruses, bacteria, aggregated proteins), with many repeating copies of a given determinant per particle, than with monomeric molecules, such as unaggregated proteins.

As with other immune responses, tolerance is specifically directed to particular determinants. For instance, rabbits made unrespon-

---

* Some Ags cannot establish unresponsiveness because of toxic side effects of high doses.

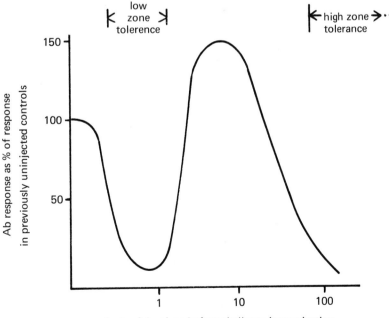

Fig. 17-27. High- and low-zone tolerance. Effect of daily injections of rats with different amounts of flagellin from *Salmonella Adelaide* on Ab response to a later challenge with 10 μg of flagellin. Ab levels are given as percent of values in control rats (no pretreatment). Low-zone tolerance is probably due to an effect on T cells. High-zone tolerance could be due to an effect on T or B cells or on both. Few Ags elicit the low-zone effect, but most elicit the high-zone effect. The responses that exceed 100% are due to the priming effects of the initial injections. [Based on Allison, A. C. *Clinical Immunobiology* 1:113 (1972) and derived from data of G. R. Shellam and G. J. V. Nossal.]

sive to the Fc fragment of human IgG can still respond to immunization with intact IgG, but the resulting Abs react only with Fab domains.

Newborn vs. Adult. After Burnet's speculation that unresponsiveness results from introduction of any Ag during fetal life, Billingham, Brent, and Medawar showed in 1953 that newborn mice can be made permanently tolerant of cells from genetically different mice (Ch. 21). It then seemed likely that some special features of the fetal lymphatic system rendered it uniquely susceptible to induction of tolerance. In fact, however, adults can also be made specifically unresponsive, particularly if immunosuppressive measures are applied at the same time as high doses of the Ag: it appears that **once Ab formation has been initiated, tolerance becomes more difficult to establish.** One reason may be this: it probably takes several days for a large quantity of injected Ag to achieve a uniformly high tolerogenic level in tissue fluids, and during this period the levels in certain tissues are transiently immunogenic, initiating Ab formation: by forming immune complexes the newly synthesized Abs accelerate degradation of the Ag (Fig. 17-25) and arrest (or reverse) the induction of tolerance. If, however, adults are first depleted of Ag-sensitive lymphocytes by nonspecific immunosuppressive measures (X-irradiation, etc.; see below) their lymphoid system comes temporarily to resemble the newborn's immature system, and they can be more easily rendered tolerant.

The easy establishment of tolerance in the fetal and neonatal period is obviously advantageous, permitting the gradual build up of self-Ags to the levels required to perpetuate tolerance during adult life.

Maintenance. Tolerance is unstable: for instance, some weeks after high-zone tolerance is induced a short burst of Ab synthesis can occur as the declining Ag reaches an immunogenic level. Persistence of Ag is thus necessary, though less is needed to maintain than to establish tolerance. Since it is usually not clear whether tolerance is due to loss or dormancy of Ag-sensitive cells it is generally not known whether loss of tolerance to a particular Ag is due to emergence of new Ag-sensitive cells or to reactivation of suppressed cells (see below).

B CELLS VS. T CELLS

Tolerance to T-dependent Ags can be due to unresponsiveness of either T or B cells. Thus an Ag fails to stimulate Ab formation in irradiated mice given bone marrow and thymus cells if either set of cells is drawn from a donor previously rendered unresponsive to that Ag. However, when prospective donors are treated with various doses of Ag at varying times before their B and T cells are separately transferred, it is apparent that **T cells become unresponsive much more readily than B cells,** i.e., the effect is obtained with lower doses of Ag and the cells remain unreactive longer (Fig. 17-28). Hence T cells are probably largely responsible for natural tolerance to most self-antigens.

This view is supported by the following relations among cross-reacting Ags. Animals tolerant of antigen I will often make Abs that react specifically with I following immunization with structurally similar Ags, such as chemically modified I (e.g., Dnp-I or X-azo-I) or with native cross-reacting I' (e.g., human serum albumin if I was bovine serum albumin): under these conditions the anti-I Abs seem to be limited to those determinants of I that are shared (or cross-react) with I'. These results suggest that anti-I B cells are still present in animals tolerant of I, and prevented from responding only by the absence of specific helper T cells: with new carrier groups on the modified or cross-reacting immunogen other helper T cells can become engaged, permitting stimulation of the persistent anti-I B cells. Similar mechanisms might be involved in some autoimmune responses (Ch. 20): self-constituents modified by, say, infection might initiate Ab formation against the unmodified, native substance.

The specificity of the resulting Ab molecules probably depends on the tolerizing dose of I: with a relatively small dose few anti-I B cells would have been eliminated and the shared anti-I Abs elicited by I' would probably correspond closely to those that would have been raised against I itself in a normal animal; but with a large tolerizing dose, many anti-I B cells would have been suppressed and the Abs that react with I, made in response to the I', would probably differ substantially from those normally induced by I.

Is there a tolerant cell? Are Ag-sensitive lymphocytes destroyed by the tolerogen or do

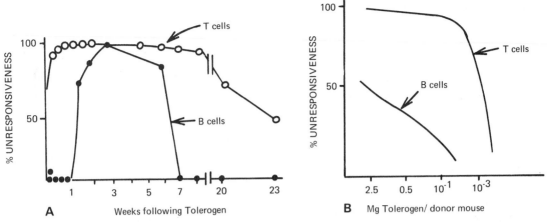

A   Weeks following Tolerogen

B   Mg Tolerogen/ donor mouse

Fig. 17-28. Induction and persistence of tolerance in B- and T-cell populations. Thymus (T) and bone marrow (B) cells were removed at various times from mice rendered tolerant with various amounts of BγG and tested, with complementary cells from normal donors, for ability to cooperate in Ab formation when transferred to irradiated, syngeneic mice. Results are as per cent of control values (untreated donors). In **A** tolerance was induced with 2.5 mg of BγG. In **B** the cells were removed 15 to 20 days after the doses of Ag shown (abscissa). Tolerance appeared sooner, lasted longer, and was established more solidly, and with lower Ag doses, in T than in B cells. [From Chiller, J. M., Habicht, G. S., and Weigle, W. O. *Science* 171:813 (1971).]

they persist as "tolerant" cells? There is evidence for both. When animals tolerant of a T-dependent Ag are thymectomized their tolerance is more persistent (Fig. 17-29): this suggests that recovery of responsiveness depends upon emergence in the thymus (or under its influence) of new T cells that are sensitive to the Ag.

The stability of tolerized B cells has been followed in animals made tolerant of T-independent Ags: spleen cells taken at various times after induction of tolerance were trans-

Fig. 17-29. Increased persistence of tolerance following thymectomy. Mice were first made tolerant by multiple injections of bovine serum albumin (BSA); then half were thymectomized. Loss of tolerance (= recovery of responsiveness) was assayed by response to a challenging injection of BSA in Freund's adjuvant. Symbols are averages for groups of five to eight mice with standard deviation: x = tolerant, thymectomized; O = tolerant, not thymectomized. Control mice (not tolerant and not thymectomized) had a titer of about 10. Nonthymectomized mice recovered responsiveness by 12 weeks; the thymectomized ones had not recovered by 24 weeks. [From Taylor, R. B. *Immunology* 7:595 (1964).]

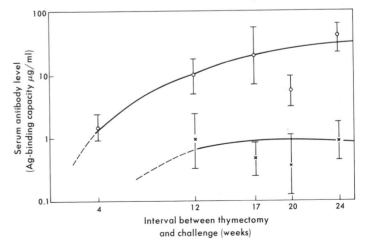

Interval between thymectomy
and challenge (weeks)

ferred to irradiated recipients, which were then stimulated with Ag. Two weeks after a tolerizing dose of pneumonococcal polysaccharide the transferred cells could already form Abs to this Ag in the surrogate host, but cells taken up to 6 months after a tolerizing dose of ievan (polyfructose) were still unresponsive. It is likely that B cells are reversibly suppressed by relatively small tolerizing doses, but are eliminated in the long-lived tolerance established by relatively large doses: tolerance probably endures until the Ag is dissipated and bone marrow stem cells generate new B cells with the appropriate specificity.

Cellular Mechanisms. It seems likely that an Ag-sensitive lymphocyte responds in all-or-none fashion (proliferation and differentiation, or tolerance) when Ag binds to its surface receptors, and that the graded responses observed in the whole animal are determined by the proportions of cells making one or the other response. For instance, with a high but not completely tolerizing dose of Dnp-protein the subsequently formed anti-Dnp Abs have unusually low affinity for Dnp; evidently the B cells with high-affinity surface receptors are preferentially tolerized.

With B cells, whose abundant Ag-binding receptors are Igs, the immunogenic pathway (cell division with differentiation toward plasma cells) seems to be triggered by cross-linking of the receptors by multivalent Ag. Hence aggregated proteins with many copies of the same determinant per particle are highly immunogenic, whereas the same Ag in disaggregated form, with only one or a few copies of a determinant per molecule, is likely to be tolerogenic: it binds without stimulating, and competitively blocks binding of the immunogenic aggregates. Univalent haptens and high levels of multivalent Ag (see Ch. 15, Ag excess in the precipitin reaction) can also be tolerogenic because they do not engage in, but block, cross-linking; their effectiveness probably depends greatly on their persistence and on whether they only temporarily suppress or somehow eliminate the cells to which they bind. Ags also exercise alternative effects on T cells; but the detailed mechanisms are totally obscure, because the nature of the T-cell surface receptor is still unclear.

Possible Additional Mechanisms. Tolerance to many self-Ags may well involve much more than a preemptive interaction that blocks the cell's Ag-driven immune differentiation. Some evidence hints at antagonistic, rather than cooperative, relations between B and T cells under some circumstances. In mice, for instance, thymectomy increases the formation of Ab to polyvinylpyrrolidone (PVP), a T-independent antigen, suggesting that certain **"suppressor" T cells** might specifically block the activity of anti-PVP B cells.

In contrast, the characteristics of **tetraparental (allophenic) mice** suggest that Abs can block T-cell activities (Ch. 20, Cell-mediated immunity). These mice are produced by mixing the cells of early embryos (at about the eight-cell blastula stage) from two genetically different sets of parents, and implanting the single combined blastula in a foster mother's uterus. The progeny are **mosaics,** with cells of genetically different origin contributing to essentially all parts of the body (skin, liver, lymphatic system, etc.). Though these remarkable animals grow and develop normally their lymphocytes can destroy cultured fibroblasts from either set of parents, but the reaction can be specifically blocked with the tetraparental animals' serum (which presumably contains some kind of blocking Abs or Ab-Ag complexes). Hence the "self-tolerance" in these mice seems to be due to opposing immune responses, i.e., each set of cells can make immune responses to the other set, with Abs (or Ab-Ag complexes) blocking potentially destructive cellular immune reactions by killer T lymphocytes (Ch. 20).

Whether it is common in natural self-tolerance for suppressor T cells to block Ab formation to self-antigens, or for blocking Abs to interfere with cell-mediated reactions against other self-antigens is still not clear. Nevertheless, it seems likely that a variety of regulatory mechanisms, with diverse fail-safe features, must have developed in evolution to guard against destructive antiself immune reactions; for without effective mechanisms for self-tolerance the potentially damaging effects of the immune response would probably have outweighed its protective benefits.

ANTIBODIES AS IMMUNOSUPPRESSIVE AGENTS

Depending upon their specificities, some Abs can block the formation of other Abs in various ways: by hindering the reaction of immunogen with appropriate cell surface receptors, or by inactivating lymphocytes, especially T cells (antilymphocytic serum).

SUPPRESSION BY ANTIBODY AS ANTIIMMUNOGEN

As noted before, if Abs are added to the immunogen before its injection, or are present in the animal as a result of previous immunization, the induction of Ab formation is likely to be blocked; inhibition is particularly pronounced when Ab is in relative excess, for the resulting Ab-Ag complexes are then degraded rapidly* (Fate of injected antigen, above).

The inhibition by excess Ab is important clinically. For instance, severe hemolytic disease of the newborn, due to maternal Abs against fetal Rh red cells, has been greatly reduced in incidence by routine injections of anti-Rh Abs into Rh⁻ mothers at the time they deliver Rh⁺ babies: the baby's red cells, entering the maternal circulation in profusion as the placenta separates, are eliminated by the anti-Rh Abs. This prevents the mother from becoming immunized and reduces the risk of an anamnestic anti-Rh response during a subsequent pregnancy with another Rh⁺ baby (Ch. 21, Rh). Another example arises from placental transfer of maternal Abs to measles, polio, etc.: these can block induction of Ab synthesis by the corresponding immunogens in the young infant. Hence active immunization of the newborn is postponed until 6 to 9 months of age, by which time all maternal Abs have been eliminated (see Fig. 17-37).

SUPPRESSION BY ANTIBODY AS ANTIRECEPTOR

Under some circumstances anti-Igs suppress the production of Igs either by eliminating B lymphocytes with the target Ig as surface receptor or by blocking their stimulation by Ag. Depending upon its specificity and the conditions under which it is administered, the attacking anti-Ig specifically suppresses the formation of Igs of the corresponding class (isotype), or allotype, or idiotype (Ch. 16, classification of antigenic determinants of Igs). These effects emphasize the importance of surface Igs for the differentiation of B cells, and perhaps even for the survival of these cells. They also suggest how immunization procedures might eventually be developed to avoid coincidental production of Abs of undesirable type (e.g., IgE Abs that cause severe allergic reactions, see Ch. 19).

Isotype Supression. Injections of newborn mice with antisera to μ chains leads to absence of serum IgM

---

* Ab-Ag complexes may have an additional, long-range suppressive effect on the corresponding Ag-sensitive lymphocytes, for such cells seem to remain unresponsive when transferred to irradiated recipients.

in the growing animal and decreases in the levels of IgG and IgA. Similar injections of anti-α or anti-γ antisera block only the production of Igs with the corresponding heavy chains (IgA and IgG, respectively). The effects persist for a few weeks, and recovery gradually ensues. Similar suppression cannot be established in adults, probably because their high levels of serum Igs neutralize the injected Abs. The broader effect of anti-μ than of Ab to other heavy chains fits additional evidence that cells with IgM on their surface are precursors of those with cell-bound IgG or IgA (Ontogeny, below).

Isotype suppression is also evident in primary spleen cell cultures, in which the addition of both sheep red blood cells (SRBC) and certain anti-Igs block production of various classes of Abs to SRBC: antisera to μ chains inhibit formation of Abs of all classes, while antisera to γ1 or to γ2 chains block only the formation of those anti-SRBC of the corresponding class. These effects (and others, see IgM-IgG shift, above) suggest that the initially reactive (virgin) Ag-sensitive cells have only IgM on the surface; once stimulated by the Ag, some of these cells apparently shift to produce surface Ig receptors with the same class of heavy chain as in the Ab molecules subsequently secreted by these cells (or their progeny).

Allotype Suppression. The first discovered case of suppression by anti-Ig was found by Dray among hybrid offspring of crosses between rabbits homozygous for different Ig allotypes (see Ch. 16, rabbit a and b allotypes of heavy chains and of κ light chains, respectively). If the newborn receives antiserum to the paternal allotype, it produces hardly any Ig of that allotype for many months; however, a compensating overproduction of the maternal allotype maintains total Ig at a normal level (Fig. 17-30).

Antiserum to the mother's allotype is not effective in the newborn, whose high levels of maternal Ig, acquired transplacentally or by suckling, neutralize the injected Ab. Antiserum to the father's allotype is suppressive only if given before a neutralizing level of this allotype has been actively produced (i.e., before the third week after birth in rabbits).

More extreme conditions are necessary to suppress both maternal and paternal allotypes; when this happens the corresponding isotype is eliminated. Thus when early rabbit embryos (8- to 16-cell stage), derived from parents homozygous for the same κ-chain allotype (b5), were implanted in the uterus of a foster mother who was injected with large amounts of anti-b5 antiserum, the resulting newborn rabbits did not form κ-containing Igs: their serum Ig levels were normal but all the light chains were λ type, which is ordinarily present in only ca. 10% of rabbit Ig molecules. In the fully suppressed rabbits it was not until 6 months after birth that blood lymphocytes appeared with the

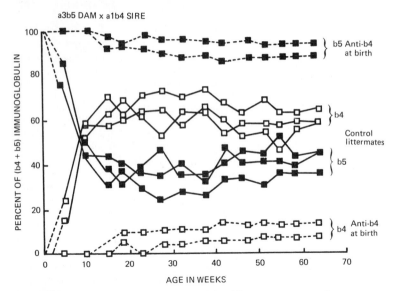

Fig. 17-30. Allotype suppression in rabbits. The parents were homozygous for different light-chain allotypes (father, b4/b4; mother, b5/b5). At birth half the offspring (b4/b5) were given 2.2 mg anti-b4 Abs (– – –); control littermates did not receive Abs (——). For over 1 year, the target allotype (b4) was virtually lacking in the treated animals' Igs while its allelic partner (b5) was overproduced; the level of total Ig in serum was normal as were the heavy chain allotypes. The changes in controls at 5 to 10 weeks are due to synthesis of the paternal allotype (b4, □) and loss of passively acquired maternal Igs (b5, ■). Relative concentrations of b4 and b5 in controls are not unusual for products of codominant alleles. Levels of individual allotypes are expressed as per cent of the sum of both allotypes (b4 + b5). [From Mage, R. G. *Cold Spring Harbor Symp Quant Biol* 32:203 (1967).]

suppressed κ (b5) chains on their surface, and the corresponding serum Igs first appeared much later, perhaps because the additional time was needed for the newly emerging cells to express a sufficiently broad repertoire of V_κ regions to be stimulated by prevalent Ags.

Since the suppressing Ab molecules are catabolized with a half life of about 6 days (Table 17-5), the chronicity of allotype suppression in rabbits (up to 3 years) is puzzling. Allotype suppression with the expected transitory existence can be elicited in most hybrid mice. However, with crosses between certain inbred strains antiallotypes evoke long-lasting suppression which appears, from adoptive transfer studies, to be due to T cells that specifically inhibit just those B cells with the target allotype. Thus cotransfer to irradiated, syngeneic recipients of spleen cells (not serum) from chronically suppressed and from normal (unsuppressed) donors resulted in suppression of the previously unsuppressed normal cells; and the block could be alleviated by prior treatment of the transferred population of suppressing cells with anti-θ serum and complement, destroying their T cells. It is possible that Ab-Ag complexes (antiallotype plus allotype) stimulate some T cells to make a long

lasting cell-mediated immune response (Ch. 20) against the corresponding allotype.

Idiotype Suppression. An animal fails to produce Ab of a particular idiotype if it has been previously immunized (actively or passively) against that idiotype. In a study in inbred mice, for example, rabbit antiserum against the idiotype of one mouse's Abs to the phenylarsonate (R) group was injected into other mice, which were then immunized with R-azoproteins: none of the resulting anti-R Abs reacted with the rabbit antiidiotype (which could, however, react with a large proportion of the anti-R Abs formed in the control mice that had been injected only with the R-azo-protein immunogen). Evidently the antiidiotype had suppressed a major anti-R clone, by eliminating it or by blocking its reaction with the immunogen; other anti-R clones were unaffected.

SUPPRESSION BY ANTILYMPHOCYTE SERUM (ALS)

Antilymphocyte heteroantisera are usually prepared in horse or rabbit against another species' thymus cells, white blood cells, or cultured lymphocytes. These antisera were developed primarily to suppress cell-mediated immune reactions and to promote acceptance of allografts (Ch. 21). Usually administered as the IgG fraction (antilymphocyte globulin, or ALG), the Abs seem to cause preferential inactivation of the long-lived pool of recirculating lymphocytes, which are primarily T cells; hence ALG dramatically prolongs survival of allografts and reduces other manifestations of cell-mediated immunity (Ch. 20). However, ALG can also reduce Ab formation in primary responses to many Ags (probably T-dependent ones), if given just before the Ag; if given a few hours later, or if given before a second ("booster") injection, Ab formation is not blocked. Because ALG hardly suppresses secondary Ab responses (which are also more resistant to X-ray and other nonspecific suppressants, see below), but can apparently greatly depress secondary cell-mediated immune responses, it is used clinically to prevent immune rejection of allografts (Ch. 21). ALG loses its effectiveness when the Fc domain is removed, suggesting that complement fixation may be involved (Ch. 18).

Clinical use of ALG is somewhat limited by its immunogenicity. It does not suppress immune reactions to itself, and about half of humans injected with horse ALS (to human cells) form Abs to the horse Igs and develop "immune-complex" disease (see Ch. 19). As is described below, the suppressive effect of ALG on T cells greatly increases susceptibility to certain infections and to tumors (Complications of immunosuppression, below, and chs. 20 and 21, Immune responses to tumors).

NONSPECIFIC IMMUNOSUPPRESSION

Whole-body X-irradiation and a variety of cytotoxic drugs (Fig. 17-31) can prevent the initiation of Ab formation; but once Ab synthesis is under way they cannot interrupt it, unless given in doses that are severely cytotoxic for cells in general. All these agents are **much more effective in blocking the primary than the secondary response:** either memory cells are more resistant than virgin Ag-sensitive cells, or the increased number of cells that can respond increases the probability that some will initiate Ab formation before they can be blocked. Some immunosuppressants act primarily as inhibitors of cell division (**antiproliferative,** e.g., the antimetabolites); others act primarily by destroying lymphocytes (**lympholytic,** e.g., 11-oxycorticosteroids); and others are both lympholytic and antiproliferative (X-rays, radiomimetic alkylating agents).

Most of the **antimetabolites** (purine, pyridimine, and folate analogs; Chs. 6 and 11) were developed as byproducts of cancer chemotherapy screening programs. Their principal action is to **block cell proliferation** (Fig. 17-31), and they are especially toxic for rapidly dividing cells: in tumors, bone marrow, intestinal and skin epithelium, as well as lymphocytes that proliferate in response to stimulation by Ag. Accordingly, the margin of clinical safety between therapeutic and toxic doses is small, but for some of these drugs it is great enough for routine clinical use (e.g., azathioprine and cyclophosphamide).

The frequency of successful kidney transplants in man is now largely due to skillful use of immunosuppressive agents: currently favored are combinations of azathioprine (an antimetabolite), prednisone (a corticosteroid), and antilymphocytic serum or its IgG fraction (ALG), which selectively destroys circulating T cells (see below and Chs. 20 and 21).

Lympholytic agents (X-rays, radiomimetic alkylating drugs, corticosteroids) cause prompt and massive destruction of lymphocytes. The chromosomal damage caused by X-rays and alkylating agents also impairs the capacity of surviving lymphocytes to undergo mitosis, blocking their normal response to subsequent antigenic stimulation.

In the following comparison of various agents it is useful to contrast their activity in the three phases of the Ab response: 1) the preinductive phase, before immunogen is administered; 2) the inductive phase, between immunogen administration and rise in titer of the corresponding serum Ab; and 3) the productive phase, when Ab is being synthesized vigorously. The **lympholytic agents are effective immunosuppressors when given in the preinductive phase, and the antiproliferative agents are most effective in the inductive phase.** All known agents appear to be ineffective in the productive phase, unless given in highly toxic doses. Though this division into phases is convenient, it is an oversimplification, for lymphoid cells do not respond syn-

Alkylating agents

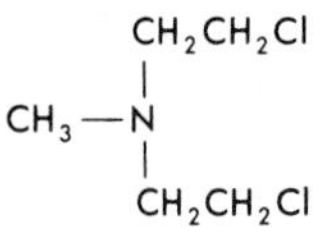

Nitrogen mustard

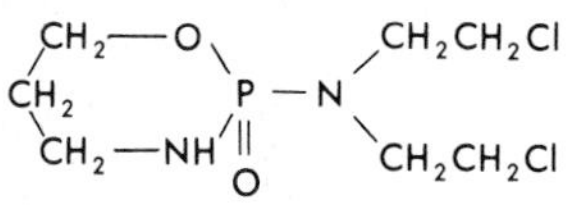

Cyclophosphamide
(Cytoxan)

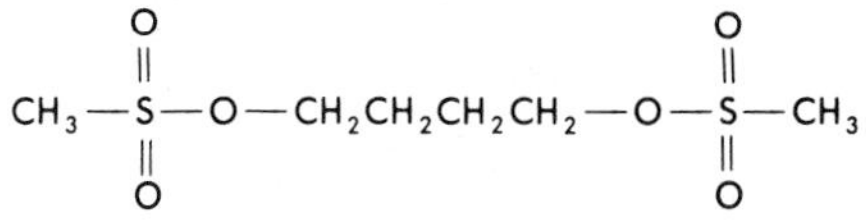

Busulfan (Myleran)

Purine analogs

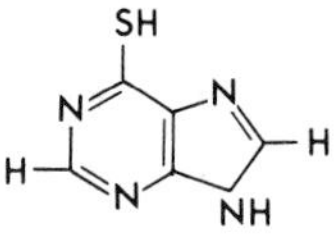

6-Mercaptopurine

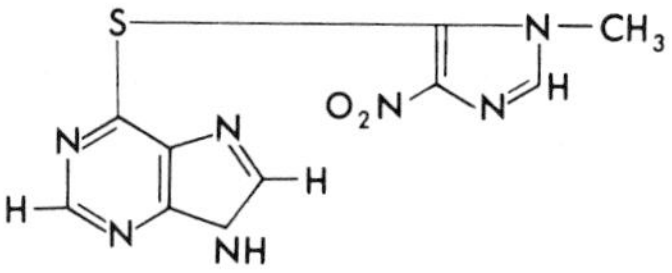

Azathioprine (Imuran)

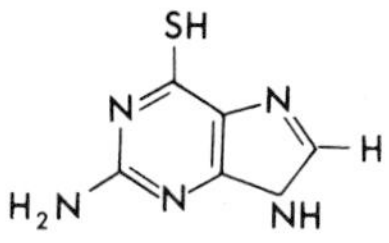

6-Thioguanine

Pyrimidine analogs

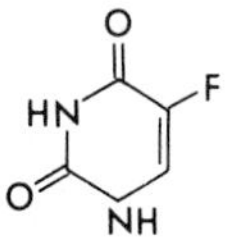

5-Fluorouracil

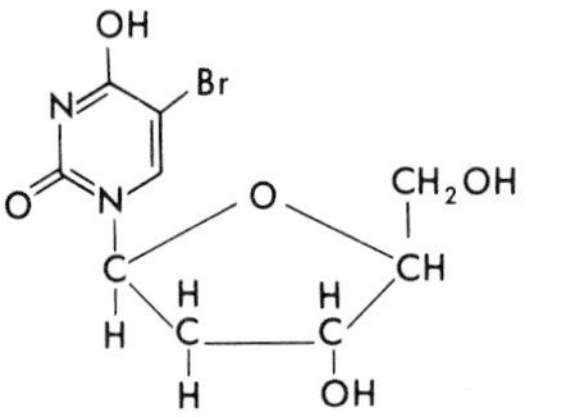

5-Bromodeoxyuridine (BUDR)

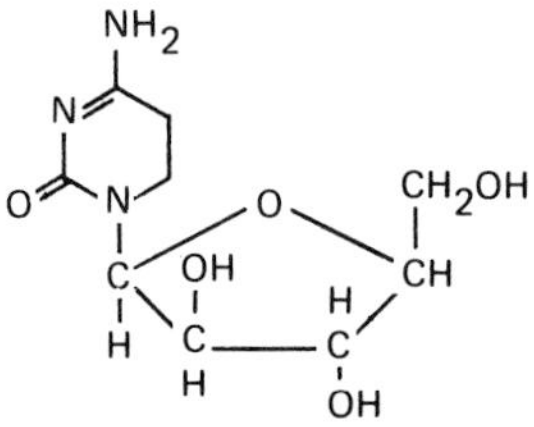

Cytosine arabinoside

Folic acid analog

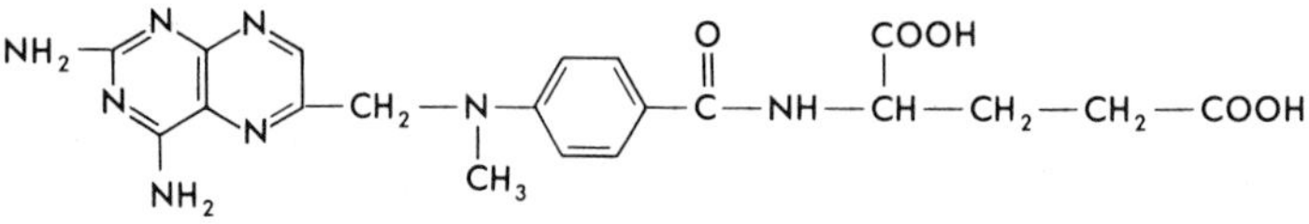

Amethopterin

Fig. 17-31. Some immunosuppressive drugs. Azathioprine (Imuran) is converted in vivo to 6-mercaptopurine by sulfhydryl or other nucleophilic groups.

chronously: the immunogen can remain active for months, and cells in all three phases may be present simultaneously.

X-rays. Whole-body irradiation with sublethal doses of X-rays (400 to 500 r) tends to suppress the response to most immunogens for many weeks, but usually not permanently. Suppression is greatest when the irradiation is given 24 to 48 hours before Ag, because massive disintegration of lymphocytes occurs promptly after whole-body irradiation. After a large dose (e.g., 500 r) active proliferation of lymphoid cells is resumed after ca. 3 to 4 weeks, and lymph nodes appear normal shortly thereafter. However, damage to chromosomes (the main tar-

gets of X-ray, Ch. 11) can be "stored": i.e., it may not be expressed until the cells attempt to divide, perhaps months or years later (Lifetime of lymphocytes, above). In the meantime the nondividing cells can apparently function normally.

When immunogen is given **after** massive irradiation it may be largely or completely eliminated before the capacity to initiate Ab formation is restored. However, if the immunogen is given just **before** irradiation the stimulated cells can apparently continue their differentiation and eventually form Abs, while already differentiated cells continue to synthesize Abs. Indeed, having begun to differentiate, the responding cells may even yield more Ab in animals irradiated 1 to 2 days after immunization (Fig. 17-32).

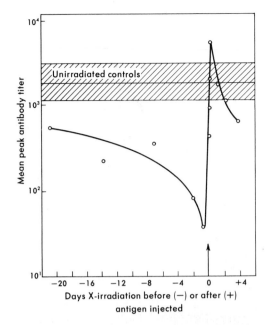

Fig. 17-32. Effect of 500-r X-irradiation of rabbits at various times before and after immunization (arrow) with sheep red cells. [Based on Taliaferro, W. H., and Taliaferro, L. G. *J Infec Dis* 95:134 (1954).]

The **secondary response** is relatively **resistant to irradiation:** the appearance of Abs may be delayed, but peak titers are usually normal. As in the primary response, Ab formation may be increased by irradiation given after the booster injection.

Alkylating Agents. Compounds such as the nitrogen mustards (Fig. 17-31) block cell division by cross-linking strands of DNA (Ch. 11). Often called radiomimetic drugs, their biological effects (such as massive destruction of lymphocytes) resemble those of X-irradiation. However, recovery is more rapid than after X-rays, and these drugs are therefore usually given at frequent intervals (e.g., daily) for sustained immunosuppression.

Corticosteroids. Large doses of 11-oxycorticosteroids cause extensive destruction of small lymphocytes. However, the surviving small T cells appear to be unusually active in some reactions, e.g., graft vs. host (Ch. 20), and even perhaps in cooperation with B cells in induction of Ab formation. Nonetheless, if given just before Ag they inhibit Ab formation in some species (rats, mice, rabbits); but at the doses used clinically a significant suppression has not been observed in man. In therapeutic doses these drugs inhibit inflammation, whether due to allergic reactions (Chs. 19 and 20) or to nonspecific irritants such as turpentine. Accordingly, they are widely used clinically to suppress allergic inflammation, especially of the delayed type.

Antimetabolites. In contrast to X-rays, which are most inhibitory when given just before the immunogen, the antiproliferative metabolite analogs, such as 6-mercaptopurine, usually suppress Ab formation best when administration is begun 2 days afterward, when the Ag-induced proliferation of lymphocytes is particularly active (Selectivity, below). The difference is readily understood: X-rays (and alkylating agents) can damage DNA whether or not it is replicating, while the antimetabolites used as immunosuppressants only damage cells with replicating DNA.

Other Immunosuppressive Drugs. Some antimicrobial drugs also inhibit Ab synthesis. **Chloramphenicol** in relatively high doses inhibits the primary response in intact animals. If added with the immunogen it also inhibits the secondary response in cultures of cells from a previously immunized animal, but after the cells are stimulated to form Abs the addition of chloramphenicol has little effect. Inhibition by chloramphenicol may be related to its ability to inhibit mitochondrial (but not cytoplasmic) ribosomes (Ch. 12).

If **actinomycin D** is added together with the immunogen the formation of Ab is substantially inhibited, because the synthesis of new mRNA is required for initiation of Ab synthesis. However, Ab formation can persist for many days in cell culture in the presence of this drug, suggesting that the corresponding mRNA is relatively stable.

Selectivity. Though immunosuppressants generally affect immune responses as a whole, rather than particular manifestations, some selective suppression is observed. For instance, as noted before, ALS seems to block cell-mediated more than humoral immunity. X-ray, corticosteroids, and antiproliferative drugs suppress IgG more than IgM production, suggesting that fewer cell divisions may be needed to initiate production of Abs of the IgM class.

The most impressive selectivity, however, is brought about by **combined administration of Ag and antiproliferative immunosuppressants** (Fig. 17-33). The clones whose proliferation has been stimulated are selectively eliminated by the drugs, as in the selective destruction of growing bacterial cells by penicillin (Ch. 6). The animal thus becomes specifically unresponsive to the Ag used, and repeated injection of that Ag can then maintain the tolerant state. The clinical utility of this approach is likely to be restricted to those situations in which the relevant Ag is known in advance of an actual response, e.g., in organ transplantation (Ch. 21).

Complications of Immunosuppression. Prolonged immunosuppression is dangerous: not only are the agents highly toxic for various cells, but they can activate latent infections and greatly increase susceptibility to serious infection with the many prevalent fungi, bacteria, and viruses that ordinarily have little pathogenicity (e.g., *Candida, Nocardia,* cytomegalovirus, herpesvirus). In addition, chronically immunosuppressed individuals, just like those with congenital immunodeficiencies (below), have an increased incidence of various cancers, especially lymphomas and reticulum cell sarcomas (see discussion of increased frequency of cancer in chronically suppressed recipients of kidney allografts, Chs. 20 and 21). Suppression of cell-mediated immunity (Ch. 20) rather than of Ab formation is probably responsible, because the most effective immune responses to most tumors seem to be cell-mediated (Chs. 20 and 21).

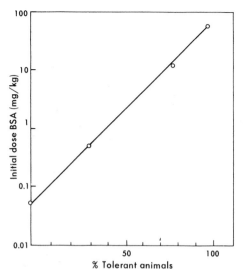

Fig. 17-33. Selective unresponsiveness produced by combined administration of Ag and an antiproliferative immunosuppressive agent. Rabbits were injected with bovine serum albumin (BSA) and 6-mercaptopurine: 1 to 3 months later many were specifically unable to make Abs to BSA, though they could respond to other Ags. The proportion of tolerant animals increased with the dose of BSA given initially with the immunosuppressant. [From Schwartz, R. S. *Progr Allergy* 9:246 (1965).]

PHYLOGENY AND ONTOGENY OF ANTIBODY FORMATION

PHYLOGENY

Invertebrates lack a lymphoid system and do not form recognizable Igs. A primitive form of cellular immunity probably provides their principal defense against invasive parasites (Ch. 20). However, invertebrates of many phyla have soluble, circulating (hemolymph) proteins that agglutinate or lyse various bacteria and vertebrate red cells; and the production of these agglutinins and lysins can be augmented by administration of the target cells. Moreover, treatment of red cells with oyster hemagglutinin enhances their phagocytosis by oyster amebocytes (motile, phagocytic cells that recognize foreign cells, see Ch. 20). Despite these superficial similarities to Ab-enhanced phagocytosis by vertebrate macrophages (Ch. 18) these invertebrate "antisubstances" (e.g., horseshoe crab and oyster hemagglutinins) seem to differ considerably from vertebrate Igs: 1) very little specificity is evident from the range of substances that induce or react with particular invertebrate agglutinins; 2) of high molecular weight (ca. 400,000), they are made of dissociable, apparently identical subunits (MW 22,000); 3) they do not show the electrophoretic heterogeneity expected of proteins with diverse specificities. It would nonetheless prove interesting if any amino acid homology were found between invertebrate agglutinins or lysins and vertebrate Igs.

In contrast to invertebrates, even the most primitive of present-day vertebrates, the **hagfish** (a cyclostome), has some capacity for immunological memory: it rejects allografts more rapidly after repeated trials (Ch. 21, Second set reaction). While these creatures have been reported to form Abs that agglutinate sheep red cells and that precipitate hemocyanin, they seem unable to make Abs to several other Ags, and their Igs have not so far been characterized. Their lymphoid system is also exceedingly primitive, and a thymus has not been identified. However, the **lamprey,** a slightly more advanced cyclostome, has a better developed lymphoid system, including a rudimentary thymus; it forms Abs to several Ags, and has recognizable Igs (Fig. 17-34).

Beginning with elasmobranchs **(sharks)** and continuing up the phylogenetic scale of complexity, essentially all features of the immune response are recognized in all vertebrates: Ab formation to a broad range of Ags, appearance of plasma cells in response to immunization, allograft rejection, and a fully developed lymphoid system.

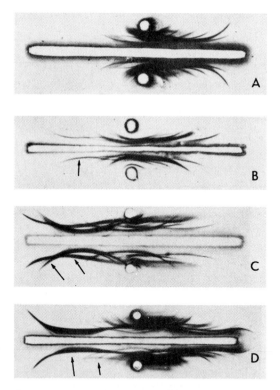

Fig. 17-34. Evolutionary development of immuno-globulins, suggested by electrophoresis of serum from selected vertebrates. Proteins with suggestive electrophoretic characteristics of Igs (arrows) were present in small amount in the lamprey **(B)**, and abundant in the bowfin, a fresh water dogfish **(C)**, and in man **(D)**. Though undetected in the hagfish **(A)**, they must also be produced in this species, which can make Abs to some Ags. [From Papermaster, B. W., Condie, R. M., Finstad, J., and Good, R. A. *J Exp Med 119*:105 (1964).]

Serological analyses indicate that the Igs of lower vertebrates are less diversified than those of mammals. However data on their amino acid sequences are scanty and tentative assignments to particular mammalian classes are based on sedimentation coefficients and electrophoretic mobilities, which are less dependable criteria (e.g., in frogs the most cathodically migrating serum proteins are not Igs).

Fish have two serum Igs (19S and 7S in sharks, 14S and 6S in bony fish), and both seem to belong to the IgM class. From the first N-terminal 10 residues it appears that at least 80% of pooled shark light chains are of κ type, with striking similarity to human κ chains. Several distinct classes of Igs are present in amphibia and in reptiles (IgM-like, IgG-like, and at least one other); the three major mammalian classes, IgG, IgM, and IgA, are present in birds. Considerable insight into evolutionary relations is emerging from amino acid sequence homologies among Ig chains (Ch. 16).

ONTOGENY

Though synthesis of Igs can be detected in mammalian fetuses, protective levels of Abs to common pathogens are not attained until some time after birth. The newborn would thus be extremely vulnerable to many infections were it not for the maternal Abs it receives before or shortly after birth. In some species the fetus receives maternal Igs only from colostrum, which is usually rich in IgA and IgG, while in others the Igs are transferred both in utero and by suckling (Table 17-10).

In man and in higher primates absorption from colostrum is probably of minor importance compared with transfer across the placenta. Maternal IgG, but not IgM, IgA, or IgE, is transmitted freely to the human fetus in utero, suggesting selective transport. Special sites on the Fc domain are evidently required: in rabbits, Fc fragments (of γ chains) are transferred as readily as intact IgG molecules and much more rapidly than Fab fragments.

The order in which Igs are produced in embryogenesis repeats the apparent evolutionary sequence ("ontogeny recapitulates phylogeny"): IgM, then IgG, and finally IgA.

The time course has been especially well studied in the chicken, where B-cell differentiation is initiated in the bursa of Fabricius. IgM-containing cells are evident in the chick embryo's bursa on day 14, and cells with IgG are not detected until 1 week later (day 21, the time of hatching). The spread of Ig-containing cells to peripheral tissues follows the same order: cells with IgM are found in the spleen on day 17 and those with IgG appear there 8 days later (4 days after hatching).

The switch of individual lymphocytes from production of IgM to IgG is suggested by the presence, just before hatching, of many cells in the bursa with both μ and γ chains, and especially from the suppressive effects of anti-μ-chain Abs, whose administration on day 13, followed by removal of the bursa at hatching, yields birds that are completely agammaglobulinemic: they are devoid of IgG and IgA as well as of IgM. If, however, injection of anti-μ and bursectomy are delayed until hatching (i.e., after the switch has taken place) the developing chicks are depleted only of IgM and they have a normal or even an elevated IgG level. (Bursectomy at an intermediate time—after IgM-producing cells have been seeded in peripheral tissues, but before IgG producers have appeared—yields many birds with persistently elevated levels of IgM and virtual absence of IgG.)

TABLE 17-10. Relation of Placental Structure and Mode of Passive Transfer of Immunoglobulins to the Fetus*

Species	No. of tissue layers between maternal and fetal circulation at term	Placental or amniotic transmission	Importance of transmission via colostrum
Pig	6	—	+++
Ruminants	5	—	+++
Carnivores	3	±	+
Rodents	2	+ (yolk sac)	+
Man	2	+++ (placenta)	—

   * In chickens, and presumably in other birds, β-globulins containing Abs are transmitted from hen to ova via follicular epithelium and are stored in the yolk sac, from which the proteins are absorbed into the fetal circulation shortly before hatching.

   From Good, R. A., and Papermaster, B. W. *Adv Immunol 4*:1 (1964); based on Vahlquist, B. *Adv Pediat 10*:305 (1958).

The differentiation of B cells from IgM to IgG production in the bursa is independent of Ag (i.e., it is not modified by administration of extrinsic immunogens); this is in sharp contrast to the Ag-driven IgM-IgG switch that seems to take place in peripheral tissues during induction of Ab formation (see above, One cell-one Ab rule, Isotype suppression, and Fig. 17-35).

   In human fetuses lymphocytes with IgM or IgG on the cell surface are detected by immunofluorescence by the tenth week of gesta-

Fig. 17-35. Scheme for successive stages in differentiation of B cells. Stem cells (from yolk sac or liver in early and late embryogenesis, respectively, or from bone marrow after birth or hatching) differentiate into IgM-bearing B cells, of which some differentiate further into IgG-bearing, and then into IgA-bearing, B cells, which are then stimulated by an appropriate immunogen to undergo further (2nd stage) differentiation into plasma cells or to proliferate and continue in circulation as Ag-sensitive memory cells. [Based on Cooper, M. D., Lawton, A. R., and Kincaide, P. W. *Clin Exp Immunol 11*:143 (1972).]

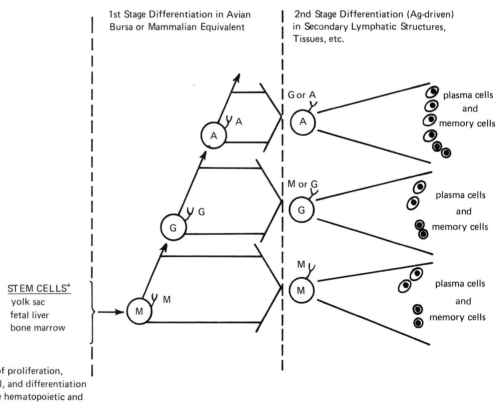

1st Stage Differentiation in Avian Bursa or Mammalian Equivalent

2nd Stage Differentiation (Ag-driven) in Secondary Lymphatic Structures, Tissues, etc.

STEM CELLS*
yolk sac
fetal liver
bone marrow

* Capable of proliferation, self-renewal, and differentiation into diverse hematopoietic and lymphoid cells.

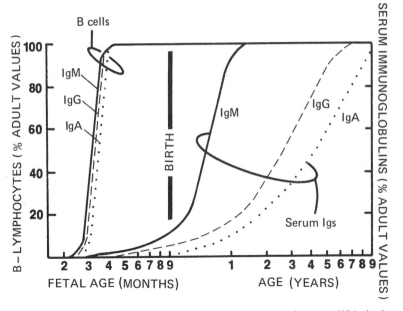

Fig. 17-36. Maturation of B cells and serum Ig levels in man. With both cells and their secreted products the ontogenetic order (IgM, IgG, IgA) recapitulates the presumptive evolutionary sequence of their appearance. [Based on Cooper, M. D., and Lawton, A. R. *Am J Pathol* **69**:513 (1972), from data of Lawton, A. R., Self, K. S., Royal, S. A., and Cooper, M. D. *Clin Immunol and Immunopathol* **1**:104 (1972)].

tion, and cells with surface IgA are detected later (12 weeks). By the fifteenth week the proportions of fetal spleen and blood cells with each Ig class is essentially the same as in the normal adult. However, active synthesis and secretion of Igs by fetal cells occur much later, perhaps because restricted diversity of Ag-sensitive cells and of foreign Ags in the sheltered fetus reduces the chances for Ag-triggering of the fetus's lymphocytes. IgM and lesser amounts of IgG normally begin to be synthesized and secreted by fetal spleen cells in about the twentieth week, but production of IgA seems to start only some weeks after birth. However, with severe fetal infection, as in congenital syphilis, Abs (of the IgM class) are formed vigorously and plasma cells are abundant in the infected 6-month fetus (Fig. 17-36).

Because IgG molecules are readily transferred from maternal to fetal blood and the other Igs are not, the newborn infant's blood contains high levels of IgG (with Gm allotype of the mother), traces of IgM (of fetal origin), and essentially no IgA. The newborn's total IgG (and total Ig) declines until ca. 8 to 10 weeks of age, when it starts to rise as the neonate's biosynthesis becomes sufficiently active. Adult serum levels of IgM are reached at about 10 months of age, of IgG at about 4 years, of IgA at about 9 to 10 years (Figs. 17-36 and 17-37), and of IgE at about 10 to 15 years.

Fig. 17-37. Changing plasma level of Igs in human infant during first year. Maternal IgG, which accounts for almost all the infant's Igs at birth, has essentially disappeared by about 6 months. [Based on Gitlin, D. *Pediatrics* **34**:198 (1964).]

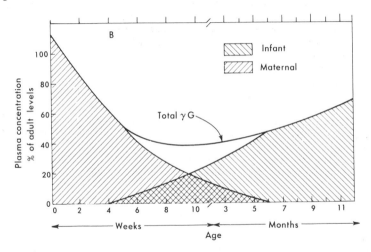

IMMUNODEFICIENCY DISEASES

Many genetic and congenitally acquired defects in ability to form Abs and to develop cell-mediated immunity have been recognized since the 1950s, when it became possible to prolong the survival of affected individuals through the use of antibiotics, Igs, and even bone marrow or thymus grafts from normal donors (Ch. 21, Allografts). These immunodeficient states help illuminate mechanisms in normal immune responses, just as mutations have clarified many other pathways. Classification of many of the clinical syndromes is unclear, but several distinctive clinical patterns are recognized (Table 17-11). Some affect only the B cell system (low levels or absence of one or all Ig classes), others the T cell system (defective cell-mediated immunity, Ch. 20), and some affect both, perhaps through defects in common stem cells. An increased incidence of cancer in these patients underscores the significance of the normal immune system in eliminating potential cancer cells (Chs. 20 and 21).

Suspected subjects with recurrent severe infections, or with close kinship to affected persons, are evaluated by procedures listed in Table 17-12. **In testing suspects for responses to routine immunization procedures it is important to avoid use of live vaccines**—e.g., attenuated viruses (polio, vaccinia, measles, ru-

TABLE 17-11.   Primary Immunodeficiency Disorders*

Probable defect in	Disease
I. B cells	Infantile X-linked aggammaglobulinemia Selective Ig deficiency (usually IgA) Transient hypogammaglobulinemia of infancy X-linked Ig deficiency with hyper-IgM
II. T cells	Thymic hypoplasia (pharyngeal pouch syndrome or DiGeorge's syndrome) Episodic lymphopenia with lymphocytotoxin

III. T cells, B cells, and stem cells	Immunodeficiency with ataxia-telangiectasia†
	Immunodeficiency with thrombocytopenia and eczema (Wiskott-Aldrich syndrome)‡
	Immunodeficiency with thymoma
	Immunodeficiency with dwarfism
	Immunodeficiency with generalized hematopoietic hypoplasia
	Severe combined immunodeficiency
	  Autosomal recessive
	  X-linked
	  Sporadic
	Variable immunodeficiency (commonest type, largely unclassified)

* Omits immunodeficiencies secondary to X-irradiation, cytotoxic drugs, lymphomas with replacement of normal by neoplastic lymphoid cells (e.g., multiple myeloma), or excessive loss of Igs through leaky lesions in intestine ("exudative enteropathy") or kidneys (nephritis, nephrosis). Severe, recurrent infections are also seen in rare children with deficiencies in some complement components (C3, C5; see Ch. 18) or in bactericidal activity of granulocytes. Cell-mediated immunity is conspicuously deficient in categories II and III, but normal in I.

† Inherited as autosomal recessive character; 80% lack serum and secretory IgA; IgM and IgG are usually normal.

‡ Inherited as X-linked character. IgM levels are usually low; IgG and IgA are usually normal or elevated. Pronounced inability to make Abs to polysaccharides.

Based on *Bull WHO 45*:125–142 (1971).

TABLE 17-12. Some Tests Used for Clinical Evaluation of Immune Status

Tests for B-cell functions	Serum Ig levels* Serum Ab levels† Biopsies examined for plasma cells by histological methods and immunofluorescence‡ Viable blood lymphocytes stained for surface Igs
Tests for T-cell functions	Skin tests for delayed-type hypersensitivity§ Lymphocyte transformation induced by plant mitogens (phytohemagglutinin or concanavalin A) or by incubation with allogeneic lymphocytes‖ Release of macrophage-inhibition factor (MIF) upon incubation of lymphocytes with common Ags¶

* Radial immunodiffusion is preferred (Ch. 15). It requires little serum (ca. 10 µl), and it is precise (±10%), sensitive (≧10 µg/ml), and not too slow (24 hr): with radiolabeled anti-Igs the sensitivity can be increased 100-fold to where, for instance, 0.05 µg/ml of IgE can be detected (Ch. 19). The distribution of Ig levels in the normal population is essentially bell-shaped and lacks the discontinuities that permit sharp definition of an Ig deficiency. By common agreement, some deficient levels are < 2 mg/ml for IgG and absence (< 10 µg/ml) of IgA.

† Commonly measured are "natural" Abs to blood group substances A and B (Ch. 21) or to sheep red cells or to *E. coli*, or induced Abs after immunization with potent, harmless and potentially helpful Ags, such as diphtheria and tetanus toxoids and *Bordetella pertussis* ("triple vaccine"), inactivated **(not attenuated)** polio vaccine, or polysaccharides from pneumococci, or *Hemophilus influenzae*, or *Neisseria meningitidis*.

‡ Plasma cells are sought in biopsies of lymph nodes that drain intracutaneous sites of injection of Ags in preceding footnote, or of the rectal mucosa, whose lamina propria layer normally contains many plasma cells (IgA-containing).

§ The Ags injected intradermally are derived from prevalent microbes: e.g., mumps virus, tuberculin (from *Mycobacterium tuberculosis*), streptokinase-streptodornase from hemolytic streptococci, and culture media supernatants from various fungi (e.g., *Candida, Trichophyton, Coccidiodes* [useful in California], or *Histoplasma* [useful in Mississippi Valley]). Skin patch tests are performed after deliberate skin sensitization with 2,4-dinitrochlorobenzene (Ch. 20).

‖ Blast transformation can be evaluated by changes in cell morphology (see Ch. 20, Fig. 20–8) or by radioautography or measurement of incorporation of ³H-thymidine into DNA. For the mixed lymphocyte culture, see Chapter 20.

¶ See Chapter 20.

bella) or bacteria (the bacillus Calmette-Guerin [BCG] variant of the tubercle bacillus) —which can cause overwhelming infections in severely affected persons. By staining blood lymphocytes with fluorescein-labeled, class-specific anti-Igs, it is possible to measure the proportion of cells with various membrane-bound surface Igs, and thus to determine whether defects occur before or after differentiation of stem cells into B cells.

Infantile X-linked Agammaglobulinemia. This X-linked genetic defect occurs in male infants who begin to suffer from recurrent bacterial (pyogenic) infections at ca. 9 to 12 months of age, when maternal Igs received transplacentally have completely disappeared (Fig. 17-37). These patients form exceedingly little if any Ab and plasma cells following deliberate immunization, and their serum Igs of all classes are greatly depressed (IgG to less than 10% and IgA and IgM to ca. 1% or less of the normal level; see Ch. 16, Fig. 16-16 F, G). Correspondingly, their blood lymphocytes lack surface Igs, as though the defect occurred in stem cell → B cell differentiation. However, differentiation into T cells seems to be unaffected, as all their cell-mediated immune responses are normal (Ch. 20). Since they generally recover without difficulty from measles, mumps, and other viral diseases of childhood, it appears that **resistance to many virus infections is due to cell-mediated immunity (T cells) rather than to serum Igs.**

Selective IgA Deficiency. This is the commonest abnormality, occurring in ca. 0.1% of all persons, often without any clinical manifestations. In some families the defect is inherited as an autosomal dominant, and in others as an autosomal recessive. IgA deficiency is also associated with two other autosomal genetic abnormalities—ataxia-telangiectasia and partial deletion of chromosome 18—and it is also frequently associated with congenital infections (rubella, toxoplasmosis), suggesting that in some cases the defect may be acquired. Despite the diversity of associated genetic and congential lesions, patients with selective IgA deficiency may have a **normal number of blood lymphocytes with surface IgA.** Moreover, the addition of a plant protein (pokeweed mitogen) that stimulates blast transformation of normal B cells can also stimulate this change in IgA-bearing cells from these patients. The defect seems, therefore, to lie in Ag triggering of terminal differentiation of the IgA-bearing B lymphocytes into IgA-secreting plasma cells. Either the cells are unable to respond to cross-linking of their surface IgA molecules by Ags, or the surface Igs are defective (e.g., they might lack good combining sites for Ag, through absence of V_H or V_L or both, or the combining sites of all IgA-bearing cells might be so uniform that the cells are unlikely to encounter an Ag and to be stimulated into secretion of IgA molecules). A block in terminal differentiation of B cells can occur in other Ig deficiencies; for example, rare children who are deficient in serum Igs of all classes but who have a normal number of lymphocytes with surface Igs of diverse classes.

However, **concordant deficiencies** can also occur: absence of serum Igs of a given class and of lymphocytes carrying surface Igs of that class suggests a block in differentiation of stem cells into B cells or of B cells with one type of Ig into B cells with another type (see Ontogeny, above, and Fig. 17-35). For instance, some individuals with "X-linked agammaglobulinemia with hyper IgM" have elevated levels of serum IgM and of lymphocytes carrying IgM but lack IgA and IgG, both as serum molecules and as surface receptors on B cells: the defect here is likely to be in the differentiation of IgM-bearing B cells into IgG- and IgA-bearing cells (see Fig. 17-35).

Thymic Hypoplasia. The most disabling immunodeficiencies are associated with T cell defects, including those due to faulty embryogenesis of the thymus. The fetus with defective development of the third and fourth branchial pouches is born without parathyroid glands and with no (or rudimentary) thymus **(DiGeorge's syndrome);** many are also born with anomalies of the great blood vessels. The disorder is not familial, and is probably due to some teratogenic agent. In some heritable cases of thymic aplasia the parathyroids develop normally (Nezelof syndrome).

If the thymic aplasia is total the infants should resemble mutant, thymus-less ("nude") mice (Thymus, above): all their lymphocytes should be B cells (with surface Igs) but Ab formation in response to T-dependent Ags should be grossly defective. In fact, however, most of the affected infants who survive long enough to be studied probably have less than total aplasia of the thymus, and their serum Igs and ability to produce Abs can be in the normal range. They also have normal frequency of plasma cells and normal germinal centers of lymphatic tissues.

However, T zones in these tissues are underdeveloped and the associated defective cell-mediated immune reactions must be severely disabling: these patients usually succumb to recurrent bacterial, viral, and fungal infections during infancy. Surprisingly, some children who survive longer seem to spontaneously recover some T cell function. In a few patients grafts of fetal thymic tissue (allografts) have been followed by dramatic improvement in clinical status.

Severe Combined Immunodeficiency. This disorder, with defects in B and in T cell function, is probably the most common of the severe heritable deficiencies. It is transmitted in some families as an autosomal recessive character and in others it is X-linked: hence reported cases are predominantly male. Severe recurrent infections due to bacteria, viruses, fungi, and protozoa begin at ca. 3 to 6 months of age and generally end fatally by the second year: death has resulted from generalized chickenpox, measles, vaccinia, and progressive BCG infection (after attempted immunization with BCG).

Serum Igs are exceedingly low and no Ab formation has been detected after trial immunization. Cell mediated immunity is also lacking (Ch. 20): skin allografts are not rejected, contact skin sensitivity to dinitrofluorobenzene cannot be induced, and delayed-type allergic skin reactions are not elicitable, even to candida Ags in infants with candida infections. The bone marrow lacks lymphocytes and plasma cells; the thymus is almost totally aplastic; and it is likely that stem cells do not differentiate into B and T cells.

Early efforts to save these infants with bone marrow transplants from normal donors invariably ended in fatal graft-vs.-host reactions (Chs. 20 and 21). However with sibling donors who have matching major histocompatibility Ags, successful transplants have been carried out, leading to long lasting restoration of B and T cell function (and only minor, transient graft-vs.-host reactions).

Some infants with severe combined immunodeficiency have normal serum Igs and some plasma cells in tissues (sometimes called Nezelof syndrome). Nevertheless they fail to form Abs in response to deliberate immunization and their clinical course is only slightly less severe.

SELECTED REFERENCES

BOOKS AND REVIEW ARTICLES

Antigen-Sensitive Cells. Their Source and Differentiation. Miller, J. F. A. P., Mitchell, G. F., Davies, A. J. S., Claman, H. N., Chaperon, E. A., and Taylor, R. B. *Transplantation Reviews 1*:3 (1969).

BENACERRAF, B., and MCDEVITT, H. O. Histocompatibility-linked immune response genes. *Science 175*: 273 (1972).

COHN, Z. A. The structure and function of monocytes and macrophages. *Adv Immunol 9*:164 (1968).

GOWANS, J. L. Lymphocytes. *Harvey Lect. ser 64*, p. 87 (1970).

GREY, H. M. Phylogeny of immunoglobulins. *Adv Immunol 10*:51 (1969).

KATZ, D. H., and BENACERRAF, B. The regulatory influence of activated T cells on B cell responses to antigen. *Adv Immunol 15*:1 (1972).

MILLER, J. F. A. P., BASTEN, A., SPRENT, J., and CHEERS, C. Interaction between lymphocytes in immune response. *Cell Immunol 2*:469 (1971).

SCHARFF, M. and LASKOV, P. Synthesis and assembly of immunoglobulin polypeptide chains. *Progr Allergy 14*:37 (1972).

SISKIND, G. W., and BENACERRAF, B. Cell selection by antigen in the immune response. *Adv Immunol 10*:1 (1969).

STEINER, L. A., and EISEN, H. N. Variations in the immune response to a simple determinant. *Bacteriol Rev 30*:383 (1966).

STERZL, J., and SILVERSTEIN, A. M. Developmental aspects of immunity. *Adv Immunol 6*:337 (1967).

WEIGLE, W. O. Immunological unresponsiveness. *Adv Immunol 16*:61 (1973).

WEISS, L. *The Cells and Tissues of the Immune System*. Prentice-Hall, Englewood Cliffs, N.J., 1972.

World Health Organization Technical Report No. 448: Factors regulating the immune response, 1969.

SPECIFIC ARTICLES

CRABBE, P. A., CARBONARA, A. O., and HEREMANS, J. F. The normal human intestinal mucosa as a major source of plasma cells containing IgA immunoglobulins. *Lab Invest 14*:235 (1965).

DAVIE, J. M., and PAUL, W. E. Receptors on immuno-
competent cells V. Cellular correlates of the "maturation" of the immune response. *J Exp Med 135*:660 (1972).

GASSER, D. L., and SHREFFLER, D. C. Involvement of H-2 locus in a multigenically determined immune response. *Nature (New Biol) 235*:155 (1972).

HENRY, C., KIMURA, J., and WOFSY, L. Cell separation on affinity columns: The isolation of immuno-specific precursor cells from unimmunized mice. *Proc Nat Acad Sci USA 69*:34 (1972).

JULIUS, M. H., MASUDA, T., and HERZENBERG, L. A. Demonstration that antigen-binding cells are precursors of antibody-producing cells after purification with a fluorescence-activated cell sorter. *Proc Nat Acad Sci USA 69*:1934 (1972).

KINCAIDE, P., LAWTON, A., BODEMAN, I., and COOPER, M. Suppression of IgG synthesis as a result of Ab-mediated suppression of IgM synthesis in chickens. *Proc Nat Acad Sci USA 67*:1918 (1970).

MAGE, R. Quantitative studies on the regulation of expression of genes for Ig allotypes in heterozygous rabbits. *Cold Spring Harbor Symp Quant Biol 32*:203 (1967).

MISHELL, R. I., and DUTTON, R. W. Immunization of dissociated spleen cell cultures from normal mice. *J Exp Med 126*:423 (1967).

MITCHISON, N. A. The carrier effect in the secondary response to hapten-protein conjugates: I, II. *Eur J Immunol 1*:10 (1971).

RAJEWSKY, K., SCHIRRMACHER, V., NASS, S., and JERNE, N. K. The requirement of more than one antigenic determinant for immunogenicity. *J Exp Med 129*:1131 (1969).

SHEARER, G. M., MOZES, E., and SELA, M. Contribution of different cell types to the genetic control of immune responses as a function of the chemical nature of the polymeric side chains (poly-L-prolyl and poly-L-alanyl) of synthetic immunogens. *J Exp Med 135*:1009 (1972).

TAKAHASHI, T., OLD, L. J., MCINTYRE, K. R., and BOYSE, E. A. Immunoglobulin and other surface antigens of cells of the immune system. *J Exp Med 134*:815 (1971).

TAYLOR, R. B., DUFFUS, W. P. H., RAFF, M. C., and DEPETRIS, S. Redistribution and pinocytosis of lymphocyte surface Ig molecules induced by anti-Ig antibody. *Nature (New Biol) 233*:225 (1971).

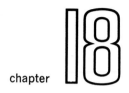

chapter 18

COMPLEMENT

Shortly after the discovery in the 1890s that immunity to diphtheria is due to serum antibodies (Abs) (Ch. 14), a curious observation led to the disclosure of another remarkable group of substances in serum that contribute to host defenses through modifying the behavior of diverse antibody-antigen (Ab-Ag) complexes. Pfeiffer observed that cholera vibrios disintegrated when injected into the peritoneal cavity of a guinea pig that had been previously immunized against the organism. The vibrios were also lysed within a few minutes in vitro when added to serum from the immunized animals. However, if the serum had been previously heated to 56° for a few minutes, or simply allowed to age for a few weeks, it lost its lytic activity, though its Abs were retained; and the addition of fresh **normal** serum to the inactivated antiserum restored its bacteriolytic capacity. Hence lysis required **both** specific Ab and a complementary, labile, nonspecific factor present in normal (as well as in immune) serum. Originally called **alexin** (Gr., "to ward off"), the unstable factor was subsequently named **complement;** it is referred to as **C.**

C is now known to consist of 11 proteins that make up about 10% of the globulins in normal serum of man and other vertebrates. These proteins are not immunoglobulins (Igs), and they are not increased in concentration by immunization. They react with a wide variety of Ab-Ag complexes, and exert their effects primarily on cell membranes, causing lysis of some cells and functional aberrations in others, e.g., degranulation of mast cells with release of histamine (Ch. 17), increased permeability of small blood vessels, directed migration of polymorphonuclear leukocytes, increased phagocytic activity by leukocytes and macrophages, and bacteriolysis.

Of these far-ranging effects, red cell lysis (hemolysis) has been analyzed in greatest de-tail, because it is so simple to measure; it also provides the basis for the C-fixation assay, an important laboratory procedure for detecting and measuring many different kinds of Ags and Abs.

THE COMPLEMENT-FIXATION ASSAY

In addition to the test Ag and antiserum the assay requires a number of standard reagents (referred to as the immunological zoo): **sheep** red blood cells, **rabbit** Abs to sheep cells (these Abs are also often called **hemolysins),*** and fresh **guinea pig** serum as a source of C. Guinea pig serum is more active than serum from other species; it is used promptly after collection, or it may be stored at $-70°$ or lyophilized.

If sheep erythrocytes in neutral isotonic salt solution are optimally coated with nonagglutinating amounts of Abs to the cells, the addition of C in the presence of adequate concentrations of Mg^{++} and Ca^{++} promptly causes the cells to lyse. The extent of lysis is evaluated qualitatively by inspection, or quantitatively by determining the concentration of supernatant hemoglobin after sedimentation of in-

---

* Rabbits immunized with intact sheep red cells form two kinds of hemolysins: **isophile Abs,** which are species specific (for determinants on red cells of sheep), and **heterophile** Abs, which are specific for the Forssman antigen, a glycolipid found in the red cells and tissue cells of many species in addition to sheep, and even in some bacteria (Ch. 21). In order to obtain more uniformly effective antiserum it is preferable to immunize rabbits with boiled stromata of sheep red cells, which evoke only the anti-Forssman (heterophile) Ab. The latter are almost entirely IgM, whereas the isophile Abs belong to both IgG and IgM classes. As noted later, the IgM are more efficient that the IgG hemolysins.

tact cells and stroma. Ab-coated ("sensitized") erythrocytes thus become indicators to detect active C. In general, when Abs combine with Ags in the presence of C some components of C are bound and inactivated. As a result, C activity, i.e., ability to lyse sensitized red cells, is lost.

C-fixation assays are therefore performed in two stages. **In stage 1** antiserum and Ag are mixed in the presence of a carefully measured amount of C and then incubated, usually for 30 minutes at 37° or overnight at about 4°. If the appropriate Ab-Ag complexes are formed C is inactivated or "fixed." **In stage 2** a suspension of sensitized red cells is added to determine whether active C has survived. **Hemolysis** indicates that C persists and, therefore, that an effective Ab-Ag reaction **has not** occurred in stage 1. Conversely, **absence of hemolysis** indicates that C has been fixed and, therefore, that an Ab-Ag reaction **has** occurred in stage 1 (positive C-fixation reaction). These steps are outlined in Figure 18-1. With a known Ag the assay can be used to detect (and measure) Abs in unknown sera; and with a standard antiserum to a known Ag it can be used to detect that Ag in complex biological materials.

Conditions of Assay. If the amount of C used in the assay is excessive, some active C may persist and cause hemolysis even though an Ab-Ag reaction has taken place in stage 1. On the other hand, if the amount of C added is insufficient, its deterioration may lead to the absence of lysis in stage 2 even if an Ab-Ag reaction has not occurred in stage 1. Accordingly, just the right amount of C is required.

Usually 5 units is an effective compromise in conventional assays (10^8 sensitized cells in a total reaction volume of 1.5 ml). The unit of C is discussed below.

The interpretation of the C-fixation assay depends on the outcome of a number of **controls.** For example, the Ag and the antiserum must be individually tested to ascertain that they are not "anticomplementary," i.e., that each does not inactivate C without the other.* To provide a margin of safety, anticomplementarity is tested with Ags or antiserum at a higher concentration than that used in the assay, and C is reduced to an amount that is just sufficient to lyse the indicator cells (Table 18-1). It is also essential to ascertain that the red cells do not lyse spontaneously, and that C survives stage 1 in the absence of an authentic Ab-Ag reaction.

Dependence on Mass and Ratio of Antibody-Antigen Complexes. The amount of C fixed depends not only on the mass of Ab-Ag complexes formed, but on their Ab/Ag ratio. When the ratio corresponds to that in the Ab-excess or the equivalence regions of the precipitin curve (Ch. 15) C is fixed most effectively.

---

* The most common artefact arises from anticomplementary properties of Ags and antisera. Particularly frequent with Ags prepared from tissue homogenates, this difficulty is especially troublesome with C-fixation assays in the serological diagnosis of diseases due to viruses, rickettsiae, and chlamydia, in which antigenic material is obtained from infected tissue. Undiluted or slightly diluted antisera are also frequently anticomplementary, usually owing to some denatured and aggregated Igs (below).

Fig. 18-1. Complement-fixation assay. Ab = antibody; Ag = the corresponding antigen; C = guinea pig complement; EA = sheep erythrocytes complexed with rabbit Abs to the cells (sensitized red cells) as indicator for active complement. C fixation has occurred in reaction (1) but not in reaction (2) or (3).

	STAGE 1		STAGE 2	
1.	Ab + Ag + C′ ⟶ Ab-Ag-C′		+ EA ⟶	No lysis
2.	Ab + C′ ⟶ Ab + C′		+ EA ⟶	Lysis
3.	Ag + C′ ⟶ Ag + C′		+ EA ⟶	Lysis

TABLE 18-1.   Complement-Fixation Test for Antibodies in Human Serum to Poliovirus*

Virus dilution	Serum dilution								Control with	
	1:10	1:20	1:40	1:80	1:160	1:320	1:640	1:1280	5 C'H$_{50}$	3 C'H$_{50}$
1:20	0	0	0	½	4	4	4	4	4	4
1:40	0	0	0	0	2	4	4	4	4	4
1:80	0	0	0	0	0	3½	4	4	4	4
1:160	0	0	0	0	0	0	4	4	4	4
1:320	0	0	0	0	0	0	2	4	4	4
1:640	0	0	0	0	0	0	1	4	4	4
1:1280	½	½	½	½	½	½	3	4	4	4
1:3200	4	3	3	3	3	3	4	4	4	4
1:6400	4	4	4	4	4	4	4	4	4	4
Control with										
5 C'H$_{50}$	4	4	4	4	4	4	4	4		
3 C'H$_{50}$	4	4	4	4	4	4	4	4		

* Assay with 5 C'H$_{50}$ units of complement; fixation at 4° for 20 hours before addition of sensitized indicator red cells. 0 = no lysis (positive C fixation); 4 = complete lysis (negative C fixation). The highest dilution of Ag (virus) that gives positive C fixation is 1:1280. A 1:640 dilution of serum gives positive C fixation with dilute virus (1:640), but with more concentrated virus the system is then in Ag excess and it is necessary to use less dilute serum. The Ag alone and the serum alone are not anticomplementary at any dilution examined, even when tested in controls with only 3 C'H$_{50}$ units of complement.

From M. Mayer *et al., J Immunol* 78:435 (1957).

When Ag is present in excess, however, fixation is less; and with Ag in extreme excess C is not fixed at all (see Fig. 18-3). Since information about optimal proportions is not generally available, C-fixation tests are best carried out by means of a "checkerboard titration," in which both Ag and antiserum concentrations are varied as shown in Table 18-1.

MEASUREMENT OF COMPLEMENT

The proportion of sensitized red cells that are lysed increases with the amount of C added (Fig. 18-2). Because 100% lysis is approached asymptotically it is convenient to **define the unit of complement (the C'H$_{50}$ unit) as that amount which lyses 50% of sensitized red cells** under conditions that are arbitrarily standardized with respect to concentration of sensitized cells, concentration and type of sensitizing Ab, ionic strength and pH of the solvent, concentrations of Mg^{++} and Ca^{++}, and temperature.

The dose-response curve of Figure 18-2 follows the von Krogh equation,

$$x = K \left(\frac{y}{1-y} \right)^{1/n}$$

in which x is the amount of C added (i.e., milliliters of guinea pig serum), y is the proportion of cells

lysed, and n and K are constants. The curve described by this equation (which was arrived at empirically) is sigmoidal when $1/n < 1$; for fresh normal guinea pig sera $1/n$ is usually about 0.2. In estimating the number of C'H$_{50}$ units per milliliter of guinea pig serum it is convenient to plot log x vs. log $(y/1—y)$; the data fall on a straight line,

$$\log x = \log K + \left(\frac{1}{n} \right) \log \frac{y}{1-y}$$

in which the intercept at 50% lysis ($y = 1—y$; log $y/1—y = 0$) gives the volume of guinea pig serum that corresponds to one C'H$_{50}$ unit.

THE QUANTITATIVE COMPLEMENT-FIXATION ASSAY

The amount of C fixed in a reaction between soluble Ag and Ab can be determined as the difference between the amount added and the amount remaining after the reaction has gone to completion. When the reaction of antiserum with increasing amounts of Ag is followed (Fig. 18-3), the amount of C fixed varies as the amount of precipitate in the precipitin reaction, increasing over the Ab-excess region to a maximum at the equivalence zone and then decreasing in the Ag-excess zone. The C reaction can thus be used as an alternative to the precipitin reaction, e.g., to measure quantitatively the concentrations of Ab or of Ag, or

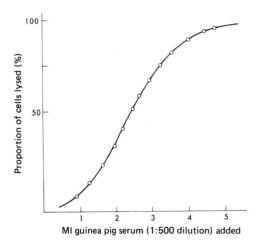

Fig. 18-2. Dose-response curve of immune hemolysis. The curve follows the empirical von Krogh equation (see text).

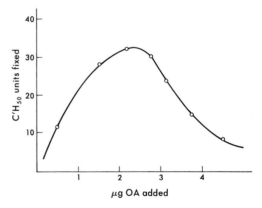

Fig. 18-3. Fixation of C by varying quantities of chicken ovalbumin (OA) and 12.5 μg Ab from rabbit antiserum to OA. Note resemblance to precipitin curves of Chapter 15, with decreasing C fixation in the region of Ag excess. [From Osler, A. G., and Heidelberger, M. *J Immunol* 60:327 (1948).]

to compare closely related Ags for their reactivity with a standard antiserum. C fixation offers the important advantage that it can be used with high precision to measure very small amounts of Ab or Ag, detecting as little as 0.5 μg of Ab. However, it measures the reactivity of only certain classes of Abs (see below), and it measures concentrations in relative rather than absolute weight units.

COMPETENT AND INCOMPETENT AB-AG COMPLEXES

The small complexes formed by Abs and univalent ligands do not fix C. But the aggregates formed with multivalent ligands of diverse chemical nature, size, and charge are effective. The almost limitless variety of effective Ags suggested that C reacts with the Ab moiety of Ab-Ag aggregates. Indeed, when Igs of an appropriate class (see below) are simply aggregated by heat or some other denaturing conditions they fix C in essentially the same way as when specifically cross-linked with multivalent Ags.

Igs from different species and of diverse classes differ greatly in ability to fix guinea pig C (which is used in most assays); e.g., cattle Igs are ineffective and those from some birds are only marginally active. Human antibodies of the IgG-1, IgG-2, IgG-3, and IgM classes are highly competent, while IgG-4, IgA, and IgE react only in a special way (Alternative

pathway for C activation, below). Since Igs of diverse classes have characteristically different heavy chains (Ch. 16), it seems likely that sites in these chains become exposed through conformational changes brought about when Ab molecules are aggregated by Ag or by denaturation.

REACTION SEQUENCE IN IMMUNE CYTOLYSIS

Various procedures destroy serum C activity, which can be restored when certain inactive preparations are recombined: hence it has long been apparent that C consists of more than one substance. From the 4 classic fractions (C'1, C'2, C'3, C'4), defined in Figure 18-4, 11 active proteins have been isolated; their properties are summarized in the same figure.

After one component (C1q) is bound by competent Ab-Ag complexes, the others react in an ordered sequence: in several steps an activated protein cleaves the next reacting member of the series into fragments, of which the largest usually also behaves as an activated proteolytic enzyme, cleaving and thereby activating the next protein in sequence. Some of the smaller proteolytic fragments have "phlogistic" activity (Gr. *phlogistos* = inflammatory): they cause inflammatory tissue changes, such as increased vascular permeability, and

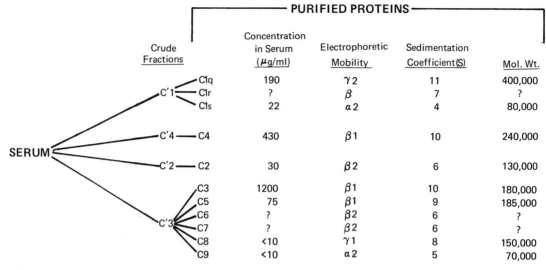

Fig. 18-4. Some properties of purified human C proteins. The four crude fractions (C′1 to C′4) were characterized originally by conditions that inactivated or removed them from fresh serum. C′1 and C′2 are extremely heat-labile: they are inactivated in a few minutes at 56° whereas inactivation of C′3 and C′4 at this temperature requires 20 to 30 minutes. C′1 is precipitated with "euglobulins" by dialysis against H_2O at pH 5, whereas C′2, a "pseudoglobulin," is soluble under these conditions. C′3 is inactivated by zymosan (see Alternate pathway for C activation, below) and C′4 by exposure to ammonia or hydrazine. C′1 to C′4 are numbered in order of discovery, which unfortunately is not the same as the order in which the components react in the C cascade (see Fig. 18-5). [Based in part on *Bull WHO 39*:935 (1968).]

attraction of polymorphonuclear leukocytes (chemotaxis). The reaction sequence is illustrated in Figure 18-5, and individual steps are discussed below. Activated C proteins with enzymatic activity are designated by an overbar (e.g., $\overline{C1}$ is the enzymatically active form of C1).

1. S + A ⇌ SA. Immune cell lysis is initiated by the specific binding of one IgM or one pair of IgG Ab molecules (A) (One-hit theory, below) to an antigenic site (S) on the cell surface, forming a "sensitized" cell. The surface Ag need not be a natural constituent of the cell membrane: in **passive hemolysis** soluble Ags or small haptens are attached artificially to the red cell membrane, and the cells are then sensitized with the corresponding Abs.

The requirement for a pair of adjacent IgG molecules implies that the effective antigenic determinants on the cell surface must be closely spaced (Fig. 18-5). Improper spacing could explain the inability of Abs to many cell surface Ags to cause lysis (for example, Abs to Rh and to some other antigens on red cells fail to sensitize for immune hemolysis; Ch. 21).

2. SA + C1 + Ca++ ⇌ SAC$\overline{1}$. With attachment to antigenic sites on the membrane, the Ab molecule probably undergoes a conformational change that

exposes sites in Fc domains of the heavy chain; these sites then interact specifically with C1. C1 exists in serum as an aggregate of three proteins—C1q, C1r, and C1s—which are associated noncovalently (in a mole ratio of 1:2:4) in a complex with Ca++. C1q, the **recognition** unit of the complex, consists of five subunits, each with one binding site for the heavy chains of those Ig classes (e.g., IgG-1, IgG-2, IgG-3, IgM) that can trigger the entire C sequence. In contrast, Abs that belong to Ig classes that do not react with C1q (e.g., IgG-4, IgA, IgE) cannot trigger the early steps in the C cascade; they can, however, activate the later-acting C components via an alternate pathway (below).

Unlike other C proteins, C1q has stable combining sites and requires no activation.* However, in binding to Igs, C1q probably undergoes a conformational change that results in modifying C1r, which in turn, converts C1s to a proteolytically active enzyme, C$\overline{1s}$, whose natural substrates are C4 and C2. (Like trypsin and some other proteases, C$\overline{1s}$ also has amino acid esterase activity, and its

---

* C1q is also unusual in its striking chemical similarity to collagen: i.e., it has a high content of glycine, hydroxyproline, and hydroxylysine, with a galactose-glucose disaccharide attached to the hydroxyl of hydroxylysine; and it can be inactivated by collagenase.

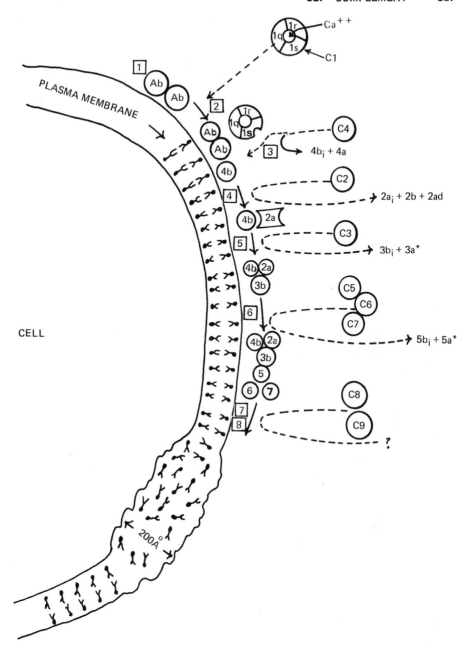

Fig. 18-5. Reaction sequence in lysis of a cell by activated C. The leaky lesions that develop after steps 7 and 8 probably correspond to "holes" (Fig. 18-6) and to local swellings of the membrane (ca. 200 A) seen in electron micrographs. The lesions could represent local perturbations in the membrane's lipid bilayer, due to a detergent-like effect of activated C8 and C9. Three activated components have enzymatic activity: C$\overline{1}$, C$\overline{4b,2a}$, C$\overline{4b,2a,3b}$. They cleave the following substrates: C2 and C4 (C$\overline{1}$), C3 (C$\overline{4b,2a}$) and C5 (C$\overline{4b,2a,3b}$). C5b,6,7, is commonly written with an overbar, as though it were an established enzymatic complex; however, its enzymatic activity has not been demonstrated. The numbers in boxes correspond to the numbered steps in the reaction sequence in text.

catalytic activities are blocked specifically by DFP, diisopropylphosphofluoridate.)

Only the C1 complexes, not the separated subunits, are activated by binding to Ab-Ag complexes. **The stability of the C1 complex depends on calcium ions (Ca^{++}), which are thus required for immune lysis of cells.** The binding of C1q, C1r, C1s (i.e., C1) to Ab-Ag complexes is reversible, and dissociated C1 can transfer to other SA sites. Chelating agents that bind Ca^{++} cause C1 complexes to come apart and to dissociate from Ab-Ag aggregates.

C1q can also form specific precipitates with soluble Ab-Ag complexes whose Ab moiety belongs to Ig classes that can bind and activate the C1 complex (IgG-1, IgG-2, IgG-3, IgM). This precipitation reaction is useful for detecting soluble immune complexes in diseases where they seem to be responsible for severe inflammatory lesions (e.g., Rheumatoid arthritis, Ch. 19).

3. $SAC\overline{1}$ + C4 → $SAC\overline{1,4b}$ + C4b + C4a. Two fragments result from the cleavage of C4 by the $C\overline{1s}$ moiety of $SAC\overline{1}$: inactive C4a (MW 15,000) and active C4b (MW 230,000). About 10% of C4b is bound by $SAC\overline{1}$, forming the next activated complex, $SAC\overline{1},4b$; the remaining C4b decays rapidly in solution ($C4b_i$). With the aid of ^{125}I-labeled C4, it has become clear that C4b binds to both the membrane-bound Ab and the membrane itself: some C4b can remain on the membrane after C1 is removed (by removing Ca^{++} with a chelating agent).

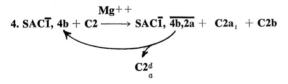

4. $SAC\overline{1}$, 4b + C2 $\xrightarrow{\mathrm{Mg}^{++}}$ $SAC\overline{1}$, $\overline{4b,2a}$ + $C2a_i$ + C2b

In the presence of Mg^{++} C2 is split by the $C\overline{1s}$ moiety of $SAC\overline{1},4b$. One fragment, C2a (MW 80,000), binds to the membrane complex, forming the next activated complex, $SAC\overline{1},\overline{4b,2a}$: the $C\overline{4b,2a}$ moiety of this complex is called **C3 convertase**, because it specifically and effectively attacks C3, which reacts next. With the formation of the C3 convertase, $C\overline{1}$ becomes unnecessary: it can be removed (by a chelating agent that withdraws Ca^{++} without affecting the remaining reactions in the complete sequence).

C2 is adsorbed on cell-bound C4b of $SAC\overline{1},4b$ before it is cleaved by $C\overline{1}$; this minimizes loss of C2a, which is readily inactivated in solution to $C2a_i$. The C2a moiety of $SAC\overline{1},4b,2a$ is also unstable (half life at 37° is 10 minutes): in dissociating from the complex (as inactive $C2_a^d$), it regenerates $SAC\overline{1},4b$ which can bind and cleave additional C2 to form more $SAC\overline{1},4b, 2a$.

5. $SAC\overline{1,4b,2a}$ + C3 → $SAC\overline{1,4b,2a,3b}$ + $C3b_i$ + C3a In this critical step the reaction is amplified, because each $SAC\overline{1,4b,2a}$ unit cleaves hundreds of C3 molecules into fragments. A small fragment, C3a (MW 7000), has pronounced phlogistic activity (see Anaphylatoxins, below). The large fragment, C3b, decays in solution (to $C3b_i$) or binds to the cell; however only those fragments that are bound in close proximity to $C\overline{4b,2a}$ can join in forming the new enzyme $C\overline{4b,2a,3b}$. The other C3b fragments, scattered over the cell membrane, are not involved in the hemolytic reaction but they contribute to immune adherence (below), which increases the cell's susceptibility to phagocytosis; i.e., C3b on the cell membrane is a potent **opsonic** agent (below).

6. $SAC\overline{1,4b,2a,3b}$ + C5·C6·C7 → $SAC\overline{1,4b,2a,3b,5b,6}$ $+C5b_i$ + C5a. In this step activated $C\overline{4b,2a,3b}$ in the $SAC\overline{1-3b}$ complex cleaves C5. A small fragment, C5a (MW 15,000), has some of the phlogistic activity of C3a (Anaphylatoxins, below); in addition, it is a powerful attractant for polymorphonuclear leukocytes (see Chemotaxis, below; and Arthus reaction, Ch. 19). About 10% of the larger activated fragment, C5b, combines with C6, and the complex then binds C7 to form the ternary complex C5b,6,7 on the cell membrane at or near the $SAC\overline{1-3b}$ complex; the remaining C5b in solution becomes rapidly inactive ($C5b_i$). Membrane-bound C5b,6,7 is the initiator of the hemolytic steps (7 and 8, below); and like C5a, it is chemotactic for polymorphonuclear leukocytes. This complex is unstable in solution, but it is possible that traces bind to non-sensitized "bystander" cells, whose subsequent reaction with C8 and C9 (below) would then lead to lysis.

7. $SAC\overline{1,4b,2a,3b,5b,6,7}$ + C8 → $SAC\overline{1-8}$. Following the binding of C8, cells with $SAC\overline{1-8}$ complexes may develop functional membrane lesions and undergo slow lysis at 37°.

8. $SAC\overline{1,4b,2a,3b,5b,6,7,8}$ + C9 → $SAC\overline{1-9}$. In this terminal step, up to six molecules of C9 are bound per $SAC\overline{1-8}$ complex (though one suffices for full activity) and the rate of cell lysis becomes greatly accelerated: small, intracellular molecules leak out of the cell and extracellular water enters rapidly, causing the cell to swell and to rupture its membrane.

Membrane Lesions. After binding C5-C9, the red cell membrane acquires circular lesions (Fig. 18-6) that could perhaps correspond to leaky foci. While these lesions could be due to a direct enzymatic attack on the membrane by activated C, it seems more likely that they

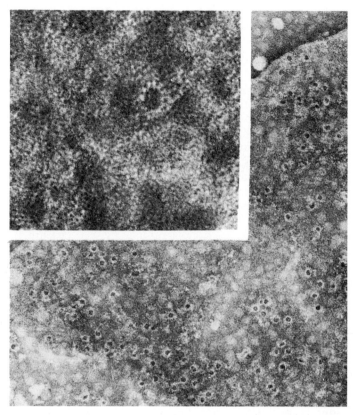

Fig. 18-6. Electron micrograph of the membrane of a sensitized sheep red cell lysed by C. Many defects ("holes") are evident. ×187,000 (reduced). Inset shows a representative lesion at greater magnification (×720,000, reduced). Preparations by R. Dourmashkin. (From Humphrey, J. H., and Dourmashkin, R. R. In *Complement.* Ciba Foundation Symposium, G. E. W. Wolstenholme and J. Knight, eds. Little, Brown, Boston, 1965.)

arise from a detergent-like action of hydrophobic patches present on activated late-acting proteins (C8,C9). Thus, membranes treated with the hydrophobic polyene antibiotic filipin (Ch. 7) develop indistinguishable circular lesions. Moreover, when completely synthetic model membranes (liposomes) with incorporated Ags are lysed by C plus Abs no covalent changes have been found in the lipids or other constituents.

Unlike red cells, nucleated cells are not usually lysed by bound, activated C but their membranes become damaged and leaky: K+ and small organic molecules (e.g., AMP) escape before macromolecules. A readily detectable change is the entry of ionic dyes that are excluded by intact cells. Hence dyes like trypan blue and eosin are often used to detect C-damaged (i.e., stained) lymphocytes and other nucleated cells.

THE ONE-HIT THEORY

The sigmoidal dose-response curve (Fig. 18-2) originally suggested that lysis depends on the accumulation of many damaged sites (S*) per cell. However, Mayer and his colleagues have provided evidence that one S* lesion per red cell is sufficient. Thus with a limiting amount of complement the extent and velocity of hemolysis is independent of the total number of sensitized cells in the reaction mixture. Moreover, with SA, or with SAC$\overline{1}$, or with SAC$\overline{1}$,4, the average number of lytic lesions per cell is linearly related to the concentration of C1, or C4, or C2, respectively. (The average number of lytic lesions per red cell is calculated from the proportion of red cells that are not lysed, by applying the Poisson distribution.† Similarly, the activation and binding of C1 is linearly related to the concentration of IgM antibodies to red cells or to the square of the concentration of the corresponding IgG antibodies (Fig. 18-7). These linear relations indicate that **the S* site is established by the binding of one IgM or one pair of IgG antibody molecules, followed by one molecule each of C1, C4, and C2.** This is sufficient to activate and bind many molecules of C3 and the remaining C components and to cause lysis.

The sigmoidal shape of the hemolytic dose-response curve (Fig. 18-2), which had constituted the principal basis for interpreting immune hemolysis as a multi-hit or cumulative process, has been reconciled with the one-hit theory by considering the properties of SACĪ,4b,2a. This complex undergoes two competing reactions (step 4, above): one hindering hemolysis, with loss of C2a; and the other, by activating C3, producing the next complex in the sequence. The loss of C2a is a unimolecular reaction, with a fixed half life at a given temperature, whereas the rate of reaction with C3 is exponentially dependent on the C3 concentration, and is greatly augmented by high concentrations of this component. Qualitatively, at least, these relations account for the sigmoidal shape of the dose-response curve.

ALTERNATIVE PATHWAY FOR COMPLEMENT ACTIVATION

Additional opportunities for C to participate in immune reactions are provided by an alternative mechanism for inducing phlogistic activities by initiating the C sequence with C3, without triggering the sequence through C1, C4, C2. In this pathway various initiators (see below) apparently react with the properdin system (see below) and bring about the formation of a proteolytically active substance ("C3 activator") that cleaves C3 in the same way as C4b, 2a (Fig. 18-7). With the forma-

tion of C3b, the remaining C proteins (C5-C9) can probably be sequentially modified as in the classic hemolytic sequence. This **bypass sequence** (C3-C9) is scarcely able to cause cell lysis, however, because C5b,6,7 decays rapidly in solution; nevertheless, the phlogistic activity of the C3-C9 sequence might be as great as in the complete C1-C9 system.

Initiators of the bypass sequence include endotoxin (lipopolysaccharide of cell walls of gram-negative bacteria), zymosan (polysaccharide from yeast cell walls), and aggregated Abs of those Ig classes (e.g., human IgG-4, IgA-1, IgA-2, IgE, and guinea pig γ1) that cannot trigger the classic hemolytic sequence because they are incapable of binding C1q. Abs that initiate the bypass sequence also differ from those (IgM, IgG-1, -2, -3) that initiate the complete sequence via C1 in the location of the relevant heavy-chain sites: from the effects of pepsin digestion (Fig. 16-6, Ch. 16), it appears that these sites are located in the Fc domain of the C1q-reactive Abs and in the F(ab′)₂ region of Abs that initiate the bypass sequence.

The Properdin System. Pillemer *et al.* argued in the 1950s that certain non-Ab, normal serum proteins, which they called the properdin system (Gr. *perdere* = to destroy), were necessary for both degradation of C3 by zymosan and for some antimicrobial activities of normal serum, e.g., killing *Shigella dysenteriae* and neutralizing some viruses. Others dismissed these proteins as natural C-fixing Abs (for zymosan and some bacterial Ags); but 15 years later properdin was purified and shown not to be an Ig (i.e., it does not react with antisera to Igs).

The steps by which aggregated Igs of certain classes and other initiators activate the properdin system are not known. Nonetheless, this system and the early-acting C1, C4, C2 components of the classic C-reaction sequence seem to represent **alternative pathways** for triggering the biologically most effective components of the C system—i.e., C3 and late-acting proteins (Fig. 18-7).

The properdin system is now known to consist of properdin itself and at least three other serum proteins, called A, B, and the 0° factor. All are needed for an as yet undefined reaction sequence, triggered by various initiators (zymosan, certain aggregated Igs), that culminates in cleavage of C3 (Fig. 18-7).

---

† $P(k) = e^{-m} \, m^k/k!$, where $P(k)$ is the proportion of cells with k lytic lesions per cell, m is the average number of lytic lesions per cell, and e is the base of natural logarithms. Unlysed cells have no lytic lesions ($k = 0$); their frequency is e^{-m} (because $0! = 1$), and $m = -2.303 \log_{10} P(0)$. For more on the Poisson distribution, see Ch. 44, Appendix.

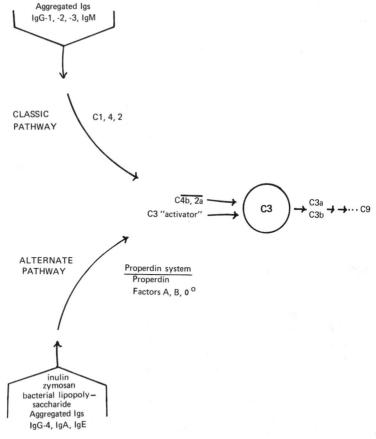

Fig. 18-7. The properdin system as the alternative pathway for activating C3 and late acting components. Different classes of immunoglobulins activate the two pathways. Cobra venom can also bring about cleavage of C3 by activating factor B of the properdin system.

Activation of factor B (also called C3 proactivator) appears to be directly involved in generating the C3-cleaving activity. The resulting C3b fragments probably account for the properdin system's antimicrobial activities: the fragments are powerful potentiators of phagocytosis (Opsonization, below), and they can probably also trigger the activation of later-acting C components (C5-C9).

Other Proteases. Besides "C3 activator" in the properdin system and C4b,2a in the classic system, C3b and C3a can be formed from C3 by certain other proteases; e.g., those released from lysosomes of degenerating polymorphonuclear leukocytes or from some bacteria (β-hemolytic streptococci), and some of those involved in blood clotting (below).

Blood Clotting and C. The activation of C probably always occurs to some extent during blood coagulation, in which plasminogen (a serum proenzyme) is converted to plasmin, a trypsin-like protease. Plasmin (like trypsin) can initiate the C sequence by converting C1 to C1, and by cleaving C3 to C3a and C3b. Kallikrein, another serum protein activated during blood clotting (see Kinins, Ch. 19), can also activate C1 to C1. A more direct connection between C and clotting has been revealed by the finding that C6 is required for normal clot formation: blood from rabbits with a genetic deficiency of C6 (see below) clots very slowly, and the addition of purified C6 corrects this defect.

OTHER REACTIONS
MEDIATED BY COMPLEMENT

Though cell lysis has dominated the study of C, the main physiological effects of activated

C are related to cellular and tissue changes associated with inflammation: e.g., increase in capillary permeability (anaphylatoxin activity), and directed migration (chemotaxis) and enhancement of phagocytic activity of polymorphonuclear leukocytes (Table 18-2). Because these phlogistic activities are generated in the immediate vicinity of the Ab-Ag complexes that activate C they lead to increased local concentrations of immunoglobulins, C, and "activated" phagocytes. The resulting destruction or containment of pathogens is probably more important to host defenses than is cell lysis itself, especially since many bacteria and probably most viruses are not susceptible to the lytic action of C (Bactericidal reactions, below).

Anaphylatoxins. This term is derived from the old observation that guinea pigs can undergo fatal shock, resembling anaphylaxis (Ch. 19), when injected with normal serum that has been incubated briefly with various substances (e.g., inulin, Ab-Ag complexes, talc). The effect was attributed to the appearance in the incubated serum of "anaphylatoxins," which have recently been identified as the small polypeptides cleaved from C3 and C5 during C activation (C3a and C5a).

The effects of C3a and C5a arise largely from their degranulation of mast cells with release of histamine; this causes (among other effects) a marked increase in capillary permeability (Ch. 19). Injection of C3a into human skin promptly elicits a wheal, and the effect can be specifically blocked by antihistamine drugs (Ch. 19).

C3a consists of the 60 N-terminal amino acid residues of C3; C5a is twice as long and probably represents the corresponding segment of C5. Both polypeptides have C-terminal arginine, indicating their origin from a trypsin-like attack of C$\overline{4b,2a}$ on C3 and of C$\overline{4b,2a,3b}$ on C5 (Fig. 18-5). The C-terminal arginine is required for anaphylatoxin activity, which is lost when just this residue is removed by a specific serum enzyme, called **anaphylatoxin inhibitor.**

Though similar in origin, activity, and structure, C3a and C5a seem to act on different mast cell receptors: isolated guinea pig ileum treated repeatedly in vitro with C3a loses its responsiveness to this substance ("tachyphylaxis"), but still responds to C5a, and vice versa. Both peptides are active at extremely low concentrations (1×10^{-8} to 5×10^{-10} M): human C5a is about 4 times more potent than C3a, but human serum contains about 20 times more C3 than C5 (Fig. 18-4).

Chemotaxis. With diffusion chambers divided into compartments by porous membranes that pass macromolecules but not cells, it has been shown that certain C derivatives in one compartment attract polymorphonuclear leukocytes from the adjacent compartment. This

TABLE 18-2. Principal Activities of Activated Complement (C) Proteins and Their Fragments

Activity	C protein or fragment
Anaphylatoxin: Histamine release from mast cells and increased permeability of capillaries	3a; 5a
Chemotaxis: Attract polymorphonuclear leukocytes	5a; $\overline{5b}$, 6, 7; ?3a
Immune adherence and opsonization: Adherence of Ab-Ag-C complexes to leukocytes, platelets, etc., increasing susceptibility to phagocytosis by leukocytes and macrophages	3b; 5b
Membrane damage: Lysis of red cells; leakiness of plasma membrane of nucleated cells; lysis of gram-negative bacteria	8; 9

chemotactic activity is exhibited by C5a, the ternary complex $C\overline{5b,6,7}$ (see step 6, above), and probably also by C3a. This activity is neither stimulated by histamine nor blocked by antihistamine drugs (see Ch. 20, Fig. 20-11).

Immune Adherence and Opsonization. The binding of C3b to Ab-Ag aggregates and to Ab-sensitized cells causes them to adhere to polymorphonuclear leukocytes, macrophages, and certain other cells (e.g., platelets, primate red blood cells). This "immune adherence" is probably responsible for the **opsonic activity** of C3b: i.e., the increased susceptibility to phagocytosis of bacteria, enveloped viruses, and other particles with Ab and C3b on their surface. An undefined serum protein can specifically inactivate and reverse the opsonic activity of soluble or cell-bound C3b.

Bactericidal Reactions. Gram-negative bacteria coated with specific antibody can be lysed by C acting through the same reaction sequence as in red cell lysis. **Gram-positive bacteria and mycobacteria, however, are not susceptible to the lytic action of complement,** and the basis for their resistance is not understood.

A cytotoxic C reaction is used in clinical diagnosis to detect Abs to the treponemes that cause syphilis. Here, however, the reaction leads not to immediate lysis but to loss of motility (*Treponema pallidum* immobilization, TPI test, Ch. 37).

Tissue Destruction. Though activation of C potentiates the defensive function of Abs, it can also cause severe damage to normal tissues. In some allergic disorders (especially those involving small blood vessels and glomeruli) the binding and activation of C by otherwise innocuous Ab-Ag complexes attracts leukocytes, whose subsequent degeneration releases lysosomal enzymes, causing local necrosis of host tissues (Arthus reaction, Ch. 19).

Immune Conglutination. A variety of Ab-Ag-C complexes are specifically precipitated by "immune conglutinin," an Ab (of the IgM class) specific for activated C3 and C4. Present in low titer in most normal sera, the level of immune conglutinin increases after various infections and after immunization with many Ags. This anti-C antibody is directed against hidden determinants in native C3 and C4, which become exposed when these proteins are activated and bound by Ab-Ag complexes. Since a given individual's activated C reacts with his own immune conglutinin, it could be regarded as autoantibody (Ch. 17).

Conglutination. Antibody–red cell–C complexes are agglutinated by a protein, **conglutinin,** which is present in the serum of certain mammals (cattle, other ruminants). The biological significance of conglutinin is not known: its formation is not increased by immunization, and it is not an Ig. It specifically binds some sugar residues of C3 (which is a glycoprotein) in a reaction that requires Ca^{++}.

COMPLEMENT DEFICIENCIES

Since C activation augments the protective role of antibodies against infectious agents, individuals deficient in C proteins should be unusually susceptible to infections. Severe, recurrent pyogenic infections have been observed in rare persons with markedly depressed serum levels of C3 (due to its excessive degradation or genetically determined absence) or with a heritable defect in C5. Surprisingly, infections have not been troublesome in human families and strains of animals with heritable deficiencies of C2 or C5 in man, C4 in guinea pigs, C5 in mice, or C6 in rabbits (Table 18-3), perhaps because a normal level of C3 and the bypass mechanism for its activation are sufficiently protective. C6-deficient rabbits give poor Arthus reactions, supporting other evidence that late-acting C components are necessary for this allergic reaction (Ch. 19).

Hereditary Angioedema. Humans with this disease are deficient not in C but in a carbohydrate-rich glycoprotein that inhibits activated $C\overline{1}$ (i.e., $C\overline{1s}$). This disorder is inherited as an autosomal dominant trait and affected individuals suffer periodically from acute and transitory local accumulations of edema fluid, which can become life-threatening when localized in the larynx, where they obstruct the tracheal airway. Serum obtained from patients during attacks has increased $C\overline{1s}$ activity (reflected in increased amino acid esterase activity) and decreased C4 and C2. Injected into skin, the serum also causes increased permeability of cutaneous blood vessels (hives, Ch. 19). The responsible factor is a small polypeptide, "C-kinin," which is split from C2 by $C\overline{1s}$; its activity resembles that of bradykinin (a nonapeptide that increases capillary permeability, see Ch. 19), but the two are distinguishable by radioimmunoassay (Ch. 15). Acute attacks seem to be triggered by activation of Hageman factor

TABLE 18-3.   Complement-Deficiency States

Primary deficiency	Species	Associated with	
		Increased susceptibility to infection	Comments
C1 inhibitor	Man	No	Become deficient in C1,C4,C2
C2	Man	No	Heritable defect with C2 about 5% of normal serum level
C3	Man	No	Heritable partial defect; two patients had severe recurrent infections
C5	Man	No	Heritable defect revealed by decrease in serum enhancement of phagocytosis in vitro; only 1 in 15 affected members in one family had recurrent infections
C4	Guinea pig	No	
C5	Mouse	No	
C6	Rabbit	No	Blood coagulation defect corrected by purified C6

(the plasma protein that initiates clotting), which causes the activation of two serum proenzymes: plasminogen and prekallikrein (Ch. 19). The resulting proteases, plasmin and kallikrein, activate C1 (and also C3), and thereby the remaining C sequence, resulting in formation of anaphylatoxin and liberation of histamine. Kallikrein, in addition, cleaves bradykinin from a serum protein substrate and thereby also releases histamine (Ch. 19). Administration of ε-aminocaproate, an inhibitor of plasmin activation of C1, reduces the frequency of attacks and antihistamines reduce their intensity.

Cobra Venom Factor. Anomalous immune reactions in C-deficient individuals help clarify the normal function of C. Since animals with genetic or congenital deficiencies (above) are not always available, soluble Ab-Ag complexes, formed in vitro, have been injected to deplete normal C levels (with simultaneous administration of antihistamines to prevent anaphylaxis due to production of anaphylatoxin and massive release of histamine; see Aggregate anaphylaxis, Ch. 19). However, the most selective and prolonged depletion (of C3) is brought about with venom from the cobra (*Naja naja* or *N. haja*). Depletion of C3 blocks certain allergic reactions (Arthus) but not others (cytotropic anaphylaxis, delayed-type hypersensitivity; Chs. 19 and 20).

The active component, cobra venom factor or CoF (MW 140,000), forms a complex with a β-globulin in serum (probably factor B of the properdin system). The complex, like C3 "convertase" (C4b,2a), cleaves C3 into a small (C3a) and a large (C3b) fragment. Intact C3 is thus eliminated and remains completely undetectable for 4 to 96 hours. Other C components are hardly affected.

CODA

The reaction of antibodies with antigens on cell surfaces is often followed by cell lysis and by extensive inflammatory changes in tissues (vasodilation, increased vascular permeability, accumulation and increased phagocytic activity of leukocytes). These changes are due to complement (C), a set of eleven proteins (C1q, C1r, C1s, C2 . . . C9) that normally exist in inactive form in serum. Except for C1q (which initiates the classical sequence of reactions), the other C proteins are converted one after the other from inactive to activated forms, some of which are enzymes whose substrate is the next protein in the sequential chain reaction. An alternative set of reactions, involving another group of four serum proteins, the properdin system, can bypass the early proteins (C1q, C1r, C1s, C2, C4) and trigger the sequence by activating C3, which then fires the other components (C5 to C9). Aggregated immunoglobulins of some classes (e.g., IgG-1, IgG-2, IgG-3, IgM) can activate the entire sequence via C1q; but others (e.g., IgG-4, IgE) seem to activate the sequence via the alternative or bypass (properdin) system.

Many of the inflammatory (phlogistic) effects of the C sequence can be accounted for by individual components or their activated products: C3b on the surface of a cell (or virus?) is a powerful opsonic agent, increasing susceptibility to phagocytosis by polymorphonuclear leukocytes and macrophages; C3a and C5a cause vasodilation and increase capillary permeability (anaphylatoxin activity); C5a, C5b·6·7, and probably C3a, attract leukocytes (chemotactic activity); C8 and especially C9 can cause severe damage to cell membranes (cytotoxic activity), resulting in lysis of some cells.

The cytotoxic effects of activated C are almost entirely confined to cells with antibodies bound to the cell membrane (sensitized cells). Neighboring cells, without bound antibody, are spared because the activated C proteins deteriorate rapidly in solution.

The importance of the C system to host defenses against microbial pathogens is brought out by the increased susceptibility to infections of rare persons with depressed serum levels of C3 and C5. But many humans, mice, and rabbits with heritable deficiencies in C2, C5, or C6 seem not to be especially troubled by infections, perhaps because a normal level of C3 is sufficiently protective. Though largely beneficial, the C system can also cause damage in tissues around otherwise benign Ab-Ag aggregates, by causing local accumulation of leukocytes whose degeneration releases destructive lysosomal enzymes. Thus C amplifies both the protective effects of Abs and their occasional capacity to cause tissue damage (hypersensitivity).

SELECTED REFERENCES

BOOKS AND REVIEW ARTICLES

ALPER, C. A., and ROSEN, F. S. Genetic aspects of the complement system. *Adv Immunol 14*:252 (1971).

GIGLI, I., and AUSTEN, K. F. Phylogeny and function of the complement system. *Annu Rev Microbiol 25*:309 (1971).

KINSKY, S. C. Antibody-complement interaction with lipid model membranes. *Biochim et Biophys Acta 265*:1 (1972).

LEPOW, I. H. Biologically Active Fragments of Complement. In *Progress in Immunology*. (D. B. Amos, ed.) Academic Press, New York, 1972.

MAYER, M. M. Highlights of complement research during the past 25 years. *Immunochemistry 7*:485 (1970).

MÜLLER-EBERHARD, H. J. Biochemistry of Complement. In *Progress in Immunology*. (D. B. Amos, ed.) Academic Press, New York, 1972.

SPECIFIC ARTICLES

ALPER, C. A., ABRAMSON, N., JOHNSTON, R. B., JANDL, J. H., and ROSEN, F. S. Increased susceptibility to infection associated with abnormalities of C-mediated functions of the 3rd component of C (C3). *N Eng J Med 282*:349 (1970).

MAYER, M. M., MILLER, J. M., and SHIN, H. S. A specific method for purification of the 2nd component of guinea pig C and a chemical evaluation of the one-hit theory. *J Immunol 105*:327 (1970).

MILLER, M. E., and NILSSON, U. R. A familial deficiency of the phagocytosis-enhancing activity of serum related to a dysfunction of the 5th component of C. *N Eng J Med 282*:354 (1970).

MÜLLER-EBERHARD, H. J. The molecular basis of the biological activities of C. *Harvey Lect* (1973).

NAFF, G. B., PENSKY, J. and LEPOW, I. H. The macromolecular nature of the 1st component of human C. *J Exp Med 119*:593 (1964).

ROMMEL, F. A., GOLDLUST, M. B., BANCROFT, F. C., MAYER, M. M., and TASHJIAN, A. H. Synthesis of the 9th component of C by a clonal strain of rat hepatoma cells. *J Immunol 105*:396, (1970).

SANDBERG, A. L., OSLER, A. G., SHIN, H. S., and OLIVEIRA, B. Biological activities of guinea pig antibodies. II. Modes of C interaction with γ1 and γ2 immunoglobulins. *J Immunol 104*:329 (1970).

SHIN, H. S., SNYDERMAN, R., FRIEDMAN, E., MELLORS, A. and MAYER, M. M. Chemotactic and anaphylatoxic fragment cleaved from the 5th component of guinea pig C. *Science 162*:361 (1968).

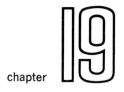

chapter 19

ANTIBODY-MEDIATED (IMMEDIATE-TYPE) HYPERSENSITIVITY

For some years after the discovery of anti-toxins and antimicrobial antibodies (Abs) the immune response appeared to be purely protective. Though it was found soon thereafter that the same mechanism could be activated by innocuous substances, such as milk proteins, it probably came as a surprise when Portier and Richet showed, in 1902, that immune responses also possess dangerous potentialities.

While studying the toxicity of extracts of sea anemones these French investigators observed that dogs given a second injection, several weeks after the first, often became acutely ill and died with a few minutes. Richet called this response anaphylaxis (Gr. *ana* = against; *phylaxis* = protection) implying incorrectly that it represented an increase in susceptibility to a toxic substance rather than the expected increase in resistance.* Almost simultaneously, however, observers in the United States and in Germany noted similar responses in guinea pigs to widely spaced injections of nontoxic antigens (Ags); and with the increasing use of horse and rabbit antisera to treat various infectious diseases in man, diverse pathological consequences of the immune response soon become commonplace.

In an attempt to organize a chaotic set of observations von Pirquet introduced the term allergy (Gr., "altered action") to cover any altered response to a substance induced by previous exposure to it. Increased resistance, called immunity, and increased susceptibility, called hypersensitivity, were then regarded as opposite forms of allergy. Through usage, however, **"allergy" and "hypersensitivity" have become synonymous: both refer to the altered state, induced by an Ag, in which pathological reactions can be subsequently elicited by that Ag, or by a structurally similar substance.**

In previous chapters the administration of an immunogen to stimulate Ab formation was called immunization. Within the context of the allergic response, however, the immunogen or Ag is often referred to as the **allergen** or **sensitizer,** and immunization as sensitization; and the immunized individual, previously called immune, is called sensitive or hypersensitive or allergic. It will also occasionally be useful to emphasize the distinction between the substance used to establish the allergic state ("inducer") and that used to evoke the allergic response ("elicitor").

Two Basic Mechanisms. Allergic responses were originally divided into two classes, immediate and delayed, on the basis of the lag in their appearance—several minutes after the administration of Ag in one, and several hours or even a few days in the other. These terms are still used, but they are now endowed with a different meaning. Not only the reactions that appear within minutes, but also some of the more slowly evolving ones, are mediated by freely diffusible Ab molecules. To emphasize this common feature both are now called **immediate type** (indicating that "immediate" is not to be taken literally). In contrast, the **delayed type** are those slowly evolving responses that are mediated by specifically reactive ("sensitized") T

---

* Magendie reported about 60 years earlier the sudden death of dogs repeatedly injected with egg albumin, and Flexnor noted shortly afterward that "animals that had withstood one dose of a foreign serum would succumb to a second dose given after the lapse of some days or weeks, even when this dose was not lethal for a control animal." These early discoverers of anaphylaxis were, however, overlooked; as often happens, valid observations were ignored until they could be accommodated within a conceptual framework.

lymphocytes rather than by freely diffusible Ab molecules; hence they are also called **cell-mediated hypersensitivity.** They constitute part of a larger group of reactions, called **cell-mediated immunity,** in which similar mechanisms are also involved in resistance to many infectious agents and to neoplastic cells.

In this chapter we consider the allergic reactions due to soluble Ab molecules, and in the next those due to sensitized lymphocytes. In allergy to drugs and in autoimmunity either reaction can be involved, and so a discussion of these clinically important subjects is postponed to the end of the next chapter.

Antibody-mediated Responses. The most important Ab-mediated responses are grouped in Table 19-1 on the basis of underlying mechanisms. The arrangement reflects the principle that mere **combination of Ab and Ag is seldom damaging unless the immune complexes trigger certain cells to release various mediators,** which serve as the immediate causes of pathological change. However, in special circumstances major aberrations follow the combination of Abs (and comple-

ment) with unusual Ags, without involving additional mediators (e.g., massive destruction of transfused red cells; Ch. 21).

ANAPHYLAXIS

Injection of a soluble Ag into a hypersensitive animal can cause an explosive response within 3 to 4 minutes. If the Ag is injected intravenously the response, called **systemic or generalized anaphylaxis,** can lead to shock, vascular engorgement, and asphyxia due to bronchial constriction; if death does not follow promptly recovery is complete within about 1 hour. If the Ag is injected into the skin the same type of reaction occurs in miniature form at the local site: called **cutaneous anaphylaxis,** it is characterized by transient redness and swelling, with complete return to normal appearance in about 30 minutes. Systemic and localized anaphylaxis occur not only in actively immunized ("sensitized") individuals, but also in those who are **passively sensitized** with certain antisera or purified Abs.

The basic mechanisms have been largely

TABLE 19-1.   Antibody-Mediated Allergic Reactions

		Mechanism	
Protype	Examples	Activated cells	Mediators released
I. Anaphylaxis	Anaphylactic shock Wheal-and-erythema responses Hayfever Asthma Hives	Mast cells Basophils* (platelets in some species)	Low moleculer weight, e.g., histamine (see Fig. 19-8)
II. Serum sickness	Arthus reaction Serum sickness syndrome Immune-complex diseases (glo-merulonephritis, ? rheumatoid arthritis, etc.)	Neutrophils*	High molecular weight, (lyso-somal enzymes)
III. Reactions to transfused blood	Red cell incompatibilities (e.g., maternal-fetal, as in Rh disease; Ch. 21) Autoantibodies to some self-Ags (Ch. 20; e.g., to platelets, or to antihemophilic globulin, caus-ing bleeding and purpura)	None	None

* The principal white blood cells (leukocytes) are polymorphonuclear granulocytes, monocytes (i.e., not fully differentiated macrophages), and lymphocytes. On the basis of affinity for various dyes the granulocytes are classified as neutrophils ($>95\%$), basophils (ca. 1%), or eosinophils (ca. 1%).

illuminated by experimental and clinical studies of passive cutaneous anaphylaxis, which can be elicited simply and safely at multiple sites in the same individual, providing ideal opportunities for controlled observations on the nature of the mediating Abs and Ags.

CUTANEOUS ANAPHYLAXIS IN MAN

The response begins 2 or 3 minutes after Ag is injected into the skin of a sensitive person: itching at the injected site is followed within a few minutes by a pale, elevated, irregular wheal surrounded by a zone of erythema (hive or urticarium). This **wheal-and-ery-thema** response reaches maximal intensity about 10 minutes after the injection, persists for an additional 10 to 20 minutes, and then gradually subsides (Fig. 19-1).

Fig. 19-1. Cutaneous anaphylaxis (wheal-and-erythema response) in man. Fifteen minutes before the photograph was taken the subject was injected intradermally with 0.02 ml containing about 0.1 μg protein extracted from guinea pig hair. Note the irregularly shaped wheal, with striking pseudopodia. The surrounding erythema is not easily visible in the photograph. No reaction is seen at the control site where 0.02 ml of buffer alone was injected.

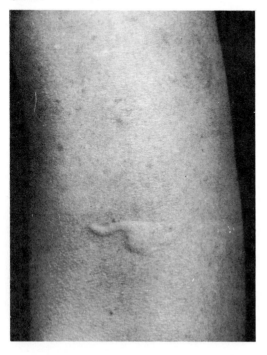

Atopy. A special group of persons, constituting about 10% of the population in the United States, is especially prone to hypersensitive responses of this type. These individuals readily become sensitive "spontaneously" (i.e., without deliberate immunization) to a variety of environmental Ags (often called **allergens),** such as airborne pollens of ragweed, grasses, and trees, and also to fungi, animal danders, house dust, and foods. When they inhale or ingest the appropriate allergen their response is prompt: most frequent and prominent among the manifestations are hayfever, asthma, and hives. The tendency to develop this form of allergy, called **atopy** (Gr., "out of place"), is heritable: it has been recognized in dogs and in cattle, and its genetic regulation is evident in inbred mouse strains (below).

Passive Transfer. Until the development of highly sensitive assays, such as passive hemagglutination (Ch. 15), the sera of atopic persons usually gave no detectable reactions with allergens in vitro. Nevertheless, these sera can, even after extensive dilution (1000-fold or more), sensitize passively the skin of normal persons. Passive sensitization is performed by injecting about 0.05 ml of serum (or serum dilution) from the sensitive donor into the skin (dermal layer) of a nonsensitive recipient. After 1 day, and up to as long as 6 weeks, injection of the corresponding Ag into the same skin site elicits the wheal-and-ery-thema response. To elicit the reaction it is usually necessary to allow a **latent period** of at least 10 to 20 hours after the injection of serum.

This transfer response is called the **Prausnitz-Küstner** or **P-K** reaction after those who first described it.* Patients are commonly tested for wheal-and-erythema responses to

---

* As described in 1921, Küstner was extremely sensitive to certain fish, but his serum gave no detectable reaction with extracts of these fish and did not sensitize guinea pigs for passive anaphylaxis. Prausnitz injected a small amount of Küstner's serum into a normal person's skin, and the injected site was tested 24 hours later with fish extract; the immediate appearance of a wheal-and-erythema response provided the basis for much of the clinical and experimental work on allergy of succeeding decades.

intradermal injections of extracts of plant pollens, fungi, food, animal danders, etc. to identify etiological Ags. P-K tests are sometimes used to avoid direct skin tests on young children or on adults with disseminated skin disease.

REAGINS AND BLOCKING ANTIBODIES

The appearance of atopic allergy depends upon the production of a special kind of Ab. Thus if ragweed extract is injected repeatedly into nonatopic human volunteers antiragweed Abs (predominantly of IgG class) appear in serum and may be detected by conventional assays, such as passive hemagglutination. However, these Abs are incapable of sensitizing human skin for wheal-and-erythema responses; instead, they combine with Ag and specifically **block** its ability to evoke this response in a sensitive person's skin (or in a normal person's skin at a P-K site). These **blocking antibodies** differ substantially from the **skin-sensitizing Abs, called reagins,** that

cause the wheal-and-erythema reaction (Table 19-2). Thus the reagins are heat-labile and do not cross the human placenta, whereas blocking Abs (like IgGs in general) are heatstable and readily cross the placenta. Most important, the sensitizing Abs persist at passively prepared (P-K) skin sites for up to 6 weeks, whereas blocking Abs diffuse away almost completely within 1 to 2 days. In addition to reagins, serum from atopic individuals usually contains some blocking Abs of the same specificity. Until the blocking Abs diffuse away they tend to competitively inhibit the reaction of injected Ag with reagin at P-K sites; the latent period in the P-K reaction probably also reflects the time required to fix reagin to tissue receptors (see Mast cells, below).

IgE IMMUNOGLOBULINS

Careful studies by the Ishizakas showed that rabbit antisera prepared against a reagin-rich serum fraction could precipitate and remove

TABLE 19-2. Comparison of Human Reagins and Blocking Antibodies To Pollen Antigens*

	Reagins	Blocking antibodies
Immunoglobulin class	IgE	IgG (predominantly)
Activity in Prausnitz-Küstner (P-K) test	Yes†	No (inhibits)
Persistence in human skin (P-K test)	Up to 6 weeks	Up to 2 days
Stability		
To heat (56°, 4 hr)	Labile	Stable
To sulfhydryls (0.1 M 2-mercaptoethanol)	Labile	Stable
Transfer across human placenta	No	Yes
Passive sensitization of guinea pigs for anaphylaxis	No	Yes†
Detection in in vitro assays	Radioimmunoassay	Hemagglutination and others
Molecular weight‡	185,000	150,000
Sedimentation coefficient ($S°_{20,w}$)	8.2	6.6
Carbohydrate‡	12%	3%
No. of amino acid residues per heavy chain‡	ca. 550	ca. 440
Heavy chains	ε	γ (predominantly)
Light chains	κ,λ	κ,λ

* Highly purified protein Ags have been isolated from ragweed and grass pollen extracts by ion-exchange chromatography. Several active fractions have been obtained from each extract, and different fractions are active in different persons. As little as 10^{-4} μg of some ragweed fractions evoke specific wheal-and-erythema responses. Fatal anaphylaxis has occurred on very rare occasions in response to skin tests with small amounts of crude extracts. Indeed, pollen antigen may be as potentially lethal (on a weight basis) for a pollen-sensitive person as botulinus toxin is for humans in general.

† Reagins are homocytotropic; blocking Abs are heterocytotropic (below).

‡ Values for reagins are those for an IgE myeloma protein.

reaginic activity from human atopic sera, even after the rabbit antisera had been completely freed of Abs to the then-known Ig classes by absorption with representative myeloma proteins (IgGs, IgA, IgM, IgD). They concluded that reagins belong to another Ig class, and this was then promptly verified by Johansson and Bennich's independent discovery in Sweden of an unusual human myeloma protein that also did not react with Abs to any of the then-known Ig classes, because of distinctive antigenic features of its heavy chain. An exchange of monospecific antisera between the two groups established that reagins and the rare myeloma protein belong to the same novel class, called IgE (Fig. 19-2).

A second IgE myeloma protein was subsequently identified in the United States, and myeloma cells from the Swedish patient were adapted to tissue culture where they continued for some time to produce their IgE. With these two crucial human proteins as immunogens, large amounts of anti-IgE sera have now

been prepared in rabbits and in goats. After absorption with human κ and λ light chains (to render them monospecific for ε chains) these antisera provide a key reagent for measurement of IgE in human sera and for diagnostic tests of human atopic allergy.

Serum IgE concentrations are measured by a form of radioimmunoassay in which anti-IgE is attached covalently to particles of an inert adsorbent which are then mixed with a standard amount of radioactive *IgE (labeled with ^{125}I) and the human serum to be tested. Unlabeled IgE in the test serum competitively reduces the specific binding of *IgE; hence radioactivity associated with the washed beads decreases in proportion to the serum IgE concentration (Fig. 19-3).

Another radioimmunoassay measures IgE antibodies of a particular specificity, e.g., to dog dander (epithelial scales). Protein extracts of the dander are coupled to Sephadex particles which are then trapped in small cellulose discs. The discs are incubated with about 0.05 ml of a patient's serum, washed, treated with radioactive anti-IgE (labeled with ^{125}I), washed, and counted. A positive test (adherent radioactivity) can detect a few nanograms

Fig. 19-2. Antigenic identity of reagins and an IgE myeloma protein. A reagin-rich fraction of human atopic serum was placed in the center well and antisera for each of the human Ig classes were placed in peripheral wells. Antisera to reagin and to the IgE myeloma gave reactions of identity. [From Ishizaka, K. *Immunoglobulins:* Biologic Aspects and Clinical Uses. E. Merler, ed. *Natl Acad Sciences,* Washington, D.C. (1970).]

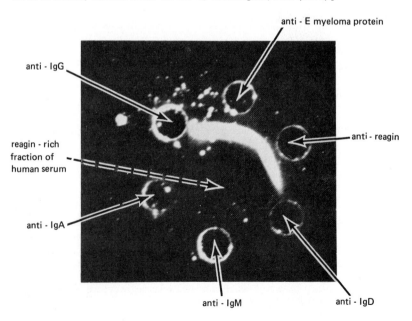

A Assay for total IgE

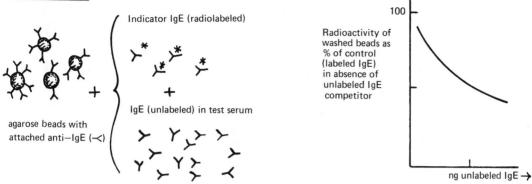

B Assay for IgE antibodies to antigen X

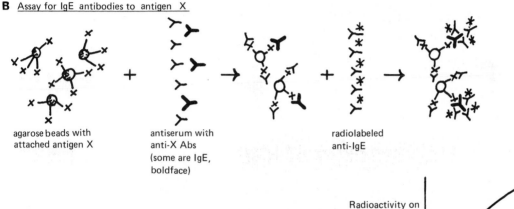

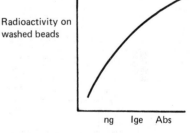

Fig. 19-3. Assays for total IgE concentration in serum **(A)** and for IgE antibodies of a particular specificity (anti-X) **(B)**. IgE molecules (in heavy type) function as Ag in the assay at top, and as both Ag and Ab in the one below.

per milliliter of IgE Abs of a particular specificity (Fig. 19-3).

In sera of atopic persons the IgE levels are often three or four times or more above the upper limit found in normal human sera, which is about 350 ng/ml. The extraordinarily low level of these biologically potent molecules (about 30,000-fold lower than the average normal concentration of IgG) ex-

plains why they were previously not detected in atopic sera that were highly active in P-K skin tests.

Chemical Properties of IgE. The IgE molecule has four chains: one pair of heavy ε chains plus one pair of κ or one pair of λ light chains. The ε chains are distinctive: they are longer than γ (approximately 540 and 440 amino acid residues, respectively), as though ε has an additional domain in its constant region (Ch. 16, Amino acid sequences), and they also have about three times more carbohydrate (Table 19-2). The differences account for the higher molecular weight of IgE than of IgG molecules. IgE and other Ig classes are compared further in the Appendix of Chapter 16.

Affinity for Mast Cells. IgE Abs have high affinity for receptors in skin: despite their extremely low concentration in serum they become attached to skin in P-K tests, and they can remain anchored for many weeks. The affinity apparently derives from sites in the Fc domain. Thus the Fc fragment of IgE myeloma protein (but not the Fab fragments) can specifically block P-K reactions, by competitively displacing reaginic Abs from skin receptors.

Immunofluorescence and radioautographs with radioactive IgE show that the tissue receptors are on **mast cells,** which are found in close association with capillaries in con-

nective tissues throughout the body. These cells are distinguished by their high content of histamine, which is concentrated in large cytoplasmic granules and is secreted as one of the key triggering events in anaphylaxis (see below, Fig. 19-9 and Chemical mediators). IgE also binds to **basophilic leukocytes** (basophils; Fig. 19-4). These cells make up ca. 1% of all blood leukocytes; they resemble mast cells in appearance and in histamine content and secretion. Other leukocytes do not bind IgE or contain histamine.

Homocytotropic vs. Heterocytotropic Antibodies. The immediate-type reactions mediated by special Abs that attach to mast cells are sometimes called **cytotropic anaphylaxis.** Because human IgE molecules (reagins) bind to human (and monkey) mast cells, but not to those of other species, they are called **homocytotropic antibodies.** Human blocking Abs, in contrast, are **heterocytotropic:** they can bind (fortuitously) to mast cells of some phylogenetically distant species (e.g., guinea

Fig. 19-4. Human IgE on the surface of a human basophil. Washed white blood cells were incubated successively (with intervening washes) with human IgE (a myeloma protein), burro antihuman IgE, hybrid 7S Abs (Ch. 16) in which one combining site was specific for burro Ig and the other for ferritin, and finally with ferritin—the iron-rich, electron-dense particles seen under brackets on the cell surface (see Ferritin-labeled Abs, Ch. 15). Basophil granules (BG is a typical one) resemble the histamine-containing granules of tissue mast cells (Fig. 19-9); basophils are the only blood leukocytes that bind IgE and contain and secrete histamine in response to specific binding of Ag or anti-IgE to the cell surface's IgE. Electron micrograph at ×77,500. [From Sullivan, A. L., Grimley, P. M., and Metzger, H. *J Exp Med 134:* 1403 (1971).]

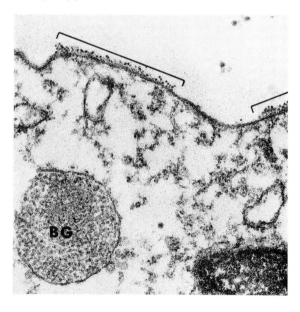
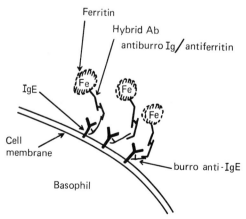

Fig. 19-5. Degranulation of mast cells and basophils and secretion of vasoactive amines by cross-linking IgE on the cell surface. The surface Abs are bound noncovalently via sites in Fc domain.

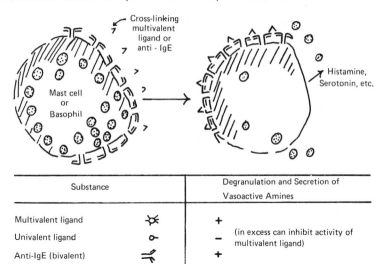

Substance		Degranulation and Secretion of Vasoactive Amines
Multivalent ligand		+
Univalent ligand		− (in excess can inhibit activity of multivalent ligand)
Anti-IgE (bivalent)		+
Anti-IgE F(ab′)$_2$ (bivalent)		+
Anti-IgE Fab′ (univalent)		− (in excess can probably inhibit activity of bivalent Ab or F(ab′)$_2$)

pigs) but not to human cells. In accord with these differences, human homocytotropic Abs can sensitize human (or monkey) skin and other tissues, but not those of guinea pigs, while human heterocytotropic Ags can sensitize guinea pigs but not humans.

Cross-linking of IgE. Aggregation of IgE molecules already bound to the mast cell surface probably initiates anaphylaxis (Fig. 19-5). Thus, when a skin site is passively sensitized with antihapten reagins the corresponding multivalent ligand can elicit a wheal-and-erythema response, but univalent ligands are usually specifically inhibitory, just as they competitively block the precipitin reaction in vitro.*

Other means of aggregating IgE on the cell surface are also effective. For example, the injection of anti-IgE Abs or their bivalent F(ab′)$_2$ fragments (but not their monovalent Fab′ fragments) can provoke wheal-and-erythema responses ("reverse cutaneous anaphylaxis"; Fig. 19-5). An injection of the aggregated Fc fragments of IgE myeloma

---

* Certain univalent ligands seem to elicit cutaneous anaphylaxis. It is unclear whether these ligands aggregate in tissues, and thus become functionally multivalent, or whether there is a special form of cutaneous anaphylaxis that can be evoked with non-cross-linked Ab-ligand complexes.

proteins (but not the monomeric Fc fragment) can also elicit the response, doubtless because they also bind to mast cells.

PROLONGED DESENSITIZATION

Atopic individuals form blocking Abs as well as reagins, especially after repeated injections of the Ag. Accordingly, such persons are commonly immunized ("desensitized") by repeated injections of small, increasing amounts of allergen, at intervals (e.g., weekly) and in doses that avoid systemic anaphylactic reactions. The level of blocking Abs, but not of reagins, often rises considerably. However, therapeutic benefits are not consistently evident, nor are they regularly correlated with the titers of blocking Abs.

Blocking Abs can be measured in atopic sera after heating (56°, 4 hours) to inactivate reagins; dilutions of the heated serum are then mixed with various amounts of Ag (e.g., pollen extract) and injected into passively sensitized (P-K) skin sites. The titer of blocking Ab is taken as the highest dilution of heated serum that inhibits the P-K reaction with a standard amount of allergen, or as the maximal amount of allergen that can be inhibited.

IgE and Intestinal Parasitism. While IgEs have obvious pathological effects, it is likely that they also have beneficial ones, contributing to their evolutionary development. A hint of benefits is suggested by the exceedingly high serum levels of IgE in persons with chronic parasitic infections: for instance, values of 3000 to 10,000 ng/ml (ca. 30 times average normal levels) are found in Africans and others with chronic intestinal roundworm infestations. With a relative abundance of IgE-producing plasma cells in the normal intestine* it is possible that IgE is especially effective in controlling intestinal parasites. The same relative abundance in the respiratory tract (which is derived embryologically from the fetal gut) probably contributes to the reactions underlying asthma and hayfever. Individuals that lack ability to synthesize IgE should provide opportunities to clarify the physiological role of IgE molecules.

---

* IgE-producing plasma cells are conspicuous in human surgical specimens of tonsils, adenoids, bronchial and intestinal mucosa; they are rare in spleen and lymph nodes. However, even in respiratory and intestinal tracts IgE-producing cells are greatly outnumbered by IgA producers.

CUTANEOUS ANAPHYLAXIS
IN THE GUINEA PIG

Cutaneous anaphylaxis can also be elicited in actively or passively sensitized guinea pigs. **Passive cutaneous anaphylaxis (PCA)** has been especially well developed by Z. Ovary into a powerful model system for evaluating abilities of various Abs and Ags to elicit anaphylactic responses. PCA and the human P-K reactions are fundamentally the same; but special measures are taken to increase visibility of the response in animal skin.

In PCA an antiserum (or purified Ab) is injected intradermally. After a latent period of several hours the corresponding Ag is injected intravenously along with a dye, such as Evans blue, that is strongly bound to serum albumin. Hence, as serum proteins rapidly pour into the dermis at the site of the reaction the response appears as an irregular circle of

Fig. 19-6. Passive cutaneous anaphylaxis in the guinea pig. In **A** the guinea pig was injected intradermally at three sites with 0.1 ml containing 1) 100 μg rabbit anti-chicken ovalbumin (Ea), 2) 10 μg anti-Ea, and 3) buffered saline. Four hours later 1.0 ml containing 2 mg Ea and 5 mg Evans blue was injected intravenously; the photo was taken 30 minutes later. Note blueing at 1 and at 2, and absence of blueing at the control site (3). In **B** a similar sequence was followed except that 30 minutes after the intravenous injection of Ea the animal was sacrificed and skinned. The photo was taken of the skin's undersurface. The amount of rabbit anti-Ea injected initially was 100μg (at 4), 10 μg (at 5), 1 μg (at 6), and 0.1 μg(at 7). The control site, which did not turn blue (8), had been injected with buffered saline. Another site (not shown) had been injected with 0.01 μg anti-Ea; it also failed to react.

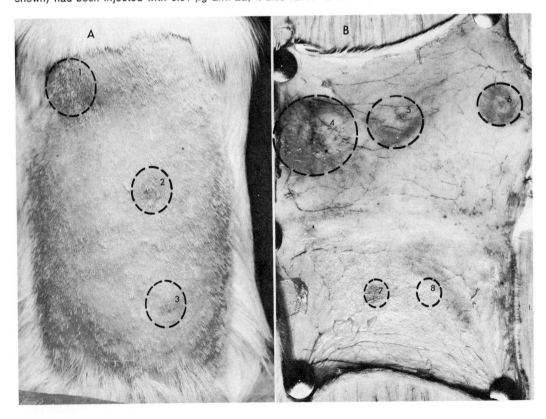

stained skin; the area is an index of the reaction's intensity (Fig. 19-6).

Two kinds of guinea pig Abs produce PCA reactions in guinea pigs: 1) reagins and 2) IgG molecules of the $\gamma 1$ subclass (Fig. 19-7). Both bind to mast cell surfaces and are **homocytotropic,** i.e., they sensitize guinea pigs but not other species. The reagins resemble human IgE: they are present at trace levels in serum (nanograms per milliliter), they persist at injected skin sites for weeks, and their skin-sensitizing activity is destroyed by sulfhydryl compounds and by heat (56°, 4 hours); they also cross-react with rabbit antisera to human IgE. In contrast, the homocytotropic $\gamma 1$ subclass of IgG is present at high levels in serum (milligrams per milliliter), is sulfhydryl- and heat-stable, and persists at injected skin sites for only 1 to 2 days.

The other major subclass of guinea pig IgG, called $\gamma 2$ (Fig. 19-7), is heterocytotropic: molecules of this subclass can sensitize mouse skin, but not guinea pig skin, presumably because they can fortuitously bind to and activate mouse mast cells.

PCA can be used to measure each of the foregoing Abs in a single sample of guinea pig serum. The response in mice measures $\gamma 2$ Abs (heterocytotropic), whereas PCA in guinea pigs measures the homocytotropic Abs: the Ag is injected into passively sensitized guinea pigs after a latent period of 3 or 4 hours to measure $\gamma 1$ molecules, and after 2 to 3 days to measure reagins. Alternatively, with PCA in guinea pigs, $\gamma 1$ molecules alone are measured in a heated test serum and $\gamma 1$ plus reagins in an unheated sample.

Many other species (rat, rabbit, dog, mouse) also have two classes of homocytotropic Abs (reagins and a heat-stable subclass of IgG, e.g., $\gamma 1$ in guinea pig and mouse and IgGa in rat); in man, however, only reagins have been identified so far. Abs of the IgM and IgA classes do not sensitize animals of the same or other species for anaphylactic responses.

GENETIC CONTROL OF REAGIN PRODUCTION

Inbred mouse strains differ in ability to produce reagins, indicating that their susceptibility to anaphylaxis, like atopy in man, is heritable. Such strains differ not only in reagin production but in over-all responses to low doses of Ag (0.1 to 1.0 μg/mouse), to which some strains make no Abs while others pro-

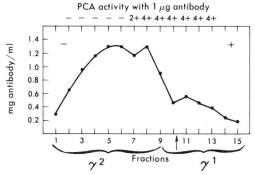

Purified guinea pig anti-Dnp-antibody

Fig. 19-7. Separation of homocytotropic from other Abs of the same specificity. Purified 7S guinea pig Abs, specific for the 2,4-dinitrophenyl (Dnp) group, were subjected to electrophoresis in starch (arrow marks point of application). Fractions eluted from 0.5-inch cuts of the starch block were tested for ability to mediate PCA in guinea pigs. The more anionic anti-Dnp molecules, called $\gamma 1$, mediated PCA, whereas the less anionic antibodies, called $\gamma 2$, did not. With a rabbit antiserum to guinea pig Igs, the $\gamma 1$ and $\gamma 2$ fractions are also distinguished antigenically. [Redrawn from Ovary, Z., Benacerraf, B., and Bloch, K. *J Exp Med 117*:951 (1963).]

duce both reagins and other Abs. Atopic persons similarly seem to differ from nonatopics primarily in ability to produce Abs (reagins and others) in response to natural exposure to trace amounts of environmental Ags, rather than exclusively in ability to form reagins.

Mouse strains that do not respond to low doses of Ag can produce reagins (and other Abs) in response to high doses (100 μg/mouse). Similarly, **with sufficient immunization nearly all persons can be actively sensitized to give wheal-and-erythema responses,** which can be elicited by the appropriate Ag in over 90% of persons injected with a sufficient quantity of horse serum (see Serum sickness syndrome, below), and in essentially all those recovering from pneumococcal pneumonia. Indeed, certain Ags, like extracts of *Ascaris* (a common nematode parasite in the intestine), seem able even with minimal immunization to sensitize nearly all persons to give wheal-and-erythema reactions.

One mouse strain (SJL) seems unable to form reagins to several Ags while able to produce Abs of other classes. Thus unlike Ir genes, which control ability to produce Abs (or cell-mediated immunity) of a particular specificity (Chs. 17 and 20), the "reagin genes" seem to regulate the ability to synthesize Abs of a particular class (IgE).

In crosses between the low-reagin strain and another strain all progeny formed high reagin titers, showing that reagin production is dominant. However, the progeny of back-crosses between the hybrids and the poor-producing parents (SJL) segregated into good, poor, and intermediate producers, suggesting that more than one gene controls reagin production.

GENERALIZED ANAPHYLAXIS

Systemic anaphylaxis in man is a rare event brought on occasionally in hypersensitive individuals by insect stings (especially bees, wasps, hornets), or by injection of horse serum or (more commonly at present) penicillin. Because of this hazard patients who receive foreign proteins (e.g., horse anti-toxin) or pencillin should first be questioned about previous allergic reactions, and sometimes tested for wheal-and-erythema responses: when horse serum is used, greatly diluted serum (1000-fold or more) should be injected, for even minute amounts of undiluted serum (ca. 0.05 ml) can precipitate systemic anaphylaxis. (For penicillin hypersensitivity and skin tests, see Ch. 20.)

Fundamental mechanisms in systemic anaphylaxis are the same as in the cutaneous wheal-and-erythema response, but certain features of the generalized reaction, which has been studied mostly in the guinea pig, are illuminating.

Mode of Administration of Antigen. Anaphylaxis depends not only on the number of Ab-Ag complexes formed in tissues but also on the **rate** at which they form, for the complexes act by causing the release of pharmacologically active mediators that are rapidly degraded (below). Intravenous injection of Ag is therefore especially effective. Inhalation of Ags dispersed in aerosols can also provoke fatal shock, but responses elicited by subcutaneous and intraperitoneal injections come on more slowly and are less often fatal.

Fixation of Antibodies. Less Ab is needed for passive anaphylaxis if a latent period intervenes between injection of antiserum and of Ag: for example, 0.18 mg of anti-egg albu-min (EA) rendered guinea pigs uniformly susceptible to fatal shock when challenged 48 hours later, whereas 12 mg was required if the Ag was injected immediately after the antiserum. The latent period is needed both for binding of cytotropic Abs to mast cells and for reducing the circulating level of unbound Abs, which lessen shock by competing with cell-bound Ab for the Ag. (Shock elicited by simultaneous injection of large amounts of Ab and Ag probably involves somewhat different mechanisms; see Aggregate anaphylaxis, below.)

The necessity for mast cell binding accounts for the inability of many Abs to mediate passive anaphylaxis. For example, guinea pigs are sensitized only by guinea pig IgE and γl, by human IgG-3, and -4 (but not by IgG-2; see Ch. 16, Appendix), and not by any Abs from chickens, goats, cattle, and horses.

Reverse Passive Anaphylaxis. Passive anaphylaxis can also be evoked by reversing the order of injections if the Ag, which is now injected first, is itself an Ig of the type that is readily bound to guinea pig mast cells (such as rabbit IgG). After a latent period the intravenous injection of antiserum, specific for the Ig used as antigen, can then cause anaphylaxis. This procedure, reverse passive anaphylaxis, is not effective with other Ags because they do not bind to mast cells. Reverse passive cutaneous anaphylaxis can be similarly carried out. It is used occasionally to evaluate an Ig's ability to bind to mast cells: the Ig under test is injected into a normal guinea pig's skin, and then antiserum to the Ig (plus blue dye) is injected intravenously.

Quantities of Antibody and Antigen Required for Anaphylaxis. The levels of Ag required are substantially greater than those necessary for precipitation in vitro: guinea pigs sensitized with 180 μg of anti-egg albumin (EA) require for a uniformly fatal response over 500 μg of EA or ca. 25-fold more than is usually needed for maximal precipitation of this amount of Ab in the EA/anti-EA precipitin reaction. Much of the injected Ag probably never has a chance to react with Abs in vivo, because it is taken up by phagocytic cells or excreted. Ags that form large complexes with circulating, soluble Abs tend to be rapidly phagocytized, and are also not efficient in provoking anaphylaxis. In fact, as suggested above, high levels of circulating Abs may protect against anaphylaxis because they compete with mast-cell-bound Abs for the Ag. Thus when an animal is passively sensitized with a small amount of antiserum and then given a sufficiently large dose of the same antiserum immediately before the Ag, fatal shock can be replaced by mild symptoms.

Acute Densensitization. Because the **speed** of complex formation determines whether anaphylaxis will occur (see above), shock can be prevented by administering Ag slowly. For example, if 100 μg of a particular Ag (injected intravenously) is required to provoke fatal shock, the same quantity given in 10 divided doses at 15-minute intervals would not elicit shock. Moreover, if the full dose were then given all at once shortly after the last small injection shock would probably still not be elicited, presumably because the supply of reactive Ab would have been depleted.

Densensitization by repeated, closely spaced injections of small doses of Ag is often resorted to clinically when it becomes necessary to administer a substance, such as penicillin or horse antiserum, to a person known or suspected to be intensely allergic to it. The procedure is effective but requires great care to avoid anaphylaxis and it has only temporary value. Several weeks afterward hyper-

sensitivity is likely to be fully restored, in contrast to the densensitization based on formation of protective ("blocking") Abs (Prolonged densensitization, above).

Species Variations. Guinea pigs are preferred for the study of anaphylaxis because they react uniformly and intensely. However, anaphylaxis has also been provoked in many other mammals, in fish, and in chickens, and it can probably be elicited in all vertebrates. The pathological manifestations differ in various species (Table 19-3) and even, as suggested above, when the Ag is injected by different routes. In a sensitized guinea pig, for example, intravenous injection leads to respiratory distress due to constriction of bronchi, and at autopsy the lungs appear bloodless and are greatly distended with air; whereas subcutaneous or intraperitoneal administration produces primarily hypotension and hypothermia, and death occurs only after many hours, with engorged blood vessels in abdominal viscera as the main pathological finding. The differences are probably due

TABLE 19-3. Anaphylaxis in Different Species

Species	Principal site of reaction (shock organ)	Pharmacologically active agents implicated	Principal manifestations
Guinea pig	Lungs (bronchioles)	Histamine Kinins SRS-A	Respiratory distress: bronchiolar constriction, emphysema
Rabbit	Heart Pulmonary blood vessels	Histamine Serotonin Kinins SRS-A	Obstruction of pulmonary capillaries with leukocyte-platelet thrombi; right-sided heart failure; vascular engorgement of liver and intestines
Rat	Intestines	Serotonin Kinins	Circulatory collapse; increased peristalsis; hemorrhages in intestine and lung
Mouse	?	Serotonin Kinins	Respiratory distress; emphysema; right-sided heart failure; hyperemia of intestine
Dog	Hepatic veins	Histamine Kinins ? Serotonin	Hepatic engorgement; hemorrhages in abdominal and thoracic viscera
Man	Lungs (bronchioles) Larynx	Histamine ? Kinins SRS-A	Dyspnea; hypotension; flushing and itching; circulatory collapse; acute emphysema; laryngeal edema; urticaria on recovery

Based mostly on Austen, K. F., and Humphrey, J. H. *Adv Immunol 3*:1 (1963).

mostly to differences in distribution or reactivity of released pharmacologically active mediators (Table 19-3).

PHARMACOLOGICALLY ACTIVE MEDIATORS

Following Dale's observations, in 1911, that injections of histamine duplicate manifestations of anaphylaxis, a number of vasoactive substances have been found to be released from tissues in response to Ab-Ag complexes. The direct action of these substances on blood vessels and smooth muscle accounts for nearly all manifestations of anaphylaxis.

Of the several active substances so far identified, two (histamine and serotonin) preexist in cells and are promptly released by appropriate Ab-Ag complexes, while the kinins and "SRS-A" are produced only after the complexes are formed. The main properties of these mediators are reviewed below (Fig. 19-8).

1) **Histamine,** formed by decarboxylation of L-histidine, is distributed widely in mammalian tissues, particularly in granules of connective tissue mast cells (which are especially abundant near blood vessels) and basophilic leukocytes of blood. As noted before (Affinity for mast cells, above), the mast cells and basophils bind on their surface only those Igs that cause anaphylaxis: human cells bind IgE (via specific sites of the Fc domain) but not other human Igs. (Mast cells can also bind appropriate heterocytotropic Abs.) The addition of Ag to tissues from a sensitized individual leads to discharge of mast cell granules and release of histamine (Fig. 19-9).

The **antihistamines** block the anaphylaxis-like effects of histamine injected in guinea pigs. (These drugs are less effective, however, against true anaphylaxis because they do not antagonize the other pharmacological mediators.) Further evidence for the role of histamine is provided by the decline of histamine in tissues, and its rise in plasma, during

Fig. 19-8. Substances that mediate anaphylaxis. Kinins are given with conventional abbreviations for amino acids with terminal α-NH$_2$ at left.

MEDIATOR	STRUCTURE	SOURCE	PROPERTIES USED FOR IDENTIFICATION
Histamine	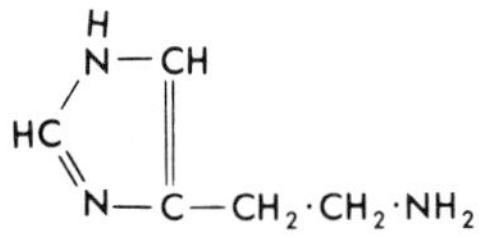 (structure)	Mast cells, Basophils, Platelets, Others?	Contracts guinea pig ileum; inhibited by antihistamines
Serotonin	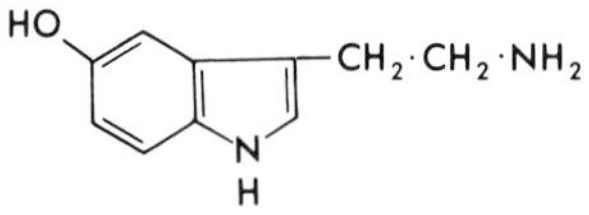 (structure)	Enterochromaffin cells, Mast cells, Platelets	Contracts guinea pig ileum and rat uterus; inhibited by lysergic acid
Kinins			
Bradykinin	Arg·pro·pro·gly·phe·ser·pro·phe·arg	Kininogen (α-globulin, plasma)	Contracts rat uterus; destroyed by chymotrypsin
Lysyl-bradykinin	Lys·arg.pro.pro.gly.phe.ser.pro.phe.arg	Tissues	
Methionyl-lysyl-bradykinin	Met.lys·arg.pro.pro.gly.phe.ser.pro.phe.arg	Tissues	
SRS-A	Acidic lipid, MW $\simeq$ 400	? Mast cells	Contracts human bronchiole; no effect on rat uterus; not inhibited by antihistamines or destroyed by chymotrypsin

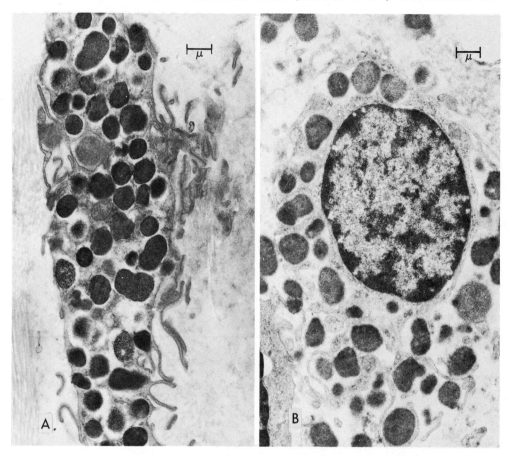

Fig. 19-9. Electron micrographs of mast cells from rat dermis. The intact cell **(A)** contains small, dense granules, each about the size of a mitochondrion. Mitochondria, which are generally scarce in mast cells, are not visible. The nucleus also is not visible in this section. The degranulating cell **(B)** contains larger, paler granules. The release of granules, associated with secretion of histamine, involves fusion of the membrane surrounding each granule with the cell membrane, releasing swollen granules into the extracellular space. ×7000. [Courtesy of S. L. Clark, Jr.; based on Singleton, E. M., and Clark, S. L., Jr. *Lab Invest 14*:1744 (1965).]

anaphylaxis. In addition, sensitized animals that are temporarily depleted of histamine by certain drugs ("histamine liberators") are not susceptible to fatal shock: when their histamine levels are restored, their susceptibility to anaphylaxis returns.

The mast cell granules that contain histamine also contain heparin, and this acidic mucopolysaccharide is responsible for the characteristic metachromatic staining with some basic dyes, e.g., toluidine blue. Heparin is released with histamine, in certain species: dogs undergoing anaphylactic shock have incoagulable blood. However, heparin does not account for the more important manifestations of anaphylaxis.

Species vary widely in their susceptibility to histamine; man and the guinea pig are exquisitely sensitive, while the mouse and rat are insensitive (Table 19-3).

2) **Serotonin** (5-hydroxytryptamine), formed by decarboxylation of L-tryptophan (Fig. 19-8), dilates capillaries, increases capillary permeability, and contracts smooth muscles in susceptible species. It is found mainly in blood platelets, intestinal mucosa, and brain.

Ab-Ag complexes cause release of serotonin in vitro from platelets in most species, and from mast cells in the mouse and rat; but it is not released

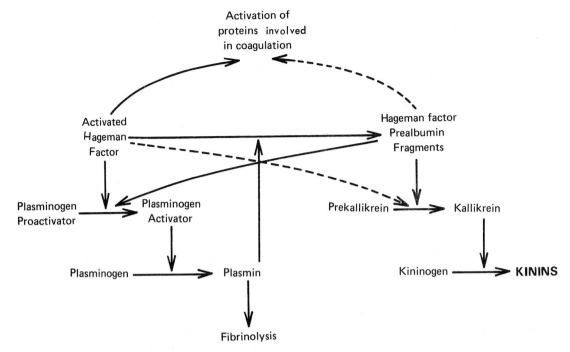

Fig. 19-10. Scheme for production of kinins. The interrelations between blood coagulation and kinin production extends to the complement proteins (C), which can be activated by plasmin and by kallikrein (see Ch. 18, Blood clotting and C). For the structure of kinins, see Figure 19-8. [Based on Kaplan, A. P. and Austen, K. F. *J Exp Med 136*:1378 (1972).]

from the brain during allergic reactions. Its effects are inhibited by lysergic acid diethylamide and by reserpine. Rats and mice are highly susceptible to serotonin, whereas humans and rabbits are highly resistant. Serotonin is probably not important in human anaphylaxis.

3) **Kinins** are basic peptides (Fig. 19-8) formed as endproducts of the sequential action of several plasma proteins (Fig. 19-10). The first, Hageman factor (HF), is activated by various negatively charged substances (footnote, p. 545), including perhaps certain Ab-Ag complexes, initiating the reaction sequence that leads to blood clotting. One component of this sequence, plasmin, cleaves from HF a fragment that converts another proenzyme, prekallikrein, into **kallikrein,*** which cleaves the basic nonapeptide **brady-**

---

* Kallikreins were discovered by mixing tissue extracts, a source of enzyme, with plasma which contains the substrate. The enzyme was named for its abundance in pancreas (Gr. *kallikreas*-pancreas); the product, bradykinin, was named for the slowness of the contraction it induces in isolated guinea pig ileum.

kinin from an α-globulin in plasma (Fig. 19-10).

Tissue kallikreins form the same peptide with a lysine or methionyllysine at the N terminus; aminopeptidases in blood remove the additional N-terminal residues, converting these kinins into bradykinin. Kallikrein also splits (via C1 acting on C4, C2; Ch. 18) another bradykinin-like peptide from complement; called **C-kinin,** the fragment has somewhat similar activities to bradykinin but differs in being susceptible to destruction by trypsin. Several mechanisms prevent dangerous accumulation of kinins, which are powerful hypotensive agents as well as inducers of bronchiolar constriction. Their activities are abolished, for instance, by 1) a plasma carboxypeptidase that removes the C-terminal arginine (see Fig. 19-8), and 2) an inhibitor of activated first component of complement (Ch. 18).

The level of bradykinin in the blood increases during anaphylaxis, causing contraction of smooth muscles, an increase in capillary permeability, and marked vasodilation. Injected into normal animals, these peptides duplicate some of the signs of anaphylaxis.

4) **SRS-A** is released along with histamine when Ag is added to lung fragments of sensitized guinea pigs. Like bradykinin, it causes slow contraction of isolated guinea pig ileum in the presence of antihistamines and is therefore called **SRS-A (slow reacting substance of anaphylaxis).** This substance is not destroyed by proteolytic enzymes (hence is not a kinin), and its action on smooth muscle is not blocked by antagonists of histamine or serotonin (Fig. 19-11). Few chemical properties of SRS-A are known: it is probably an acidic lipid, MW ca. 400.

SRS-A appears to be synthesized as well as released following the immune reaction, for it has been found in tissues of animals only during anaphylaxis. It appears to be important in human allergy: it is released from lung fragments of ragweed-sensitive persons by ragweed pollen extracts in vitro, and it is a powerful constrictor of isolated human bronchioles. Moreover, human allergic bronchospasm is hardly benefited by antihistamines, suggesting that another mediator is a major factor.

Two additional mediators may be involved in anaphylaxis. Ags also stimulate release from lung fragments of allergic individuals of **ECF-A** (eosinophil chemotactic factor of anaphylaxis), which attracts eosinophils, but not other leukocytes, through millipore filters (see Fig. 20-11, Ch .20). This factor could account for the characteristic infiltration of eosinophils at sites of repeated reaginic reactions in atopic individuals (e.g., in nasal and bronchial mucosa of persons with recurrent allergic reactions of the respiratory tract). The role of **prostaglandins** is anaphylaxis is uncertain.

Some of the ubiquitous prostaglandins seem to inhibit Ag-initiated histamine release from sensitized basophils, perhaps through increasing intracellular levels of cAMP (Modulation, below). However, other prostaglandins seem to cause vasodilation and increased permeability of venules. It is possible that some prostaglandins promote allergic inflammation while others are inhibitory.

The manifestations of anaphylaxis vary among species (Table 19-3) because of differences both in the amount of the various mediators that they release and in the responses of their smooth muscles and blood vessels to these substances (Table 19-4).

Because the pharmacologically active mediators are rapidly degraded and excreted they act only transiently. Their failure to accumulate, and their slow resynthesis, account for the efficacy of repeated, closely spaced injections of small doses of Ag in bringing about temporary desensitization (Acute desensitization, above).

ANAPHYLACTIC RESPONSES IN ISOLATED TISSUES

Many organs from sensitized animals respond to Ag in vitro. In the Schultz-Dale reaction the isolated uterus from a sensitized guinea pig contracts promptly when incubated

Fig. 19-11. Assays for histamine and SRS-A. Standards and test samples were added to an isolated strip of guinea pig ileum, whose contractile response was recorded on a moving strip of paper (kymograph). Antihistamines block response to histamine. Methysergide can be added to block serotonin and chymotrypsin to degrade kinins. Note the latent period and slow response to SRS-A and the faster response to histamine. Time scale is about 30 seconds (vertical markers). (Based on Orange, R. P. and Austen, K. F. in *Immunobiology*, [R. A. Good and D. W. Fisher, eds.] Sinaver, Stamford, 1971.)

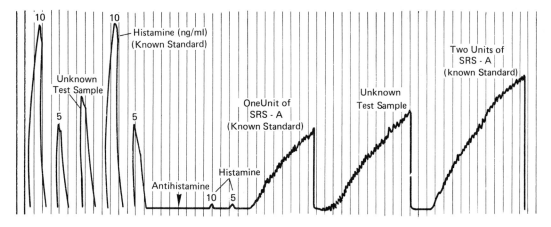

TABLE 19-4. Species Variation in Tissue Levels and Susceptibility to Histamine and Serotonin

Species	Lung content (μg/gm)		Bronchiolar sensitivity (minimal effective dose in μg)	
	Serotonin	Histamine	Serotonin	Histamine
Cat	<0.2	34	0.01	2
Rat	2.3	5	0.01	>5
Dog	<0.1	25	0.05	0.3
Guinea pig	<0.2	5–25	0.4	0.4
Rabbit	2.1	4	>8	0.5
Man	<0.3	2–20	>20	0.2

From various sources summarized in Austen, K. F., and Humphrey, J. H. *Adv Immunol 3*:1 (1963).

with Ag, which doubtless reacts with cytotropic Abs on tissue mast cells and causes release of mediators (Fig. 19-12). Similar reactions are obtained with isolated segments of ileum, gallbladder wall, and sections of arterial wall. These responses can also be elicited with tissues from passively sensitized animals, and with isolated normal tissues that are sensitized simply by incubation with antiserum. Because of the high affinity of reagins for the mast cell surface, the isolated tissues retain reactivity after extensive washing.

In response to Ag, minced fragments of lung from sensitized individuals release measurable amounts of histamine, SRS-A, and ECF-A. The liberation of histamine is complete within 5 minutes, whereas SRS-A is not detected for several minutes and its concentration then rises slowly. In one of the simplest in vitro reactions Ag elicits the release of histamine from washed leukocytes of atopic persons and the degranulation of basophils (demonstrated by staining smeared cells; see Fig 19-9): extremely small amounts of Ag suffice (e.g., 10^{-13} mg/ml of purified ragweed Ag). The degranulation has been used as a diagnostic assay for penicillin allergy (see Ch. 20, Allergy to drugs). Human basophils can also be passively sensitized with atopic sera and with purified human IgE.

The release of vasoactive amines from mast cells appears to be due to secretion rather than to cell lysis. Thus releasing cells remain impermeable to ionic dyes that can penetrate into killed but not into living cells, and the release requires an intact glycolytic pathway and is controlled by intracellular levels of cyclic AMP (Modulation, below). The clinical benefits of some drugs (sodium cromoglycate, diethylcarbamazine) in preventing bronchospasm in asthma are probably due to inhibition of secretion of vasoactive amines: these drugs do not hinder combination of Ab and Ag or the response to histamine.

Modulation. Cyclic AMP (cAMP) inhibits mediator release from Ag-stimulated mast cells: both **the rate and extent of release are enhanced when intracellular cAMP levels are low and are reduced when the levels are**

Fig. 19-12. Smooth muscle contraction in vitro in response to Ag (Schultz-Dale reaction). A uterine horn, excised from a guinea pig 13 days after a sensitizing injection of a horse serum euglobulin, was suspended in Ringer's solution to which various protein fractions from horse serum were added (arrows): at A, 1 mg of pseudoglobulin was added; at B, 10 mg of pseudoglobulin; at C and at D, 10 mg of euglobulin (the immunogen). Following the specific response at C the muscle was almost totally desensitized, because the tissue-bound Abs were saturated with Ag or because the content of vasoactive amines was depleted. Time scale markers at 30-second intervals. R = changes of Ringer's solution. [From Dale, H. H., and Hartley, P. *Biochem J 10*:408 (1916).]

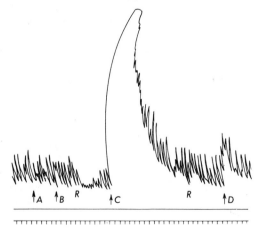

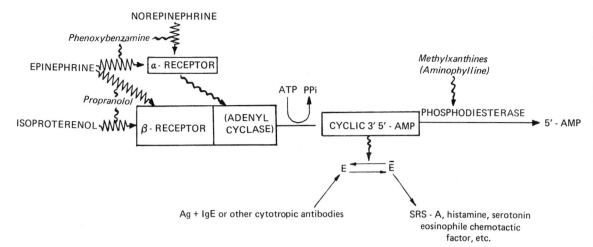

Fig. 19-13. Schematic view of the modulating effect of the cyclic-AMP system on the immunological release of SRS-A and vasoactive amines. Stimulation of α and β receptors on the cell surface membrane supposedly inhibits and enhances, respectively, the enzyme (adenyl cyclase) that generates cAMP (cyclic 3',5'-AMP). E and $\bar{E}$ are inactive and activated forms of a hypothetical proteolytic enzyme, whose existence is suggested because release of mediators requires Ca^{++} and is blocked by diisoprophylphosphofluoridate (which specifically phosphorylates and blocks a group of proteases with esterase activity). Curved lines ($\sim$) refer to inhibition, jagged lines ($\mathcal{W}$) to stimulation. (Based on Austen, K. F. *Sixth International Symposium on Immunopathology.* Schwabe, Basel, 1970.)

high. Hence drugs that stimulate adenylcyclase, the enzyme that synthesizes this nucleotide, or that inhibit the phosphodiesterase that degrades it, block the release of histamine and SRS-A (isoproterenol, epinephrine, aminophylline; Fig. 19-13). These drugs have been used clinically for control of anaphylaxis and allergic bronchospasm for many years (i.e., before this mechanism of action was suspected). The modulating effects of cAMP and of cyclic GMP (which blocks the effect of cAMP) suggest a possible explanation for the influence of emotional states on the intensity of acute allergic reactions (asthma, hayfever, hives, perhaps atopic eczema).

AGGREGATE AND CYTOTOXIC ANAPHYLAXIS

All passive cytotropic responses need a latent period for attachment of cytotropic Abs to mast cells. In contrast, there are other forms of passive anaphylaxis that do not involve IgE or other cytotropic Abs and that do not require a latent period. One class, **"aggregate anaphylaxis,"** seems to be caused by relatively large amounts of **soluble** Ab-Ag complexes interacting with complement (C)

(see below). For example, in a normal guinea pig a single intradermal injection of such complexes, prepared by dissolving a specific precipitate in a concentrated solution of Ag, can evoke passive cutaneous anaphylaxis; and fatal shock can follow intravenous injection of antisera that have been incubated for a few minutes with soluble Ag.* Even some heat-aggregated Igs, without any Ag, can elicit cutaneous anaphylaxis, suggesting that the essential role of the Ag is simply to cross-link certain classes of Ab molecules. Effective soluble immune complexes are those that fix C (e.g., with average molar composition of about Ag_3Ab_2); those that do not fix C are ineffective (e.g., the Ag_2Ab complexes that form in extreme Ag excess; Ch. 18).

Another form of acute allergic reaction,

---

* Normal serum becomes similarly toxic after incubation with suspensions of various particles (kaolin, talc, barium sulfate, inulin, agar), which apparently activate Hageman factor, plasmin, kallikreins (Fig. 19-10), and C with formation of anaphylatoxin (Ch. 18). The response to these incubated sera (without Ag) is sometimes called "anaphylactoid" shock.

called **cytotoxic anaphylaxis,** sometimes follows the injection of Abs to natural constituents of cell surfaces (prototype III, Table 19-1). For example, guinea pigs injected with rabbit Abs to the Forssman Ag, a constituent of all guinea pig cells, undergo acute shock. Acute hemolytic **transfusion reactions** in man are also sometimes associated with shock and could be considered a form of cytotoxic anaphylaxis (Ch. 21).

COMPLEMENT AND ANAPHYLAXIS

Aggregated homocytotropic Abs (e.g., human IgE, guinea pig IgE-like reagins and γl) can activate C3 via the alternate pathway that bypasses the early-acting C components (Ch. 18). It is doubtful, nonetheless, that any C activation is necessary in cytotropic responses, for cytotropic cutaneous anaphylaxis is not altered in animals depleted of C3 (by cobra venom, see Ch. 18).

However, C fixation is probably essential for aggregate anaphylaxis; there is a consistent correlation between ability of aggregates to fix C in vitro and ability to evoke this form of anaphylaxis (see above), in which the release of histamine is probably caused by the anaphylatoxin formed in the C reaction sequence (Ch. 18).

ARTHUS REACTION

Shortly after the discovery of anaphylaxis, Arthus, a French physiologist, described a substantially different kind of Ab-dependent allergic reaction. When rabbits were inoculated subcutaneously each week with horse serum there was at first no noticeable response, but after several weeks each injection evoked a localized inflammatory reaction. Similar responses were soon described in man and in many other vertebrates, and were called **Arthus reactions.** These reactions are not limited to the skin: they can take place when Ags are injected into the pericardial sac or synovial joint spaces. **The principal requirement is the formation in tissues of bulky immune aggregates that fix C and attract polymorphonuclear leukocytes: lysosomal enzymes released by the cells cause tissue damage, characteristically with destructive inflam-**

mation of small blood vessels ("vasculitis").

Patients with serum sickness or with certain forms of glomerulonephritis (below) develop similar lesions in small blood vessels and in kidney glomeruli, respectively; and those with high serum levels of Abs to the thermophilic *Aspergillus* that thrives in decaying vegetation, or to molds used to produce cheese, develop severe localized lung lesions of Arthus type when they inhale these fungi or fungal spores (farmer's lung or cheesemaker's lung).

The main features are illustrated by the passive cutaneous form of the Arthus reaction, in which an antiserum is first injected intravenously into a nonsensitive recipient and the corresponding Ag is then injected into the skin. Alternatively, in the **reverse passive Arthus reaction** the antiserum is injected in the recipient's skin and the Ag is then injected into the same dermal site or intravenously.

Time Course. After intradermal injection of Ag the Arthus response comes on more slowly than cutaneous anaphylaxis and is much more persistent. Local swelling and erythema appear after 1 to 2 hours, followed by punctate hemorrhages. The changes are maximal in 3 to 4 hours and are usually gone in 10 to 12 hours; but severe reactions, with necrosis at the test site, subside more slowly (cf. tuberculin skin reaction, Ch. 20).

Type and Amount of Antibody. The higher the level of precipitable Abs the more intense and persistent the lesion. Abs of almost any class of Igs, and from almost any species, can mediate the reaction, and even the injection of Ab-Ag complexes formed in the test tube can evoke the response, though with less intensity than when the aggregates form in situ. The passive Arthus reaction requires a large amount of Ab, ca. 10 mg when injected intravenously in a rabbit and ca. 100 μg when injected into the skin. In contrast, a few nanograms of reagin (almost 100,000-fold less) is sufficient for passive cutaneous anaphylaxis in man (Prausnitz-Küstner reaction, above).

Though most Igs appear to be effective, different types account for different features of the Arthus reaction: in guinea pigs, for instance, γl Abs induce the edematous changes, and γ2 Abs appear to be responsible for the hemorrhage and necrosis (see Fig. 19-7).

Histopathology. In anaphylaxis the inflammatory changes are limited to vasodilation and exudation of plasma proteins; inflammatory cells are not conspicuous. The Arthus response, however, is characterized by classical inflammation: blood flow through small vessels is markedly retarded; thrombi rich in platelets and leukocytes form within small blood vessels; erythrocytes escape into the surrounding connective tissue; and after several hours the skin site becomes edematous and heavily infiltrated with polymorphonuclear leukocytes (Fig. 19-14). Finally, localized patches of necrosis appear in walls of affected small blood vessels. As the lesion begins to subside, after 4 to 12 hours, neutrophils become necrotic and are replaced by mononuclear cells and eosinophils. Within a

Fig. 19-14. The passive Arthus reaction in a rat, showing localization of Ag and complement in the wall of an affected blood vessel. The skin site was excised 2 to 3 hours after an intradermal injection of 300 μg of rabbit Abs to bovine serum albumin (anti-BSA) and an intravenous injection of 6 mg of BSA. (The Ab was injected intradermally, and the Ag intravenously, to conserve Abs.) **A.** Note intense polymorphonuclear leukocyte infiltration in and around the wall of a small blood vessel adjacent to skeletal muscle. **B.** The section was stained with fluorescent rabbit Ab to a purified component of rat C (C3; see Ch. 18). **C.** The section was stained with fluorescent anti-BSA to localize the aggregated Ag in the blood vessel wall and in the adjacent perivascular connective tissue. The same result would be obtained by staining the aggregated Ab (rabbit anti-BSA) with fluorescent anti-rabbit Ig. [From Ward, P. A., and Cochrane, C. G. *J Exp Med 121*:215 (1965).]

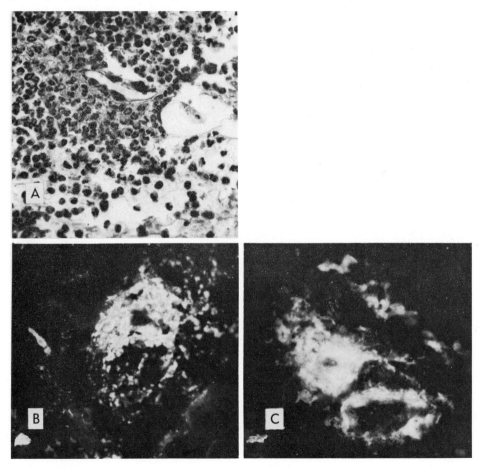

few days, the phagocytized immune complexes are degraded and inflammation disappears.*

The response in the cornea emphasizes the role of blood vessels. The injection of Ag into an immunized rabbit's normal cornea, which is devoid of functional blood vessels, can result in concentric opaque rings of Ab-Ag precipitates, like bands in gel precipitin reactions in vitro (Ch. 15), but little or no inflammation is observed. If, however, functional blood vessels are present (e.g., as a sequel of some earlier trauma to the cornea), then the Ag can elicit an Arthus response in the cornea, as in any other tissue.

Role of Complement and Granulocytes. At the site of the local reaction immunofluorescence reveals Ab-Ag aggregates with C

___

* In gross and microscopic appearance the Arthus reaction resembles the **Shwartzman reaction,** in which hemorrhagic and necrotic inflammatory lesions are evoked with the endotoxin of gram-negative bacteria (Ch. 26). Two skin injections, spaced about 1 day apart, are generally used to elicit the Shwartzman reaction: one injection consists of endotoxin and the other can be endotoxin or any of a wide variety of immunologically unrelated substances, such as agar, starch, or even Ab-Ag precipitates. An immune mechanism does not appear to be a fundamental feature of the Shwartzman phenomenon.

components (C3) localized in blood vessel walls, between endothelial cells and the internal elastic membrane (Fig. 19-14). The aggregates are also evident within granulocytes in perivascular connective tissue. If an animal's C activity has been greatly reduced (e.g., by depleting C3 with cobra venom; Ch. 18), or if its level of circulating polymorphonuclear (PMN) leukocytes has been depressed (e.g., by an anti-PMN serum or by nitrogen mustards), no inflammatory reaction appears, even though the immune complexes form in blood vessel walls.

It has been suggested therefore that the Arthus reaction depends on the following sequence: 1) Ag and Ab diffuse into blood vessel walls, where they combine and form complexes and fix C; 2) the resulting chemotactic factors (C5a and C5b,6,7; see Ch. 18) attract PMN leukocytes, which ingest the aggregates and release lysosomal enzymes; 3) the enzymes cause focal necrosis of the blood vessel wall and the other inflammatory changes. From the release of acid-soluble peptides (from radiolabeled Ags) it is evident that lysosomal enzymes degrade the immune complexes, whose disappearance is associated with subsidence of inflammation.

Increased permeability of the blood vessel endothelium (due to vasoactive amines released from mast cells or basophils or plate-

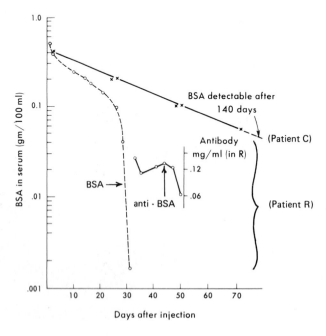

Fig. 19-15. Serum sickness syndrome in man following the injection of 25 gm of BSA at zero time. Patient R had serum sickness from day 24 to 31; patient C did not exhibit serum sickness or form Abs to BSA. [Data of F. E. Kendall; From Seegal, B. *Am J Med* 13:356 (1952).]

lets) seems to aid the penetration of Ab-Ag complexes into blood vessel walls (see Serum sickness syndrome, below). However, antihistamines have little (if any) clinical benefits on Arthus lesions.

SERUM SICKNESS SYNDROME

From about 1900 to 1940 several types of bacterial infection in man were treated routinely by injecting patients with a large volume of antiserum prepared in horses or rabbits. The recipients often developed, from 3 days to 2 or 3 weeks later, a characteristic syndrome called serum sickness. Heterologous antisera are now used much less in medicine (e.g., for tetanus, rabies, and prevention of allograft rejection with horse antisera to human lymphocytes), but the syndrome is also encountered as an allergic reaction to penicillin and other drugs (Ch. 20).

The syndrome includes 1) fever, 2) enlarged lymph nodes and spleen, 3) erythematous and urticarial rashes, and 4) painful joints. The disease usually subsides within a few days. In the few patients who have died at the height of the illness, autopsy has disclosed vascular and perivascular inflammatory lesions like those of the Arthus reaction.

The mechanisms have been analyzed in rabbits and in humans injected with large amounts of purified foreign protein. The opportunity to make detailed observations in man arose in connection with attempts, during World War II, to use bovine serum albumin (BSA) as a plasma expander in the treatment of traumatic shock (Fig. 19-15).

Mechanisms. The illness usually becomes evident 7 to 14 days after the initial injection of Ag. During this interval the Ag level declines, but it is still high enough after Ab production starts to form the small soluble Ab-Ag complexes (in Ag excess) that initiate focal vascular lesions (in coronary arteries, glomeruli, etc.; Fig. 19-16). Serum sickness is thus usually observed only after exceptionally large amounts of foreign protein are injected, e.g., 25 gm BSA in man, or 1 gm in a rabbit. However, in a previously sensitized person, with an accelerated (anamnestic) Ab re-

Fig. 19-16. Representative cardiovascular and renal lesions in experimental serum sickness in the rabbit. The Ag was BSA (see Fig. 19-17). **A.** Medium-sized coronary artery: endothelial cell proliferation, necrosis of media, polymorphonuclear leukocyte infiltration through all layers, and mononuclear cells in the media and adventitia are evident. **C.** An affected glomerulus showing increase in size, proliferation of endothelial and epithelial cells, and obliteration of capillary spaces. **B.** Section through a normal glomerulus of a control rabbit for comparison with **C**: note the much lower density of glomerular cells and patency of capillaries. (From Dixon, F. J. In *Immunological Diseases.* M. Samter, ed. Little, Brown, Boston, 1965.)

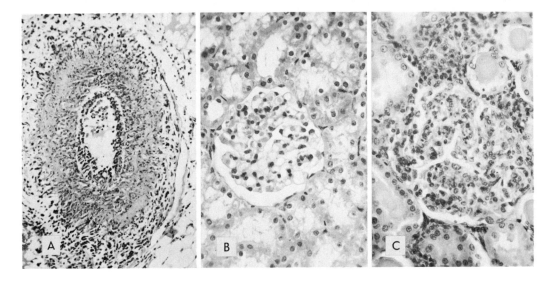

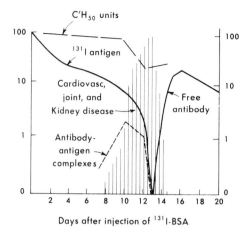

Fig. 19-17. Serum sickness in the rabbit. Changes in serum levels of free Ag (^{131}I-labeled BSA), free Ab (anti-BSA), Ag-Ab complexes, and complement activity (C'H$_{50}$ units, see Ch. 18) following the injection of rabbits at zero time with 250 mg of ^{131}I-BSA per kilogram of body weight. Ordinate (log scale) refers to ^{131}I-BSA in total blood volume, as per cent of amount injected; anti-BSA as micrograms of Ag bound per milliliter of serum; C activity as per cent of normal serum. All animals had cardiovascular, joint, and kidney lesions (Fig. 19-16), shown by shaded area, on day 13. (From Dixon, F. J. In *Immunological Diseases*. M. Samter, ed. Little, Brown, Boston, 1965.)

sponse, the reaction appears earlier and therefore requires much less Ag: e.g., 3 or 4 days after 1 ml of horse serum.

As the manifestations of serum sickness appear, the decline in level of free Ag is accelerated (Figs. 19-15 and 19-17). During this period soluble Ab-Ag complexes can be detected in serum if ^{131}I-labeled BSA (*Ag) is used as Ag (for example, ammonium sulfate at 50% saturation precipitates the *Ag-Ab complexes, but not the free *Ag). As Ab-Ag complexes form they fix C, which is depressed at the height of the illness (Fig. 19-17); and, as in the Arthus reaction, the most abundant C component (C3) can be detected by immunofluorescence in immune aggregates within the focal blood vessel lesions (Fig. 19-14). As the complexes disappear free Abs become detectable and inflammatory lesions regress.

The injection of preformed complexes (made in vitro) also elicits the characteristic lesions in rabbits. The most effective complexes are those prepared in moderate Ag excess (Ag$_3$Ab$_2$). Complexes formed at equivalence or in extreme Ag excess (Ag$_2$Ab) are ineffective: the former are generally particulate and tend to be rapidly cleared from the circulation, and the latter fail to fix C (Ch. 18).

Vasoactive Amines. Increased vascular permeability seems to be necessary for the penetration of immune complexes from plasma through endothelium into the blood vessel wall, and vasoactive amines probably aid at this step.

Thus vascular deposition of injected preformed complexes is diminished in rabbits that are treated with antihistamines and antiserotonins or are depleted of platelets (which are the major circulating reservoir of vasoactive amines in rabbits). The immune complexes probably contain enough cytotropic Abs to activate blood basophils, which are thought to produce (in rabbits) a soluble factor that clumps and lyses platelets, releasing vasoactive amines. These amines could also be released by platelets that are clumped on Ab-Ag-C complexes (immune adherence due to the bound C3b fragment, Ch. 18). The pathogenetic steps are summarized in Figure 19-18.

Relation to Other Allergic Reactions. Serum sickness involves both Arthus and anaphylactic elements (Table 19-1). The focal vascular lesions and the requirement for immune complexes and for C suggest that the syndrome is essentially a disseminated form of the Arthus reaction, with the same injected substance, given in a single large amount, serving first as immunogen and then as reacting Ag. However, the role of homocytotropic Abs seems larger than in the Arthus reaction, since urticarial skin lesions are also prominent in serum sickness. Moreover, after a person has recovered from the disease he will generally give a wheal-and-erythema response to intradermal injection of the responsible Ag. The amines probably contribute also to development of the focal vasculitis, as in the Arthus reaction.

Multiplicity of Antigens. The overlapping kinetics of Ag disappearance and Ab appearance explain some of the confusion that arose in earlier studies of serum sickness due to foreign sera. For example, just before, during, and for some weeks after clinical manifestations had run their course both horse serum proteins and Abs to these proteins were detectable in a given patient's serum. In addition, even after a single injection of horse serum a patient

1. Ab-Ag complexes fix C, causing either release of a leukocyte factor that acts on platelets or immune adherence (Ch. 18) that clumps and damages platelets.

2. Platelets lyse, releasing vasoactive amines (histamine, serotonin).

3. Permeability of vascular endothelium increases.

4. Ab-Ag complexes penetrate into blood vessel walls or form within the walls, fixing C and forming chemotactic factors (C5a, $\overline{C5b, 6, 7}$) for polymorphonuclear leukocytes (neutrophils).

5. Neutrophils penetrate into blood vessel walls, ingesting immune complexes and releasing lysosomal enzymes.

6. Lysosomal enzymes damage neighboring cells and connective tissue elements, leading to more inflammation.

7. If immune complexes are formed in an acute episode ("one-shot" serum sickness) the lesions abate as complexes are degraded.

8. If immune complexes are formed repeatedly (as in persistent viremia, malaria, some other forms of human glomerulonephritis) chronic inflammatory disease can develop in small blood vessels and kidney glomeruli.

Fig. 19-18. Pathogenesis of lesions in and around blood vessels in serum sickness in rabbits.

might suffer a series of attacks of serum sickness, separated by illness-free intervals. These effects were evidently due to the multiplicity of Ags in horse serum; each bout of illness represented the response to a particular Ag and the patient's serum under these circumstances resembled the supernatants of a precipitin reaction performed with horse serum as the Ag (Ch. 15; Fig. 15-9).

IMMUNE-COMPLEX DISEASES

Glomerulonephritis. The pathogenesis of experimental Arthus and serum sickness lesions probably accounts for some forms of glomerulonephritis, a kidney disease in which obstructive inflammatory lesions of glomerular blood vessels can lead to renal failure. Immunofluorescence of biopsies usually reveals lumpy deposits of Ig and C3 (probably Ab-Ag-C complexes) beneath the glomerular endothelium (Fig. 19-19). The deposits resemble those of serum sickness, especially the

chronic experimental model of Dixon *et al.*, in which Ag is administered almost daily for many weeks at a rate that approximates Ab synthesis and provides continuous production of immune complexes.

Ags have been identified in human glomerular lesions in special circumstances. *Plasmodium malariae* Ags have been recognized by immunofluorescence in kidneys of patients with the chronic nephritis associated with malaria, and Abs to malarial Ags have been eluted from kidney biopsies (at pH 2 to 3 to dissociate Ab-Ag complexes, see Appendix, Ch. 15).

Similarly, Abs to single- and double-stranded DNA have been eluted from kidney tissue of patients with systemic lupus erythematosus; these patients often have high serum levels of Abs to nucleic acids and develop progressive glomerulonephritis with lumpy glomerular deposits containing Ig, C, and DNA (see Ch. 20, Autoimmune diseases).

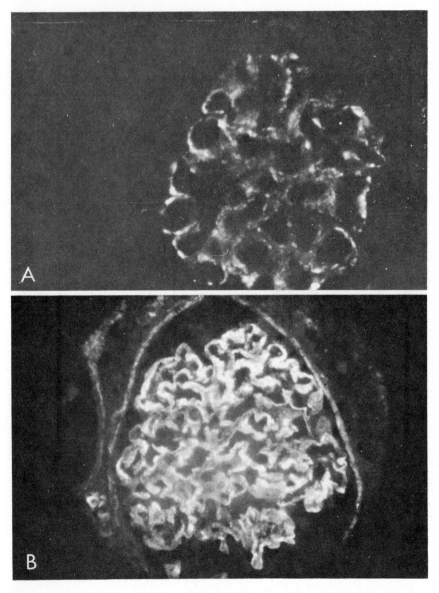

Fig. 19-19. Immune complexes in glomeruli revealed by immunofluorescence. Kidney biopsies from patients with glomerulonephritis were stained with fluorescein-labeled Abs to human Igs. **A** Lumpy deposits due to Abs-Ag-C in glomerulus from a patient with systemic lupus erythematosus. **B** Linear deposits due to Igs attached specifically to the glomerular basement membrane (Goodpasture's syndrome; see Autoimmune diseases, Ch. 20). (Courtesy of Dr. C. Kirk Osterland.)

Most cases of human glomerulonephritis occur as a sequel to infection with β-hemolytic streptococci (especially Type XII, the "nephritogenic" strain; see Ch. 26), but streptococcal Ags have not been consistently detected in the associated glomerular deposits of Ig and C, perhaps because reactive sites are usually covered by antistreptococcal Abs; the specificity of the Abs eluted from affected kidneys has not yet been determined.

Viral Complexes. Observations with mice suggest that chronic viral infection may be a source of immune-complex disease. Animals

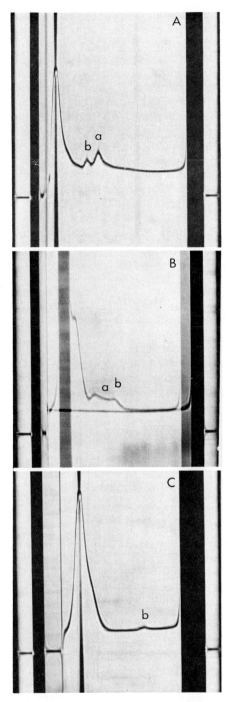

infected at birth with lymphocytic choriomeningitis (LCM) virus become chronic carriers of the virus, but they are not tolerant of it (see Ch. 17, Pseudotolerance). Instead, they produce large amounts of antiviral Abs that do not neutralize infectivity. Virus- antivirus-C complexes in serum are revealed by a reduction in titer of infectious virus when specific precipitates are formed by addition of antisera to mouse Igs or to mouse C components (usually anti-C3; see Ch. 18). Progressive renal disease in these mice is associated with inflammatory vascular lesions and lumpy glomerular deposits containing LCM virus, antiviral Ig, and C.

Immune-complex disease with glomerulonephritis also occurs in mice as a result of neonatal infection with murine leukemia viruses, murine sarcoma virus, Coxsackie B virus, and polyomavirus; and similar lesions seem to be responsible for the high mortality rate in an economically important disease of mink that probably also derives from a neonatal viral infection (Aleutian mink disease).

Antikidney Antibodies. In a rare form of human glomerulonephritis immunofluorescence reveals not lumpy but "linear" glomerular deposits of Ig that follow the basement membrane continuously (Fig. 19-19). The pattern resembles that seen in the experimental nephritis produced with heteroantisera to basement membrane (e.g., the so-called Matsugi nephritis produced in rabbits with duck antisera to rabbit kidney). Some monkeys inoculated with Igs eluted from human kidneys with linear deposits have developed glomerulonephritis, suggesting that the human lesion could be due to autoantibodies to glomerular basement membrane, or to the cross-reacting membranes in lung (see Ch. 20, Goodpasture's disease).

Rheumatoid Arthritis. In this common, chronic inflammatory disease of joints the fluid in joint (synovial) cavities contains high levels of Ig (much of it synthesized locally in synovial membrane) and C-fixing aggregates of Igs, as well as granulocytes and C components that attract granulocytes (C5a,

Fig. 19-20. Immune complexes in human serum. Sera were diluted with buffered saline and subjected to velocity sedimentation at about 50,000 RPM in the analytical ultracentrifuge. **A** Serum from a patient with rheumatoid arthritis showing at *a* specific complexes (22S) of "rheumatoid factor" of the IgM class with IgG (ligand); the 19S at *b* represents unbound IgM immunoglobulins. **B** Serum from a patient with rheumatoid arthritis showing a less common pattern with polydisperse immune complexes involving "rheumatoid factor" of the IgG class with normal IgG (ligand) (*a*); the normal (unbound) 19S IgM peak is at *b*. **C** Control: serum from a normal person; *b* represents the normal IgM peak. No complexes are evident. (Courtesy of Dr. C. Kirk Osterland.)

C5b,6,7). Hence the joint fluids contain all the ingredients for an Arthus reaction. However, the actual Ags remain unknown (as in most human diseases that are suspected to arise from immune complexes).

The IgG in joint fluid might conceivably function as Ag for the characteristic **rheumatoid factors** of rheumatoid arthritis, which are IgM and IgG molecules that react specifically with antigenic determinants on Fc domains of various IgGs (see Ch. 16, Human Gm allotypes). The IgG-IgM and the IgG-IgG complexes could then initiate the C-granulocyte-lysosomal enzyme sequence that results in Arthus inflammation (Fig. 19-18). Alternatively, the IgGs could function as Abs that bind special Ags in affected joints, such as DNA (and probably other, unidentified Ags): the rheumatoid factors would then not be essential participants but would have arisen secondarily as Abs to new antigenic sites that appear on conformationally altered IgG molecules in immune complexes. Indeed, IgM molecules that behave like rheumatoid factors are found in diverse situations where immune complexes are present at high levels for protracted periods (e.g., experimental chronic serum sickness, see above).

Evidence for Persistent Soluble Immune Complexes. In rheumatoid arthritis, glomerulonephritis, systemic lupus erythematosus, and other chronic diseases where immune complexes are probably pathogenic their presence is often revealed by the formation of precipitates when sera, or joint fluids in rheumatoid arthritis, are simply stored at 4°. These **cryoprecipitates** contain IgM (probably anti-antibodies), IgG, and sometimes additional components that could represent Ags (e.g., single-stranded DNA in patients who form anti-DNA, such as those with systemic lupus or with rheumatoid arthritis).

The presence of soluble immune complexes can also be revealed by: 1) ultracentrifugation (Fig. 19-20); 2) appearance of breakdown products of C3 (recognized by immunoelectrophoresis with specific antisera); 3) increased levels of "immune conglutinins," which are Abs (of IgM class) to antigenic sites that appear on activated C3 and C4 components of C (Ch. 18); 4) precipitation with C1q, a stable subunit of the first C component, which reacts specifically with soluble immune complexes if the Ab moiety of the complex belongs to certain Ig classes (e.g., IgG-1 and IgM in man; Ch. 18); and 5) certain highly avid monoclonal IgMs with rheumatoid activity (e.g., from patients with Waldenström's macroglobulinemia; see Ch. 16).

Autoimmune diseases will be discussed further in the next chapter.

SELECTED REFERENCES

BOOKS AND REVIEW ARTICLES

AUSTEN, K. F., and BECKER, E. L. (eds.). *Biochemistry of the Acute Allergic Reaction.* Oxford, Blackwell, 1968, 1971.

BECKER, E. L. Nature and classification of immediate-type allergic reactions. *Adv Immunol 13*:267 (1971).

BECKER, E. L., and HENSON, P. M. In vitro studies of immunologically induced secretion of mediators from cells, and related phenomena. *Adv Immunol.* In press.

BENNICH, H., and JOHANSSON, S. G. O. Structure and function of human IgE. *Adv Immunol 13*:1 (1971).

BLOCH, K. J. The anaphylactic antibodies of mammals including man. *Prog Allergy 10*:84–150 (1967).

COCHRANE, C. G. Immunologic tissue injury mediated by neutrophilic leucocytes. *Adv Immunol 9*:97–162 (1968).

COCHRANE, C. G., and KOFFLER, D. Immune complex disease in experimental animals and man. *Adv Immunol 16*:186 (1973).

ISHIZAKA, K., and ISHIZAKA, T. Biologic function of IgE antibodies and mechanisms of reaginic hypersensitivity. *Clin Exp Immunol 6*:25 (1970).

OSLER, A. G., LICHTENSTEIN, L. M., and LEVY, D. A. In vitro studies of human reaginic allergy. *Adv Immunol 8*:183 (1968).

SAMTER, M. (ed.) *Immunological Diseases.* Little, Brown, Boston, ed. 2. 1971.

Symposium: Cellular mechanisms and involvement in acute allergic reactions. *Fed Proc 28*:1702–1735 (1969).

UNANUE, E. R., and DIXON, F. J. Experimental glomerulonephritis: Immunologic events and pathogenetic mechanisms. *Adv Immunol 6*:1 (1967).

VON PIRQUET, C. F., and SCHICK, B. *Serum Sickness.* (Engl. trans. B. Schick.) Williams & Wilkins, Baltimore, 1905.

ZVAIFLER, N. J. The immunopathology of joint inflammation in rheumatoid arthritis. *Adv Immunol 16*:265 (1973).

SPECIFIC ARTICLES

COCHRANE, C. G., Mechanisms involved in the deposition of immune complexes in tissue. *J Exp Med 134*:75S–89S (1971).

HENSON, P. M. Interaction of cells with immune complexes: Adherence, release of constituents, and tissue injury. *J Exp Med 174*:114S–135S (1971).

ISHIZAKA, K., ISHIZAKA, T., and HORNBROOK, M. M. Physico-chemical properties of human reaginic antibody. IV. Presence of a unique immunoglobulin as a carrier of reaginic activity; V Correlation of reaginic activity with gamma E-globulin in antibody. *J Immunol 97*:75–85, 840–853 (1966).

JOHANSSON, S. G., and BENNICH, H. Immunological studies on an atypical (myeloma) immunoglobulin. *Immunology 13*:381–394, 1967.

JOHANSSON, S. G., BENNICH, H., BERG, T., and HÖGMAN, C. Some factors influencing the serum IgE levels in atopic diseases. *Clin Exp Immunol 6*:43 (1970).

KOCHWA, S., TERRY, W. D., CAPRA, J. D., and YANG, M. L. Structural studies of IgE. I. Physicochemical studies of the IgE molecule. *Ann NY Acad Sci 190*:49 (1971).

KOFFLER, D. AGNELLO, V., THOBURN, R., and KUNKEL, H. G. Systemic lupus erythematosus: Prototype of immune complex nephritis in man. *J Exp Med 174*:169S–179S (1971).

LEVINE, B. B. Atopy and mouse models. *Int Arch Allergy 41*:88–92 (1971).

LEVINE, B. B., CHANG, H., and VAZ, N. M. Production of hapten-specific reaginic antibodies in the guinea pig. *J Immunol 106*:29–33 (1971).

MCCLUSKEY, P. T. The value of immunofluorescence in the study of human renal disease. *J Exp Med 184*:242S–255S (1971).

MCPHAUL, J. J., and DIXON, F. J. Characterization of human anti-glomerular basement membrane antibodies eluted from glomerulonephritic kidneys. *J Clin Invest 49*:308 (1970).

ORANGE, R. P., AUSTEN, W. G., and AUSTEN, K. F. Immunological release of histamine and slow-reacting substance of anaphylaxis from human lung. I. Modulation by agents influencing cellular levels of cyclic 3',5'-adenine monophosphate. *J Exp Med 134*:136S–148S (1971).

WINCHESTER, R. J., KUNKEL, H. G., and AGNELLO, V. Occurrence of γ-gloublin complexes in serum and joint fluid of rheumatoid arthritic patients: Use of monoclonal rheumatoid factors as reagents for their demonstration. *J Exp Med 134*:286S—295S (1971).

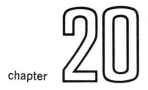

chapter **20**

CELL-MEDIATED HYPERSENSITIVITY AND IMMUNITY

GENERAL PROPERTIES OF CELL-MEDIATED IMMUNE RESPONSES

Following the discovery of anaphylaxis a bewildering variety of other allergic responses were recognized. Though classification proved difficult it became clear in the 1920s that anaphylactic, Arthus, and serum sickness reactions differed from a special group, called delayed-type, in which the responses always evolved slowly and passive transfer could not be achieved with antisera. It gradually became apparent much later that these **delayed-type hypersensitive** responses are mediated by specifically reactive lymphocytes, now known to be T cells, rather than by conventional, freely diffusible ("humoral") antibody (Ab) molecules: hence they are now also referred to as **cell-mediated hypersensitivity.**

Delayed-type hypersensitive skin responses have long been used to diagnose infectious diseases and to screen populations for those with previous or current infections (Table 20-1). Moreover, these responses appear to be responsible for a number of autoimmune diseases; and in the form of allergic contact dermatitis they constitute one of the commonest skin diseases of man. However, the practical significance of these responses extends beyond allergic reactions, for similar mechanisms (independence of humoral Abs and dependence upon specifically reactive lymphocytes) underlie many other immune reactions, including resistance to a variety of infectious agents,* rejection of grafted cells from genetically different individuals of the same species (allografts), and resistance to most tumors. Thus, all these responses, including delayed-type hypersensitivity, are now called **cell-mediated immune reactions** (Table 20-2). The principal differences between these responses and those due to conventional Ab molecules (humoral immunity) are summarized in Table 20-3. Though the distinctions are fundamental, many clinical reactions are actually mixtures, with both Ab- and cell-mediated reactions to the same Ag occurring in the same individual and even in the same inflammatory lesion.

Various forms of cell-mediated immunity, best studied in different species, illuminate different aspects of their common mechanisms; and no one manifestation can be used to illustrate all the fundamental features. For instance, the peculiar specificity requirements are best appreciated in skin reactions, which are recognized readily in guinea pigs but only with difficulty in mice, rats, and chickens; while the effects of neonatal thymectomy (and bursectomy in chickens) are effectively studied in the latter species but not in guinea pigs.† Hence an understanding of the basis for the diagram that summarizes the essentials of all of these reactions (Fig. 20-1) requires an appreciation of the key manifestations of diverse cell-mediated reactions.

---

* **Bacterial** or **infectious allergy,** older terms for delayed-type hypersensitivity, are misleading synonyms, for despite the frequent association of these reactions with chronic bacterial infections, microbial antigeus (Ags) can also evoke immediate-type hypersensitivity and nonmicrobial Ags can elicit delayed-type responses.

† Newborn guinea pigs appear to have fully differentiated lymphocytes; hence the effects of thymectomy are probably as difficult to discern in them as in adult mice, rats, etc.

TABLE 20-1. Some Delayed-Type Skin Reactions Used as Diagnostic Tests and for Epidemiological Surveys

Disease	Type of etiological agent	Antigenic preparation used in skin test
Tuberculosis	Bacteria	Tuberculin
Leprosy	Bacteria	Lepromin
Brucellosis	Bacteria	Brucellin
Psittacosis	Bacteria	Heat-killed organisms
Lymphogranuloma venereum	Bacteria	Extract of chorioallantoic membrane of infected chick embryo
Mumps	Virus	Noninfectious virus from yolk sac of infected chick embyro
Coccidioidomycosis	Fungus	Concentrated culture filtrate
Histoplasmosis	Fungus	Concentrated culture filtrate
Blastomycosis	Fungus	Concentrated culture filtrate
Leishmaniasis	Protozoan	Extract of cultured *Leishmania*
Echinococcosis	Helminth	Fluid from hydatid cyst
Contact dermatitis	Simple chemical	Patch tests with simple chemicals

TABLE 20-2. Cell-Mediated Immune Responses

Delayed-type hypersensitivity
Resistance to many infectious agents (especially intracellular parasites)
Resistance to most tumors
Rejection of allografts
Graft-vs.-host reaction
Some drug allergies
Some autoimmune diseases

TABLE 20-3. Basic Differences Between Humoral and Cell-Mediated Allergic Reactions

Property	Humoral	Cell-mediated
Time course in already sensitized individual	Minutes to hours	One or more days
Histology of inflammatory lesion	Edema, polymorphonuclear leukocytes (granulocytes)	Mononuclear cells*
Transfer with	Serum (Abs†)	Lymphoid cells (T lymphocytes†)
Specificity	Small determinants, ranging from a benzenoid molecule to a hexasaccharide or a hexapeptide	Large molecules, usually proteins (especially on cell surfaces)

* A noncommittal term for lymphocytes and macrophages, which cannot be readily distinguished in the light microscope in ordinary histological preparations.

† The active, unit reacting specifically with Ags. Lymphoid cell preparations are heterogeneous cell populations from lymph nodes, spleen, or blood; predominantly lymphocytes, they also include many macrophages (or monocytes, the immature macrophage in blood), some granulocytes, red cells, and probably a rare plasma cell.

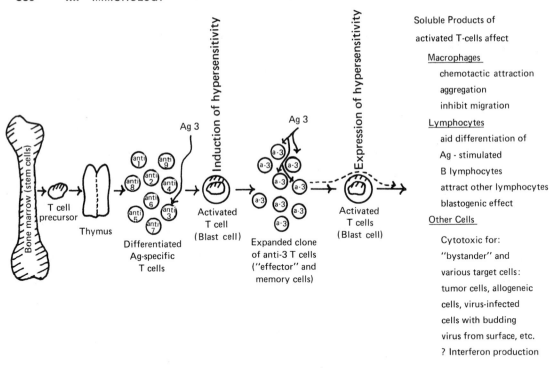

Fig. 20-1. Essentials of cell-mediated immune responses. Precursor cells differentiate into mature Ag-sensitive T cells, which can be specifically activated by the corresponding Ag to 1) proliferate into an expanded clone (includes specific "memory" and "effector" cells; whether they are the same is uncertain), and 2) produce soluble factors that affect a variety of other cells.

DELAYED-TYPE HYPERSENSITIVITY

RESPONSES TO INFECTIOUS AGENTS AND TO PURIFIED PROTEINS

The response to proteins of the tubercle bacillus has been studied longer than other cell-mediated responses because of its suspected role in tuberculosis; it serves as a general model for delayed-type allergic reactions to soluble proteins and to microbial Ags.

Koch observed in 1890 that viable tubercle bacilli inoculated subcutaneously into guinea pigs evoke a much more intense inflammatory reaction in previously infected than in uninfected animals (Koch phenomenon). Moreover, filtrates of cultures of *Mycobacterium tuberculosis,* even after concentration by boiling,* elicited an inflammatory reaction many

hours after injection into tuberculous but not into normal animals. Similar preparations from other bacterial and fungal cultures elicit similar delayed-type responses in those infected with the corresponding organisms (Table 20-1).

Cutaneous Reaction. After 0.1 μg of tuberculin* is injected intradermally into a sensitized individual no change is observed at the inoculated site for at least 10 hours. Erythema and swelling then gradually appear and increase progressively; maximal intensity and size (up to ca. 7 cm diameter) are reached in 24 to 72 hours, and the response then subsides over several days.

In highly sensitive humans 0.02 μg of tuberculin can cause necrosis, ulceration, and scarring at the

---

* After concentration by boiling and removal of debris, the culture filtrate was called tuberculin (now called **old tuberculin** or **OT**). In modern preparations the active proteins are concentrated from autoclaved cultures by precipitation with ammonium

sulfate; the somewhat purified product is **purified protein derivative** or **PPD**. A standard batch, PPD-S, has been designated as the basis for the international unit: 1 tuberculin unit (TU) equals 0.02 μg of total protein (see Ch. 35 for further details).

bonds with skin protein in vivo (see Fig. 20-4), and the complexity of the derived molecules obscured the unusual specificity requirements of this and other cell-mediated responses (Carrier specificity, below).

Induction. Contact skin sensitivity is usually induced by percutaneous application or intradermal injection of the sensitizer. The skin can be bypassed only by administering the sensitizer in complete Freund's adjuvant. It has been suggested that skin lipids might exert an adjuvant effect comparable to the mycoside of *M. tuberculosis* (above).

Elicitation. Beginning 4 or 5 days after the sensitizing exposure an application of the sensitizer almost anywhere on the skin surface of man or guinea pig elicits delayed inflammation.*

Guinea pigs are tested with a drop of a dilute solution on the skin (after hair has been removed), followed by light massage. Humans, however, are tested with a **patch test:** a 1-cm piece of filter paper soaked with a dilute solution of sensitizer is placed on the skin, covered with tape, and left for 24 hours. The area of contact is examined a few hours after the patch is removed, and the response is scored again the next day.

Since sensitizers are potential irritants (because they react indiscriminately with most proteins; see below), they must be used at concentrations that avoid nonspecific inflammation, which are determined by testing nonsensitized individuals: with many potent sensitizers 0.01 M solutions are suitable.

Most simple sensitizers are relatively hydrophobic and readily penetrate the intact skin. They are usually administered in solvents that are partly nonvolatile, such as 1:1 acetone-corn oil, to prevent excessive concentration by evaporation. Hydrophilic sensitizers penetrate the skin less well, and relatively high concentrations are required (e.g., 0.5 M penicillin). These substances probably penetrate human skin via sweat ducts, and their penetration of guinea pig skin, which lacks sweat glands, can be augmented by addition of nonionic detergents to the solvent.

The **time course** of the contact skin response is the same as that of the tuberculin reaction:

---

* Allergic contact dermatitis can be elicited on the ears of mice, but it cannot be evoked elsewhere on the skin in this species, or in many others, perhaps, as has been suggested, because of anatomical differences in small cutaneous blood vessels.

erythema and swelling appear at ca. 10 to 12 hours and increase to a maximum at 24 to 48 hours. Unusually intense reactions produce necrosis, and complete recovery of the skin site can take several weeks, even without necrosis.

Histologically, the dermis (deep layer of skin) at the site of contact is invaded by mononuclear cells, as in delayed-type responses to tuberculin (cf. Figs. 20-2 and 20-3). The epidermis (superficial layer of skin), however, looks different: it is hyperplastic and is invaded by mononuclear cells. In addition, **intraepidermal vesicles** regularly form in human (but not in guinea pig) skin; they sometimes coalesce to form large blisters filled with serous fluid, granulocytes, and mononuclear cells (Fig. 20-3).

Reactions with Proteins in Vivo. In accord with the general requirements for immunogenicity (Ch. 17), the actual immunogens are not the simple substances themselves, but the covalent derivatives they form with tissue (skin) proteins in vivo. For instance, among a group of 2,4-dinitrobenzenes those that can form stable, covalent derivatives of protein -SH and -NH_2 groups in vivo are sensitizers, while those that cannot form such derivatives are not (Fig. 20-4).†

Persistence. Once established in guinea pig or human, contact skin sensitivity probably persists for years, though it tends to wane. A patch test to evaluate its persistence can boost the level of sensitivity.

The persistence of sensitizers in tissues is evident in the "flare reaction." In this phenomenon a small amount of sensitizer, applied percutaneously as a diagnostic test to the skin of an insensitive person, causes no reaction; but 10 to 20 days later the test site flares up with a typical contact skin reaction. At that time repetition of the test anywhere on the skin elicits the characterisitc allergic response. Evidently enough sensitizer remains at the first site to provide an effective test dose when the subject be-

---

† Some macromolecules, such as denatured nucleic acids, become immunogenic on forming noncovalent complexes with proteins; the complexes are extremely stable because they involve many noncovalent bonds per interacting molecule. However, the simple inducers of contact sensitivity can form only a few noncovalent bonds per molecule and hence they definitely must form covalent derivatives.

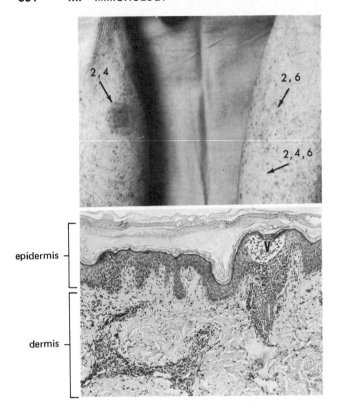

epidermis

dermis

Fig. 20-3. Allergic contact dermatitis in man. The subject was sensitized to 2,4-dinitrofluorobenzene (DNFB) and then tested with 2,4-dinitrochlorobenzene (2,4), 2,6-dinitrochlorobenzene (2,6), and 2,4,6-trinitrochlorobenzene (2,4,6). The positive response was evident at 24 hours and photographed at 72 hours. Specificity is shown by the strong reaction to 2,4-dinitrochlorobenzene, and the absence of reactions to the 2,6 and 2,4,6 analogs. DNFB and all the analogs tested form dinitrophenyl (or trinitrophenyl) derivatives of skin proteins in vivo. Histology of the skin reaction is shown below. Note the characteristic intraepidermal vesicle (V) and the dense infiltration of dermis and epidermis by lymphoid cells. Epidermal cells around vesicles generally have a foamy cytoplasm ("spongiosus").

comes sensitive a few weeks later. The flare reaction thus resembles serum sickness (Ch. 19), though more extended in time and involving cell-mediated, rather than humoral, allergy.

SPECIFICITY

The determinants of specificity are still incompletely defined, but they appear to be larger and more complex than those involved in Ab-mediated reactions. For instance, guinea pigs sensitized with 2,4,6-trinitrophenyl-bovine γ-globulin (Tnp-BγG) respond more intensely to the immunogen than to the unsubstituted protein (BγG), and not at all to Tnp conjugated onto unrelated carriers, such as ovalbumin (Tnp-Ea). Hence the response appears to be specific for the total immunogen (Tnp plus carrier protein) or a large part of it: **delayed-type responses are carrier-specific.**

In Ab-mediated reactions, in contrast, the determinants are both smaller and better defined, in vitro and in vivo: for example, anti-Tnp Abs, produced in response to Tnp-BγG, form precipitates with Tnp-Ea, bind Tnp-lysine, and mediate anaphylactic and Arthus

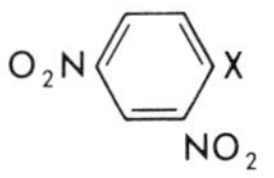

Substituents (X) in C-1 of $O_2N\langle\bigcirc\rangle X$ with NO_2	Reaction with protein in vivo		
	with ϵ-NH_2 of lysine residues	with SH of cysteine residues	Ability to induce and elicit contact skin sensitivity
X = −F	+	+	+
−Cl	+	+	+
−Br	+	+	+
−SO₃	−	+	+
−SCN	−	+	+
−SCl	−	+	+
−H	−	−	−
−CH₃	−	−	−
−NH₂	−	−	−

Fig. 20-4. Correlation among C-l substituted 2,4-dinitrobenzenes between ability to form 2,4-dinitrophenylated proteins in vivo and ability to induce and to elicit contact skin sensitivity. (Based on Eisen, H. N. in *Cellular and Humoral Aspects of the Hypersensitive States,* H. S. Lawrence, ed. Hoeber, New York, 1959).

responses with Tnp conjugated onto almost any protein (Table 20-3).

The need for large and complex antigenic units is also suggested by the apparent requirement that agents triggering cell-mediated responses must be immunogenic: for instance, with hapten conjugates of poly-L-lysines of varying lengths, only oligomers with more than seven lysines can both establish and elicit delayed hypersensitivity, whereas smaller nonimmunogenic oligomers react perfectly well with Ab molecules raised against the larger conjugates.

The requirement for large antigenic units helps clarify the specificity of contact skin allergy: for instance, an individual who has been sensitized with Tnp-BγG, and who gives delayed-type responses to an injection of this conjugate, will not respond to a contact test with Tnp-chloride (TNCB or picryl chloride), which readily forms Tnp conjugates with skin proteins in vivo. Conversely, guinea pigs sensitized with TNCB give delayed-type skin reaction to this substance, but not to conjugates of Tnp on BγG or other common proteins. It appears, therefore, that self-proteins of skin, specifically modified by covalent attachment of particular sensitizer groups (such as Tnp) are the actual antigenic units in contact skin responses.

The simple group, however, seems also to be required: for example, guinea pigs with contact skin sensitivity to TNCB do not give contact skin reactions to the corresponding 2,4-dinitrophenyls

(such as the chloro- or fluoro-derivatives, DNCB or DNFB), which readily form Dnp conjugates in vivo, probably by reacting with the same amino and sulfhydryl groups of the same skin proteins as TNCB (Fig. 20-4). Hence, both the specific haptenic and carrier groups seem to be needed (see also Fig. 20-3).

Why are the agents that trigger delayed-type responses larger and more complex than those that react with Abs? One possibility is that the binding sites of receptors on T lymphocytes (see below) are structurally different from binding sites of Abs; another is that triggering the cellular responses requires more than merely binding of Ag: the cell's membrane presumably undergoes a perturbation that results in "activation" and release of diverse products (see below). It is also possible that the triggering of delayed-type responses requires cell-cell cooperation, though the cells are likely to be T lymphocytes with or without macrophages (see below), rather than T and B cells (and macrophages) as in induction of secondary responses in Ab formation, where the need for carrier specificity is also prominent (Ch. 17). Indeed it is possible that large multideterminant ligands and "carrier specificity" are characteristic requirements of all cellular responses to Ags, whether involved in delayed-type hypersensitivity or induction of Ab synthesis, rather than a distinguishing difference between cell-mediated and humoral immunity.

OTHER CELL-MEDIATED IMMUNE RESPONSES

RESISTANCE TO INFECTIOUS AGENTS

Many bacteria survive phagocytosis and even multiply within phagocytic cells (e.g., tubercle bacilli, leprosy bacilli). Clinical and experimental observations have shown, however, that macrophages from individuals with such infections have augmented ability to kill the infecting bacteria and also many other antigenically unrelated ones. Though the antimicrobial activity of these altered macrophages is nonspecific, their conversion into "angry killers" is due to a specific immunological process: when an animal is primed by infection with one organism and then cured and later reinfected with a small number of bacteria of the same type, its macrophages promptly become nonspecific killers, but a similar small number of antigenically unrelated bacteria as a challenge would not have triggered the conversion of macrophages into killer cells. Like other cell-mediated immune reactions the specific ability to activate macrophages can be transferred—not with antisera but with lymphocytes whose specific reaction with Ag releases soluble factors that probably cause differentiation of macrophages into angry killers (below). Modified cells are more phagocytic, and have more lysosomes and lysosomal enzymes than normal macrophages (Figs. 20-5, 20-6).

Fig. 20-5. Comparison of resting **(A,C)** and activated **(B,D)** macrophages. All are peritoneal cells from normal **(A,C)** or infected mice **(B,D)** 14 days after injection of tubercle bacilli (BCG, bacillus Calmette-Guerin). In the phase-contrast photographs **(C,D** ×1900) the activated macrophages **(D)** are larger (the field is almost filled by one-half a cell), more spread out, and have increased content of organelles, especially lysosomes (dense, spherical bodies); the translucent spherical bodies represent ingested culture medium (pinocytotic vesicles). In the electron micrographs **(A,B;** magnification uncertain) the dense spherical lysosomes (L) are abundant in activated cells and rare in resting cells, most of whose organelles are mitochondria (M). **[A,B** from Blanden, R. V., Lefford, M. J., and Mackaness, G. B. *J Exp Med 129*:1079 (1969); **C,D** courtesy of Dr. G. B. Mackaness.]

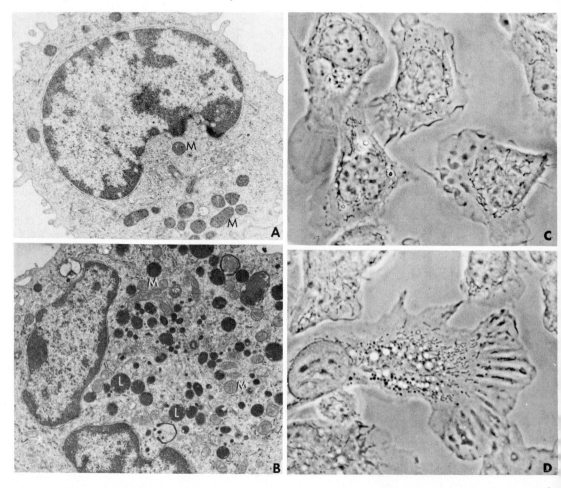

Fig. 20-6. Increased bactericidal activity of activated macrophages. *Salmonella typhimurium* coated (opsonized) with anti-*Salmonella* antibodies are ingested and killed more rapidly and in greater numbers by activated than by normal macrophages. [From Mackaness, G. B. *Hosp Practice,* 73 (1970).]

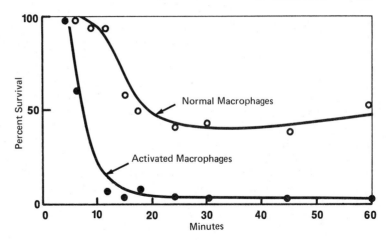

Besides its protective role in infections with intracellular bacteria (tuberculosis, leprosy, brucellosis), this type of cell-mediated immunity is probably important in many viral, fungal, and protozoan infections. The evidence comes not only from a lack of Ab protection in experimental infections, but from the greater severity of clinical infections in those with diminished cell-mediated immunity due to heritable or acquired defects (Clinical deficiencies, below) or to certain immunosuppressive agents (antilymphocyte serum, below). Activated macrophages are also important in some other cell-mediated immune responses (Accessory cells; Tumor immunity, below).

REJECTION OF ALLOGRAFTS

Cells, tissues, or organs that are transferred from a donor to a genetically different recipient of the same species are called **allografts.** Because of extensive polymorphism of certain surface glycoproteins (Ch. 21) the grafted cells almost invariably contain on their surfaces histocompatibility or transplantation Ags that are lacking on host cells (and vice versa).*

---

* Chapter 21 deals in detail with the principles governing survival of transplanted cells. It is necessary to repeat here (see also Chs. 17 and 21) that cell surface histocompatibility Ags, like Ig allotypes, are genetically segregating alloantigens (Gr., *allos,* other): they are present in some and absent in other members of the same species. Genetically identical (syngeneic) individuals (monozygotic twins or members of highly inbred animal strains) have identical histocompatibility Ags and accept grafted cells freely from each other. Genetically different

The resulting host response leads to destruction of the allograft through a delayed-type hypersensitivity reaction, which depends on specific lymphocytes (below) and seems usually to be independent of Abs.

When one allograft is followed by another from the same donor the second rejection occurs more rapidly than the first (Ch. 21, Second-set reaction). The acceleration is specific: it does not occur with another allogeneic graft, donated by a third party, to the same recipient. As with delayed-type tuberculin hypersensitivity, the site of the allograft rejection is characterized by chronic infiltration with lymphocytes and macrophages, and the capacity for the second-set reaction can be transferred by living lymphocytes, but not by antiserum. Moreover the intensity and speed of graft rejection do not correlate with the level of serum Abs to transplantation Ags; indeed, these Abs are often undetectable.

Under special circumstances, however, certain allografts can be rejected wholly, or partly, as a result of reactions with conventional Abs. In contrast to "solid" tissue and organ grafts, dispersed allogeneic lymphocytes can be lysed by the combined action of Abs to their transplantation (or other surface) Ags, plus complement (C). The rejection of tissue allografts can also sometimes be speeded up by transfer of massive amounts of antiserum from hyperimmune animals, but the histological appearance is then anomalous, with edema, vascular occlusion, and granulocytes, rather the usual mononuclear in-

---

(allogeneic) individuals of the same species reject each other's grafts, owing to the host immune response against histocompatibility Ags on the grafted cells.

filtrate. Abs to vascular endothelium can also accelerate rejection of kidney allografts, probably through occlusion of nutrient blood vessels (Ch. 21, Effect of blood group incompatibilities on kidney allografts).

GRAFT-VS.-HOST REACTION

This form of the allograft reaction occurs when lymphocytes are transferred from an immunologically competent donor (normal adult) to an allogeneic incompetent recipient (e.g., newborn). These reactions have increasing clinical importance because of therapeutic attempts to transfer normal thymus or bone marrow cells to immunodeficient humans [e.g., infants with genetic defects (see Ch. 17 and below), patients with leukemia treated with cytotoxic drugs and whole-body X-irradiation]. The recipient exhibits loss of weight, skin rash (in guinea pigs and man), increase in spleen size, stimulation of macrophage activity (below); chick embryos receiving allogeneic lymphocytes from adult chickens develop characteristic focal lesions on the chorioallantoic membrane. The intesity of the reaction is generally proportional to the number of transplanted lymphocytes, and a sufficient number can cause the recipient's death.

Nodules appear in many organs, but are most numerous in the spleen. Cells from mouse donors with the easily recognized T6 chromosomes show that a typical nodule starts with proliferation and blast transformation of donor lymphocyes (see below and Ch. 17), followed by massive proliferation of host fibroblasts.

TUMOR IMMUNITY

Clinical observations have long hinted at immunity against tumors, e.g., cancers disappear spontaneously from rare patients, and unusually slow-growing tumors are often prominently infiltrated with lymphoid cells. Almost all carefully studied tumor cells are now known to have distinctive surface Ags that are lacking or masked on normal cells (Ch. 21). Considerable evidence shows that these tumor-specific Ags are immunogenic in the **autochthonous host** (the one in whom the tumor arises), and that cell-mediated responses are especially capable of restricting tumor growth.

1) In a classic study by Klein and coworkers, a sarcoma induced in a mouse by methylcholanthrene was excised and carried by successive transplants in syngeneic mice while the surgically cured autochthonous host was immunized with his X-irradiated sarcoma cells.* The immunized animal was then able to reject a graft of his own tumor, but was not resistant to another sarcoma.

2) Under standard tissue culture conditions a patients' tumor cells usually form fewer colonies if incubated with his own lymphocytes than if incubated with lymphocytes from other persons (Hellstrom).

3) Oncogenic polyomavirus causes tumors to appear in adult mice only if the animals' ability to make cell-mediated responses has been eliminated, e.g., by thymectomy and antilymphocyte serum (ALS; see below, Ch. 17, and Table 20-4). Moreover, humans with defective cellular immunity have an abnormally high incidence of various cancers: in chronically immunosuppressed recipients of kidney allografts, malignant lymphomas, particularly reticulum cell sarcomas, appear ca. 4000 times more frequently (ca. 0.5%) than in the population at large (same age and sex distribution).

The role of cell-mediated immunity in resistance to tumors is also evident in the behavior of **transplanted tumors.** Tumor cells usually have the same histocompatibility Ags as normal cells (Ch. 21) of the autochthonous host and hence are rejected (like normal tissue allografts, Ch. 21) when transplantetd to allogeneic recipients. However, tumor grafts can flourish and eventually kill recipients that are syngeneic with the autochthonous donor. The number of cells required for a successful (i.e., lethal) syngeneic graft increases if the recipient has been previously immunized against that tumor (Fig. 20-7).

For instance, 1000 tumor cells might suffice to produce progressive tumors in 50% of unimmunized syngeneic recipients (TD_{50} = 1000 cells/recipient), whereas this number might produce only a rare tumor in recipients who were previously immunized with that tumor, or even with its isolated tumor-specific Ag. This resistance can, however, be overcome by a larger inoculum, which might range from perhaps 3 to 1000 times the TD_{50} dose. Tumors vary greatly in virulence: TD_{50} doses can range from 10 to 10^6 cells per unimmunized recipient. This wide variation, and the effect of immunization (Fig. 20-7), suggest that **progressive growth of a tumor (as graft or as indigenous clone) requires a critical mass above which it can grow more rapidly than it can be destroyed by the immunity it elicits.**

---

* X-irradiation (e.g., 750 r) blocks cell division by damaging DNA (Ch. 11) but leaves the cell Ags intact.

TABLE 20-4. Increased Incidence of Tumors (Due to Polyomavirus) in Mice with Impaired Cell-Mediated Immunity

Preliminary treatment of adult mice, CBA strain*	Treatment 7 wk later†	No. of mice	Percent that develop tumors
Normal rabbit γ-globulin (control)	None	24	0
Thymectomy + ALS*	None	14	100
Thymectomy + ALS	Inject lymphoid cells from normal CBA mice	10	90
Thymectomy + ALS	Inject lymphoid cells from CBA mice immunized with polyomavirus	11	0

* Polyomavirus was injected after thymectomy and the first of three biweekly injections of ALS (γ-globulin fraction of rabbit antiserum to mouse lymphocytes).
† Ten days after final injection of ALS.
Based on Allison, A. C. *Proc R Soc Lond* (*Biol*) *177*:23–39 (1971).

The resistance induced by immunization is specific for the tumor used as immunogen, and sometimes for closely related tumors (e.g., those raised in other animals with the same oncogenic virus, Ch. 63). It can usually be transferred with viable lymphocytes but not with serum. Indeed, **passively transferred serum can sometimes decrease the recipient's resistance:** i.e., transfer of antiserum plus tumor cells can result in a higher incidence and earlier appearance of tumors, perhaps because Abs bind to surface Ags on the tumor cells, preventing either induction of cell-mediated immunity or its expression (attachment of specifically reactive lymphocytes: see below and Ch. 21, Enhancement).

Current efforts to increase clinical resistance to established tumors include injections of avirulent tubercle bacilli (BCG strain) into human skin tumors, or painting the tumors with 2,4-dinitrochlorobenzene, a potent skin sensitizer (DNCB, Fig. 20-4). The ensuing delayed-type allergic reaction within the tumor may increase destruction of tumor cells by providing "angry" macrophages (see Resistance to infectious agents, above) or cytotoxic

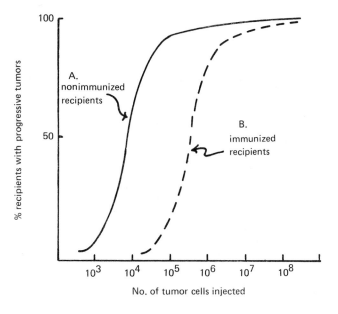

Fig. 20-7. Dose-response curves for growth of transplanted tumors. Recipients were syngeneic with the autochthonous host. Besides use of X-irradiated cells as immunogen, resistance can sometimes be induced with a subthreshold inoculum (e.g., 100 cells, curve A): before it reaches the critical mass the tumor is eliminated by the immunity it induces. A recipient will often also become resistant to another graft of the same tumor if its first tumor graft is excised after about 1 week's growth.

factors (Products of activated lymphocytes, below); or tubercle bacilli and allergic inflammation may have an adjuvant effect on the immunogenicity of the tumor-specific Ags (Ch. 17, Adjuvants).

Surveillance. All of the foregoing suggests that cell-mediated immunity probably functions continuously in normal individuals as a **surveillance** mechanism, destroying newly arising neoplastic clones before they exceed a critical mass. Occasional clones probably develop into clinically significant tumors because 1) their cell surface tumor-specific Ags have exceptionally low immunogenicity, 2) the host may lapse in its ability to make cell-mediated immune responses to Ags in general, 3) tumor variants may emerge with high growth rates or increased resistance to cytotoxic effects of immune reactions (below), and 4) "blocking" Abs to tumor Ags can sometimes prevent attack by specifically reactive lymphocytes (below and Ch. 21, Enhancement). Selective pressure of immune surveillance may account for feeble immunogenicity of distinctive tumor-specific Ags of most well-established tumors in their autochthonous hosts. Immunity to tumors is discussed further (Ch. 21).

PHYLOGENY AND ONTOGENY

As was noted before (Ch. 17) all species of vertebrates have both cell-mediated and humoral immunity at birth or hatching or shortly afterward. Invertebrates do not form Abs (Ch. 17) and their defenses against invasive parasites are probably based on primitive forms of cell-mediated immunity. Metchnikoff's classic description of motile, phagocytic cells (amebocytes) engulfing a penetrating thorn in a sea star indicated that macrophage-like cells of invertebrates could recognize and react against foreign objects; and amebocytes of a marine worm are now known to phagocytize various foreign cells (but not their own). Suggestive evidence for rejection of skin allografts has also been found in earthworms (but not in other invertebrates).

Since ontogeny generally recapitulates phylogeny, the time sequence for acquisition of diverse immune responses during fetal development of vertebrates should clarify evolutionary sequences. However, the evidence is not easily interpreted: fetal lambs become capable of rejecting allografts at 75 days of gestation (halfway through pregnancy), but they make Abs to certain Ags before 60 days and to other Ags only after birth (Ch. 17). Human fetuses also synthesize Igs (Ch. 17), but delayed-type skin reactions seem not to be elicitable until some months after birth, perhaps because of immaturity in accessory cells (below) or in the skin itself, rather than in the immunologically specific cells.

CELLULAR BASIS FOR CELL-MEDIATED IMMUNITY

Conventional Ab molecules are excluded from a role in these reactions because countless attempts to transfer the capacity for delayed-type skin reactions with serum have failed, and the few reported successes have not been corroborated. Moreover, these reactions, and allograft rejection, can be elicited in individuals who are almost devoid of serum Igs: e.g., children with immunodeficiency disorders (X-linked agammaglobulinemia, Ch. 17), mice treated from birth with Abs to μ chains (Ch. 17).

T LYMPHOCYTES AS MEDIATORS

Though suspected from the early 1900s, cells were first shown to mediate delayed-type allergy in 1942, when Chase transferred delayed sensitivity to tuberculin from sensitive to normal guinea pigs with viable lymphoid cells. Since then similar results with many other Ags, and with other forms of cellular immunity,

have established that **transfer by viable cells from lymph nodes, spleen, or peritoneal exudates is an essential characteristic of cell-mediated immune reactions.** However, it is not an exclusive property: similar populations of lymphoid cells from an intensively immunized animal can continue to form Abs in the recipient (or even in tissue culture, Ch. 17) and thus can probably also occasionally transfer immediate-type allergy.

The cell suspensions ordinarily used to transfer sensitivity are usually referred to as "lymphoid cells," to emphasize that they are crude mixtures of lymphocytes (themselves highly heterogeneous), macrophages, and other cells (erythrocytes, granulocytes). After fractionating a mixture by sedimentation Gowans demonstrated that **small lymphocytes** are the active cells in the graft-vs.-host reaction.

Extirpation experiments then showed that **the active small lymphocyte is a T cell:** for example, allograft survival is greatly prolonged in neonatally thymectomized chickens or mice but not in bursectomized chickens (Ch. 17, Table 17-4). Moreover, lymphoid cell populations enriched for T cells (by passage over glass beads to remove B cells, Ch. 17) require fewer cells to transfer cell-mediated reactions, while populations enriched for B cells (by destroying most of the T cells with Abs to the θ surface antigen, Ch. 17) are less active.

The association of T cells with cell-mediated immunity and of B cells with humoral immunity is in accord with zonal effects within the lymph nodes that drain sites of injected Ags: when the stimulus leads to delayed-type hypersensitivity (e.g., painting the skin with a contact sensitizer) the regional lymph node's T zones become greatly hyperplastic, and when the stimulus causes Ab formation with little or no cell-mediated immunity proliferation of lymphocytes is largely confined to B-cell areas (Ch. 17, see germinal follicles in Figs 17-15 and 17-16).

MACROPHAGES AS NONSPECIFIC ACCESSORIES

Macrophages are even more abundant than lymphocytes at sites of delayed-type reactions or allograft rejections, and are required. Thus lethally irradiated animals (900 r) developed cell-mediated responses only when both lymphocytes and bone marrow cells were transferred. Administration of ^{3}H-thymidine to the marrow donor showed that rapidly dividing "promonocytes" in bone marrow (tagged in DNA) are precursors of blood-borne monocytes (immature macrophages, Ch. 17) which infiltrate the developing skin lesion and differentiate there into mature macrophages with abundant lysosomal enzymes (see Fig. 20-5). **The macrophages act nonspecifically, for nonsensitized and sensitized donors provide equally effective marrow cells. The lymphocytes, however, are effective only if obtained from a sensitized donor.**

Relatively few specific T cells are needed to initiate an allergic response. After adoptive sensitization of a normal recipient with labeled lymphocytes (from an actively sensitized donor who had been treated with ^{3}H-thymidine) fewer than 10% of the mononuclear cells in the recipient's skin lesion were labeled, whereas

over 90% were labeled when normal recipients were given ^{3}H-thymidine and sensitized lymphocytes were then transferred from an unlabeled donor. Studies with cultured cells (below) show that on reacting with Ag the sensitized lymphocytes release substances that cause the chemotactic accumulation and differentiation of macrophages. It is likely that the accumulated macrophages can behave as the "angry killers" that destroy diverse, antigenically unrelated bacteria in cell-mediated immunity to infections (Figs. 20-5 and 20-6).

GENETIC CONTROL

The ability of guinea pigs to develop delayed-type hypersensitivity to some Ags is governed by a genetic locus that seems to determine specific binding of Ag by lymphocytes. Thus with hapten–poly-L-lysine (PLL) conjugates as Ag animals of an inbred "responder" strain (2) can develop delayed skin sensitivity but those of a "nonresponder" strain (13) cannot. The nonresponders, however, are able to exhibit delayed skin reactions to the PLL conjugates if adoptively sensitized with lymphoid cells from an immunized responder*: hence the nonresponder is defective in the induction of sensitivity, rather than in its expression.

Breeding experiments show that the responder phenotype is governed by a single, dominant autosomal gene: e.g., all F_1 hybrids (2 × 13) are responders ($PLL+/PLL-$), as are 50% of the progeny of the back-cross between the heterozygotes and nonresponders ($PLL-/PLL-$). The PLL gene is linked to the locus that specifies potent histocompatibility alloantigens on guinea pig cells.† The PLL gene's product may be a histocompatibility Ag; or it may be the elusive Ag-binding receptor on T cells, for antisera produced in nonresponders to histocompatibility Ags of the responder strain block specific reactions of the responder's T lymphocytes (such as Ag-induced blast transformation), but their B cells, whose receptors are clearly immunoglobulins (Ch. 17), are not affected.

---

* Though the transferred lymphocytes are allografts they can mediate delayed-type hypersensitivity in the recipient for about 1 to 2 weeks; i.e., until they are destroyed by the recipient's immune response to their histocompatibility Ags.

† The corresponding locus in mice, *Ir-1*, is linked to the locus for the most potent histocompatibility alloantigens in this species (*H-2;* see Ch. 17, Genetic regulation of Ab formation; also Ch. 21). *Ir-1* probably also specifies delayed-type allergic reactions, but those elicited with soluble proteins are difficult to discern in mice.

RELATION TO HELPER CELLS IN ANTIBODY FORMATION

The T lymphocytes that specify cell-mediated immune responses have many properties in common with those that serve as helper cells in Ab formation:

1) The reactions with Ag appear to be specific for larger determinants ("carrier-specific") than those of conventional Abs.

2) Both require macrophages as nonspecific accessory cells in carrying out their respective activities (delayed-type allergic reactions and modulation of the B-cell response to immunogen).

3) Both can function without dividing: i.e., X-irradiation does not block their activities, though it inhibits their induced proliferation (Nonspecific suppression, below).

4) Recognition of Ag by both cells might be specified by the same genetic locus (called *Ir-1* in mice and *PLL* in guinea pigs), which could conceivably code for their Ag-binding receptors (see Ch. 17, Genetic control of Ab formation).

However, the effector T cells of cell-mediated immunity react specifically with the concerned Ag, whereas helper function can be less specific. For instance, T cells triggered by diverse Ags can modulate nonspecifically the B cell responses to other Ags (see Ch. 17, Allogeneic effect, and Antigenic promotion and competition).

The ability of Ag-sensitive T lymphocytes to engage in both functions would provide a basis for the old view that delayed-type hypersensitivity is a preliminary stage in the induction of Ab formation: the initial proliferation of T cells in response to an immunogen could contribute to the subsequent differentiation of neighboring B cells. Delayed-type hypersensitivity reactions might thus serve as an "adjuvant" in the formation of Abs to T-dependent Ags. Some conventional adjuvants probably also exercise their effects by attracting (and activating) many T cells: thus Freund's complete adjuvant promotes Ab formation to many T-dependent Ags, but not to T-independent ones, such as pneumococcal polysaccharides (Ch. 17).

TRANSFER FACTOR

Though cell-mediated responses are readily transferred with living lymphocytes, disrupted cells are ineffective in all animal species tested except man, in whom Lawrence found that extracts of blood leukocytes can apparently transfer the cell-mediated responses of the leukocyte donor. Recipients become reactive to Ag 1 to 7 days after receiving the extract and sensitivity can persist for years, even when the extract is prepared from as little as 5 ml of blood (corresponding to about 10^7 total lymphocytes).

The active component, "transfer factor," has been difficult to characterize since it can be assayed only in humans. It is dialyzable, stable on prolonged storage, and has a molecular weight of less than 10,000; it is inactivated by heat (56°, 30 minutes) but not by trypsin, RNase, or DNase. Clinical trials indicate that transfer factor may be effective even in those with deficient cell-mediated immunity (below). For instance, patients with disseminated *Candida* infections (chronic mucocutaneous candidiasis) lack delayed skin responses to *Candida* proteins, but after receiving transfer factor from *Candida*-sensitive donors their previously intractable infections sometimes subside, and some of them manifest delayed-type skin reactions to *Candida*. Similar events have occurred in patients with disseminated vaccinia, as well as in children with congenital cell-mediated immunodeficiencies (Wiskott-Aldrich syndrome, below).

Transfer factor seems to lack antigenicity; it is not inactivated by anti-Igs; and it seems too small to be an informational molecule, such as mRNA. Possibly it is an immensely potent nonspecific adjuvant, enhancing induction of cell-mediated immunity to prevalent Ags or to those injected intradermally to evaluate its effects. Clarification of the nature and mode of action of transfer factor is likely to illuminate fundamental mechanisms of cellular immunity.

CELL-MEDIATED IMMUNE REACTIONS WITH CULTURED CELLS

The reactions of cultured cells have been intensively explored to develop assays for measurement of cell-mediated immunity and to analyze mechanisms. In contrast to methods for measuring Abs and Ab-mediated reactions, assays for cell-mediated responses are cumbersome and imprecise. Nonetheless, the in vitro analyses clearly emphasize several phases: specific reaction of Ag with sensitized T lymphocytes stimulates their differentiation into blast cells and their secretion of factors that act nonspecifically on a variety of other cells. The products of activated lymphocytes ("PALs" or "lymphokines") have not so far been obtained in sufficient quantity or purity for detailed analysis; hence they are consid-

TABLE 20-5. Products of Activated Lymphocytes

Product	Activity
A. Affects macrophages	
Migration-inhibition factor (MIF)	Inhibits migration of normal macrophages
Aggregation factor (AF)	Agglutinates suspended macrophages
Chemotactic factor (CF)	Causes migration of macrophages toward increasing concentration of the factor
B. Affects lymphocytes	
Blastogenic or mitogenic factor (BF or MF)	Induces normal lymphocytes to differentiate into blast cells (increasing their incorporation of thymidine into DNA)
Potentiating factor (PF)	Enhances blast transformation in Ag-stimulated cultures
Helper factor	Enhances differentiation of Ab-forming cells in culture
C. Affects cultured cells	
Lymphotoxin (LT)	Damages or lyses various cultured cell lines (human Hela, mouse L)
Proliferation inhibitory factor	Blocks proliferation of cultured cells without lysing them
Interferon (?)	Inhibits viral multiplication in cultured cells
D. In vivo effects	
Skin reactive factor	Produces indurated skin lesions in normal guinea pigs
Macrophage disappearance factor	Intraperitoneal injection causes macrophages to adhere to peritoneum

Courtesy of Dr. Barry R. Bloom.

ered below only in terms of their effects on various target cells in vitro (Table 20-5).

BLAST TRANSFORMATION

Transformation Due to Antigen. The addition of Ag to cultured lymphocytes from sensitized individuals causes a small proportion of the cells to differentiate into large, rapidly dividing blast cells (Fig. 20-8). The morphological changes (which include conversion of nuclear chromatin from heterochromatin to euchromatin, and the development of conspicuous nu-

cleolus and polyribosomes; see Ch. 17) are associated with increased synthesis of protein, RNA, and especially of DNA, as though cells were preparing to enter mitosis. The peak of the response occurs ca. 5 days after Ag is added, and the changes are most conveniently revealed by increased incorporation of ^{3}H-thymidine into DNA.

Similar changes are brought about with lymphoid cells from individuals who are primed for Ab production but lack obvious cell-mediated hypersensitivity for the stimulating Ag (e.g., from persons with immediate-type hypersensitivity to plant pollens,

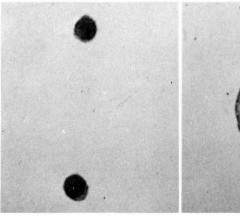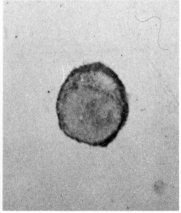

Fig. 20-8. Blast transformation of lymphocytes. Small (resting) lymphocytes at left; the same after stimulation by Ag or a plant mitogen (lectin) at right. (Based on Hirschhorn, K. *Human Transplantation.* Rapaport, F. T., and Dausset, J., eds. Grune and Stratton, New York, 1968.)

penicillins, etc.; Chs. 17 and 19). Nevertheless, the reactions seem to occur more regularly and with greater intensity among cells from those with delayed-type hypersensitivity.

Transformation by Mitogens. Certain plant proteins that react specifically with various sugars of glycoproteins on the lymphocyte surface can also induce differentiation into blast cells. The changes seem to be the same as those induced by Ag, but the **plant "mitogens"** act nonspecifically: prior sensitization of the donor is unnecessary, and the majority of lymphocytes of a given class react.

B and T cells respond to different mitogens: for example, soluble concanavalin A (Con A) and phytohemagglutinin (PHA) transform T cells, but when these plant proteins are attached to insoluble particles (Sephadex beads) they also stimulate B cells (Fig. 20-9). **Pokeweed mitogen** (at low dose and in insoluble form) stimulates B and T cells. Though not

Fig. 20-9. Evidence that lymphocytes responding to phytohemagglutinin (PHA) are predominantly T cells. Injection of antilymphocyte serum (ALS) on day 0 abolished cells that respond by blast transformation to PHA; recovery of responsiveness to PHA was not observed in thymectomized mice, but was almost complete by day 20 in normal mice. [Based on Tursi, A., Greaves, M. F., Torrigiani, G., Playfair, J. H. L., and Roitt, I. M. *Immunology* 17:801 (1969).]

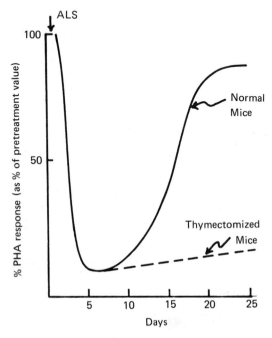

of plant origin, **lipopolysaccharide** of cell walls from Enterobacteriaceae transforms B cells exclusively.

The time course of events triggered by PHA spreads out over 4 or 5 days in culture. Within 5 minutes an increased turnover of phosphatidyl inositol of the cell membrane is noted, followed a few minutes later by acetylation of histones; increased synthesis of RNA is measurable at 2 hours but morphological changes are not detected until 20 hours, and increased incorporation of thymidine into DNA is measurable only after 2 to 4 days' incubation with the mitogen (or Ag).

Transformation by Mixed Lymphocyte Culture. Small lymphocytes can also be transformed by culturing together the cells from genetically different individuals of the same species: because of extensive polymorphism at loci for cell surface proteins, the two cell populations are virtually always different antigenically, and they stimulate each other to undergo blast transformation. If individual X is made tolerant of individual Y, but not vice versa, Y's cells will undergo blast transformation in the mixed culture, but not X's. (The distinction between X and Y can be made in the "one-way reaction" through prior incubation of one or the other set of cells with mitomycin C; the drug blocks DNA synthesis without affecting the surface Ags and one can thus tell which cells stimulate and which respond.)

The results of mixed cultures help predict the histocompatibility "matching" and fate of human allografts (Ch. 21), but the high proportion of reactive cells in nonsensitized individuals (ca. 3%) raises some doubts about the immune mechanisms involved, especially since the proportion is not increased in sensitized individuals and it seems to be even lower with combinations of lymphocytes from different species, where the antigenic incompatibilities must be greater.

Specificity of Blast Transformation. The specificity of T cells has been demonstrated in cultures of cells from individuals who are sensitive to several Ags: if cells are stimulated by one Ag to incorporate bromodeoxyuridine (a light-sensitive analog of thymidine) and then are killed selectively by exposure to visible light, further response to that Ag is eliminated without affecting other cells in the same culture that are sensitive to other Ags.

If a given T cell can react with only one Ag, and the repertoire of Ags that evoke cell-mediated responses is as great as in Ab formation, the cells that respond to a given Ag should represent a very small fraction of an individual's lymphocytes. However, incubation with an Ag for a few days will often convert as many as 1% of an individual's lymphocytes into blast cells, and the proportion can reach 5% or more. These values could reflect death and lysis of nondividing cells in the culture, proliferative increase of Ag-activated cells (whose generation time is probably ca. 8 hours) and, most of all perhaps, recruitment of nonsensitized cells by the "blastogenic" factor released from authentically sensitized cells in response to Ag stimulation (below). The high proportion of blast cells elicited by single Ags has not been accounted for. Whether T cells are as restricted in specificity as B cells (Ch. 17) and Ab molecules is still uncertain.

Virus Plaque Assay for Cell-mediated Immunity.
The number of Ag-activated lymphocytes can be counted by a novel plaque assay that is reminiscent of the hemolytic plaque assay for counting Ab-secreting cells (Ch. 17). This assay depends upon the capacity of Ag- (or mitogen)-activated T cells to support the replication of many viruses (mumps, measles, polio, vesicular stomatitis virus, etc.) that fail to multiply in resting lymphocytes. Each activated lymphocyte can then serve as an **infectious center,** producing a distinct cytopathic plaque when plated on a monolayer of virus-susceptible indicator cells (e.g., mouse L cells).

About 1 per 1000 lymphocytes from tuberculin-sensitive guinea pigs forms a plaque in culture after 24 hours' incubation with tuberculin, and the number increases linearly over several days, whether or not antimitotic agents are present (e.g., vinblastine). The infected cells therefore differ from blast cells, which increase exponentially and are prevented from increasing by the presence of antimitotic agents. Since X-irradiated (nondividing) lymphocytes can also mediate delayed-type hypersensitivity in adoptively sensitized animals the effector cell in vivo may be more like the responding lymphocyte in the virus plaque assay than the cell undergoing blast transformation.

The removal of glass-adherent cells abolishes the ability of Ag to establish infectious centers, suggesting that a macrophage is also required. This result fits the observation that the number of plaques formed is proportional to the square of the number of cultured lymphoid cells, indicating that two cells are necessary to form one center. Function of the macrophage in this reaction is obscured, as in blast transformation, where it seems also to be required.

PRODUCTS OF ACTIVATED LYMPHOCYTES

Effects on Macrophages. Ag-stimulated lymphocytes are associated with macrophages not only in many reactions in vivo but also in vitro. It has been known for over 40 years that the addition of Ag inhibits the outward migration of macrophages in cultured lymphoid cells from a donor with delayed-type hypersensitivity to that Ag (Fig. 20-10); in contrast, cultures from donors who lack this form of allergy are unaffected, even if the donor can make Abs to the Ag, or has immediate-type hypersensitivity to it. The response exhibits the "carrier specificity" that characterizes delayed-type skin reactions to hapten-protein conjugates (legend, Fig. 20-10), supporting the belief that it is an authentic cell-mediated immune reaction in culture.

Inhibition of macrophage movement is due to a **migration-inhibition factor** (MIF), which is released when Ag interacts with sensitized T lymphocytes. Thus if only 1% of the cells in a mixed culture are lymphocytes from a sensitized donor, migration of macrophages in the nonsensitive major population can still be inhibited by addition of Ag. Culture supernatants of Ag-stimulated sensitized lymphocytes have a similar effect. Peripheral blood lymphocytes from sensitive humans also release MIF on incubation with Ag.*

The culture supernatants of Ag-activated T cells can also **attract** macrophages: when separated by microporous filters from macrophages, these mobile cells move along the resulting gradient toward the supernatant (Fig. 20-11). But when mixed, the active supernatant blocks motility, apparently without killing the macrophages: net movement ceases because there no longer is a gradient for the cells to follow. In addition, the immobilized macrophages stick to each other, paralleling perhaps the disappearance of these cells from peritoneal cavity (and of monocytes from blood) when tuberculous guinea pigs are injected with large amounts of tuberculin. All three activities—inhibition of migration, chemotactic attraction, aggregation—could be due to the same substance (MIF).

PHA (above) not only stimulates blast transformation of T cells but causes release of MIF. De-

---

* Because of the difficulty in obtaining human macrophages the human culture supernatants are assayed with guinea pig macrophages (obtained from the peritoneal cavity 1 to 2 days after injecting thioglycollate or another irritant).

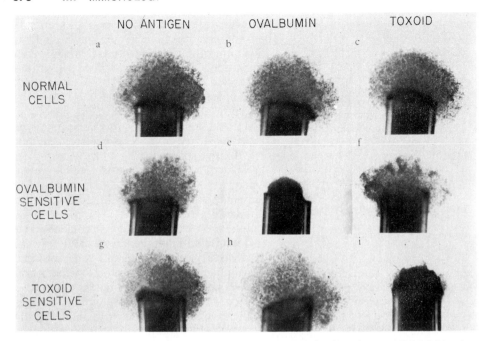

Fig. 20-10. Inhibition of macrophage migration: a response in vitro that parallels delayed-type hypersensitive reactions in vivo. Peritoneal exudate cells (predominantly macrophages and lymphocytes) are cultured in capillary tubes in presence or absence of Ags (ovalbumin, diphtheria toxoid). An Ag blocks outward migration of macrophages from the cell population derived from guinea pigs sensitive to that Ag. The response is also carrier-specific: for example, Dnp-guinea pig albumin (Dnp-GPA) blocks migration of cells from animals sensitized with Dnp-GPA, but not cells from those sensitized with Dnp or another protein, say Dnp-BγG. [From David, J. R., Al-Askari, S., Lawrence, H. S., and Thomas, L. *J Immunol 93*:264 (1964).]

Fig. 20-11. A two-compartment chamber demonstrates chemotaxis: the movement of cells along a concentration gradient of an attracting substance (chemotactic factor). Movement of macrophages from one chamber to and through the pores of a Millipore filter reveal chemotactic activity in culture supernatants of Ag-activated T lymphocytes (left). In the control (right) the uniform mixing of the culture supernatant with macrophages immobilizes the cells, as in the macrophage inhibition assay of Figure 20-10. Culture supernatants of Ag-activated lymphocytes are also chemotactic for normal lymphocytes (probably owing to another attractant).

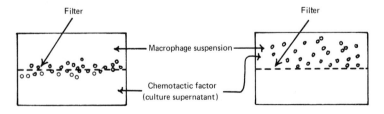

spite this aid to purification only trace amounts of impure MIF have been obtained: the active substance appears to be a polydisperse relatively heat-stable glycoprotein (MW between 35,000 and 65,-000).

Macrophages modified by MIF are "sticky" (i.e., they are more adherent to glass and to each other) and they exhibit increases in 1) movement of the surface membrane ("ruffled borders"), 2) phago-cytic activity, 3) O_2 consumption, 4) lipid biosynthesis (perhaps related to increased activities at the cell membranes), 5) glucose degradation via the hexose monophosphate shunt (related to lipid biosynthesis), and 6) H_2O_2 production. All these changes are consistent with the differentiation of macrophages into "angry killers" of ingested bacteria, but so far increases in lysosomal enzymes and in bactericidal activity have not been definitely established in MIF-modified macrophages.

Effects on Cultured Cell Lines. Supernatants from activated lymphocytes (stimulated by reaction with Ag, or plant mitogen, or with allogeneic cells in mixed lymphocyte cultures) can destroy or inhibit growth of various cultured cell lines (HeLa cells, L cells, etc.). The active substance, called *lymphotoxin* (LT), could account for necrosis of normal "by-stander" cells at sites of delayed-type allergic skin reactions and in the severe inflammatory reaction around some chronic infections (e.g., tuberculosis).

Release of LT is not consistently associated with blast transformation; it precedes the characteristic increase in synthesis of DNA, and it is brought on by some mitogen inducers of blast transformation (e.g., PHA) but not by others (Con A).

Human lymphocytes stimulated by prolonged incubation with Ag (> 3 days) seem also eventually to produce **interferon,** which can block viral infection of other cells.

Effect on Lymphocytes. Prolonged incubation of sensitized lymphocytes with Ag releases a **"blastogenic"** factor, whose addition to other cultures increases both proliferation of non-sensitized lymphocytes and the Ag-induced transformation of sensitized lymphocytes. Accordingly, the large number of transformed cells that appear with time in an Ag-treated culture probably represents **recruitment of nonsensitized lymphocytes** by the "blasto-genic" factor from a much smaller number of authentically sensitized cells, activated specifically by the Ag. Culture supernatants of Ag-

activated lymphoid cells are also chemotactic for lymphocytes (Fig. 20-11).

Effect on Skin. Culture supernatants of Ag-treated lymphocytes produce localized inflammation in guinea pig skin. The reaction has little if any erythema, and its course is slightly more rapid than that of a typical delayed-type reaction: the indurated lesion appears at 3 hours, is maximal at 6 to 12 hours, fades at 24 hours, and is prominently infiltrated with mononuclear cells. The skin activity could be due to the combined effects of some of the factors discussed above.

CYTOTOXIC MECHANISMS

A variety of cell-mediated reactions can destroy target cells (i.e., those with the relevant surface Ag) and also bystander cells, which happen to be in the immediate vicinity of a specific reaction between a T lymphocyte and its Ag. One model system indicates that target

Fig. 20-12. Contact killing of target cells by sensitized lymphocytes. The target cells, cultured mastocytoma cells from C57Bl mice or lymphoma cells from DBA mice, were labeled with ^{51}Cr; released radioactivity measured their lysis. The sensitized lymphocytes were obtained by graft-vs.-host reactions: i.e., the transfer of spleen cells from C57Bl mice to X-irradiated DBA mice (yielding C57Bl anti-DBA cells), or from DBA to X-irradiated C57Bl mice (yielding DBA anti-C57Bl cells).

The cultures contained 1) anti-DBA lymphocytes plus labeled DBA and unlabeled C57Bl target cells; 2) anti-C57Bl lymphocytes plus labeled C57Bl and unlabeled DBA target cells; 3) anti-DBA lymphocytes plus labeled C57Bl and unlabeled DBA target cells; 4) anti-C57Bl lymphocytes, plus labeled DBA and unlabeled C57Bl target cells. [Based on Brunner, K. T., Nordin, A. A., and Cerottini, J. C. *Int Adv Immunol* (1970).]

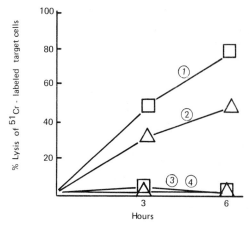

cells are destroyed by specific contact with T lymphocytes ("contact killing"); another suggests that a toxic substance, released by Ag-activated T cells, lyses target and bystander cells; in a third it appears that normal lymphoid cells destroy target cells that are coated with Ab molecules (Ab-dependent cell mediated cytotoxicity). Each of these mechanisms is defined by a model in vitro system; which ones are important in vivo is still unclear.

Contact Killing. In this system thymus cells are injected into X-irradiated allogeneic recipients, where they home to the spleen and proliferate in a graft-vs.-host reaction (above). When subsequently isolated from the spleen these cells (now "educated" against host alloantigens) lyse cultured cells carrying the host's histocompatibility Ags (target cells). If the active spleen cells are added to a mixture of cells of various origins only the target cells are lysed (Fig. 20-12), suggesting that killing depends upon specific cell–cell contact, rather than on release of a soluble cytotoxic factor. Cytotoxicity is prevented by anti-θ and by ALS (see above, and Ch. 17), but not by anti-Igs, indicating the T lineage of the killer lymphocytes.

A linear relation between the number of added lymphocytes and the proportion of target cells that lyse suggests that the reaction is "one-hit" (i.e., a single sensitized T cell can kill a target cell); moreover as many as 1% of the lymphocytes in a highly sensitized individual appear to be specific killers for a particular type of target cell. A soluble cytotoxic substance has not been detected in this system (Fig. 20-12), perhaps because too few lymphocytes are used (see below).

Cytotoxicity by Released Lymphotoxin. In this system, incubation of a more concentrated suspension of lymphocytes with their Ag, or with PHA, releases into the medium a toxic substance (**lymphotoxin,** see above), that can damage or lyse a wide variety of cells (e.g., human HeLa cells, mouse L cells, and other cultured cell lines).

Antibody-dependent Cell-mediated Cytotoxicity. This system differs fundamentally from T-cell-mediated immune reactions: target cells with Ab molecules bound specifically to their surface Ags are destroyed by normal lymphoid cells (i.e., from nonsensitized donors). The active cells (from spleen, lymph nodes, blood, but not thymus) are not T cells, and they adhere to glass. They seem to be B lymphocytes, or macrophages, or "A" cells (adherent mononuclear lymphoid cells whose lineage is obscure). Like B lymphocytes (Ch. 17), the cytotoxic cell evidently has surface receptors for the Ab moiety of Ab-Ag complexes, recognizing perhaps an altered conformation in the Fc domain that results from Ab binding to Ags on target cells. Complement is not involved in binding the Ab or in the destruction of the target cell.

INTERFERENCE WITH CELL-MEDIATED IMMUNITY

TOLERANCE: SUPPRESSION BY ANTIGEN

Similar conditions lead to unresponsiveness for cell-mediated reactions and for Ab formation: in general, **an Ag tends to be tolerogenic under conditions where it is not immunogenic** (Ch. 17). Thus unresponsiveness is more readily established in neonatal than in immunologically mature adults. In fact, current interest in tolerance was largely stimulated by Billingham, Brent, and Medawar's dramatic demonstration of allograft tolerance in newborn mice; the injection of living cells from one inbred strain into newborn mice of a second strain established enduring and specific tolerance in the recipients for allografts from the first strain (Ch. 21). As is discussed in Chapters 17 and 21, the inoculated cells can continue to multiply throughout the recipient's lifetime; hence they probably maintain tolerogenic levels of histocompatibility alloantigens.

It is also possible that this induced form of unresponsiveness is actually pseudotolerance, resulting from production of blocking Abs (see Tetraparental mice, below; and Ch. 21, Enhancement).

Variations in **route** of administration are also important. Guinea pigs fed 2,4,6-trinitrochlorobenzene (picryl chloride) became specifically unable to develop contact skin sensitivity to this potent sensitizer, or to form anti-Tnp Abs to picryl proteins, while remaining normally responsive to other Ags. Similarly, unresponsiveness to neoarsphenamine can be established by injecting this substance intravenously, rather than intracutaneously (an immunogenic route). The large doses presumably correspond to high-zone tolerance (Ch. 17); low-zone tolerance in cell-mediated immunity has not yet been demonstrated. Since T cells are more readily and more persistently tolerized than B cells, tolerance should be more easily established for cell-mediated responses than for Ab formation; but so far a difference seems not to have been clearly demonstrated.

Immune Deviation. Administration of Ag under some conditions (adsorbed on alumina gel, or sometimes in solution) seems to induce Ab formation without intervening delayed-type hypersensitivity. When this happens the cell-mediated sensitivity is not likely to be induced by a subsequent injection of the same Ag under what would ordinarily be effective conditions (e.g., incorporation in complete Freund's adjuvant). This effect borders on selective tolerance in respect to cell-mediated immunity and the mechanism is obscure. It may not be due entirely to interception of Ag by the Abs formed as a result of the first inoculum, because the phenomenon has not been regularly reproduced with antisera. If it could be consistently achieved, this "immune deviation" could have considerable clinical value in enhancing survival of allografts (Ch. 21).

Desensitization. In contrast to the establishment of tolerance, where Ag acts as tolerogen *before* it has a chance to function as immunogen, desensitization is established by administering the Ag *after* an individual has already been sensitized to it. Partial desensitization probably occurs whenever a sensitized individual is tested simultaneously at many skin sites with the same Ag: the reaction at each site is usually less intense than after a single test is applied, probably because the number of sensitized T cells is limited. Similarly, in overwhelming infections (such as miliary tuberculosis or disseminated fungal or protozoan infections) delayed-type hypersensitive skin responses can no longer be elicited, probably because the large amount of released Ag saturates sensitized lymphocytes. Comparable events occur in certain industries, where workers with allergic contact dermatitis sometimes lose skin sensitivity after prolonged and intense exposure to the sensitizer. However, deliberate desensitization by repeated administration of Ag or simple sensitizers has been difficult to achieve regularly in patients without frequently precipitating severe allergic reactions. Moreover, any desensitization that is achieved is short-lived (e.g., 5 to 10 days).

It is reported that American Indians formerly chewed poison ivy leaves as prophylaxis or treatment of poison ivy dermatitis. Recently a similar approach, refined by feeding the purified catechol responsible for poison ivy sensitization, has been found to be of dubious value: the presence of the catechol in feces occasionally produces in sensitized individuals an unusually severe perianal contact dermatitis, once referred to as the "emperor of pruritus ani."

SUPPRESSION BY ANTIBODIES

Antibodies as Antiimmunogen. The effects of Abs on cell-mediated immunity are variable: some complexes with Ab reduces the Ag's immunogenicity and others enhance it (see also Ch. 17 for parallel variations in induction of Ab formation). The differences probably derive from variable effects of Abs with different heavy chains, and of Ab·Ag complexes with different mole ratios (below).

In the most provocative effect antisera block cell-mediated rejection of tumor grafts, resulting in **"immune enhancement"** of tumor growth. This effect could arise in two ways: Ab molecules covering tumor-specific antigenic sites on the surface of tumor cells could block induction of cell-mediated immunity **(afferent enhancement)** or block its expression (i.e., attack by sensitized lymphocytes or **efferent enhancement**). The latter mechanism appears to operate in many cancer patients: in tissue culture the patient's tumor cells usually form fewer colonies if incubated with his own lymphocytes than with those from other persons, and his own serum (but not other sera) can specifically block his lymphocytes' inhibitory activity (Ch. 21, Tumor immunity). Abs to histocompatibility Ags may similarly prolong survival of allografts of normal cells (Ch. 21, Enhancement).

Observations on **tetraparental (allophenic) mice** suggest that "blocking" Abs might be similarly involved in natural self-tolerance. These animals are produced by dissociating early embryos (at about the eight-cell stage) from two genetically different sets of parents, mixing the cells, and implanting the single combined blastula in a foster mother's uterus. The progeny are genetic mosaics with cells of both origins contributing to essentially all organs and tissues. The lymphocytes of these remarkable animals **can destroy cultured fibroblasts from either parent.** Nevertheless, the animals grow and develop normally, apparently because their serum contains Abs (or Ab·Ag complexes) that specifically block the cytotoxic reaction. Hence natural tolerance in these genetic mosaics seems to be due not to absence of an immune response but to two canceling ones: serum Abs block the destructive potentialities of cell-mediated immunity. In general, however, injections of antisera into sensitized individuals cannot be depended upon to block delayed-type hypersensitivity reactions to soluble Ags.

Antilymphocyte Sera (ALS).

The antisera made in one species against the thymus cells of another are particularly destructive against the latter's recirculating pool of lymphocytes, which are mostly T cells (Ch. 17): studies with ^{51}Cr-labeled cells show, however, that lymphocytes in lymph nodes and in other secondary lymphatic organs are much less affected. The differences could account for ALS's selective depression of cell-mediated immune reactions (i.e., circulating T-cell effectors of cell-mediated responses are abolished, but T cells in lymphatic organs persist and remain able to support Ab production). Treatment of recipients with ALS therefore leads to greatly prolonged survival of allografts. However, Abs are made against the serum proteins of ALS (including the antilymphocyte Abs themselves). The resulting risk of anaphylaxis and the serum sickness syndrome limits the clinical usefulness of these antisera in the prevention or treatment of rejection of allografts (Ch. 21).

Antisera to θ, one of the distinctive surface alloantigens on mouse thymus cells (Ch. 17), selectively inactivate T cells; accordingly these antisera are effective inhibitors of all cell-mediated reactions in appropriate strains of mice, blocking both induction and expression of responses. As noted before, θ is an alloantigen in mice; anti-θ antisera are not yet available in other species.

NONSPECIFIC SUPPRESSION

The cytotoxic agents that block Ab formation by preventing mitotic division (of cells in general), or by causing massive destruction of lymphocytes, were considered in Chapter 17. No new principles are involved in their application to cell-mediated immunity. The agents that block proliferation of lymphocytes (X-rays, alkylating drugs, purine and folate analogs; Ch. 17, Fig. 17-31) block induction, but not expression of cell-mediated immunity: evidently **Ag-sensitive T cells and macrophages can generate inflammatory responses without themselves undergoing cell division.**

The agents most widely used clinically to inhibit cell-mediated allergic responses are the 11-oxycorticosteroids. In therapeutic doses they act as nonspecific suppressors of inflammation, but they probably **do not block induction** of the sensitive state. Indeed it is possible that mature T cells are particularly resistant; for the small proportion of mouse thymus cells (ca. 5%) that resist steroid action are both more mature than the others (they have less θ and more histocompatibility Ags) and more effective in carrying out a graft-vs.-host reaction.

The survival of human kidney allografts depends upon skillful use of immunosuppressants. ALS (horse antiserum to human lymphocytes) is usually administered for the initial 2 weeks, while prednisone (a corticosteroid) and imuran (a purine analog; Ch. 17, Fig. 17-31) are usually given continuously. These measures prolong graft survival, but the resulting suppression of all cell-mediated immune responses increases susceptibility to overwhelming infection by prevalent "opportunistic" bacteria and fungi, and increases the risk of cancer (Ch. 17, Immunosuppression in Ab formation; also Ch. 21).

CLINICAL DEFICIENCIES

The fundamental distinctions between cell-mediated and Ab-mediated immunity have come to be appreciated partly from clinical experience with patients having massive defects in one or the other. Defects in B cells, leading to deficiencies in Igs and in Ab formation, were considered in Chapter 17 along with clinical procedures for evaluating suspected immunodeficient states (see especially Tables 17-11 and 17-12). Some T cell deficiencies are considered here.*

Thymic Aplasia. The principal form of this rare disorder, the **DiGeorge syndrome,** arises from defective embryonic development of the third and fourth pharyngeal outpouchings that give rise to the thymus, parathyroid, and thyroid glands (Ch. 17); hence hormonal deficiencies (hypoparathyroidism, rarely also hypothyroidism) are present in addition to profound immune defects. Another form of thymic aplasia, inherited as an autosomal recessive trait, occurs without associated hormonal deficiencies (Nezelof syndrome). Infants with either

---

* As was indicated before (Ch. 17), live (attenuated) vaccines must be avoided in evaluating immune responses of infants with suspected deficiencies: disseminated infections following immunization with BCG (an attenuated strain of tubercle bacilli) and vaccinia have been fatal in severely affected infants.

form suffer from severe recurrent infections; they also lack delayed-type skin hypersensitivity to Ags of prevalent microbes, and fail to develop contact skin sensitivity to potent sensitizers, such as 2,4-dinitrochlorobenzene (DNCB, Fig. 20-4). Their blood lymphocytes are nearly all B cells (with normal distribution of surface of Igs; Ch. 17), with absent T cell function: for instance, they respond poorly to stimulation with phytohemagglutinin (PHA) or to allogeneic cells in mixed lymphocyte cultures (see Ch. 17, Table 17-12; also Ch. 21).

Since many Ags are T-dependent, these infants would also be expected to form Abs poorly in trial immunizations and to have low serum Ig levels (especially IgG). However their serum Igs are usually in the normal range, as is their ability to form Abs to diverse Ags, including proteins that are expected (from responses in mice) to be T-dependent. It is likely that thymic aplasia is not complete in infants who survive beyond 1 or 2 years after birth; indeed, in some who survive longer there seems to occur a spontaneous recovery of some T-cell functions (such as stimulation of thymidine uptake by PHA).

Severe Combined Deficiency Disease. Infants with this disease suffer from crippling absence of both T and B cell functions, probably because hematopoietic stem cells fail to differentiate normally (see Ch. 17, Table 17-11). Most attempts to reconstitute the defective system with transplants of allogeneic

bone marrow cells and T lymphocytes (peripheral blood leukocytes) from normal donors have resulted in fatal graft-vs.-host reactions. However, in a few instances where the donor was a sibling with well-matched histocompatibility Ags (see Ch. 21, HL-A matching) the graft-vs.-host reactions were minimal and prolonged recovery of all immune functions has been achieved. With female donor and male recipient the female sex chromatin (Barr body) demonstrated long-term persistence of donor cells in the recipient (see Ch. 21, Chimeras).

Acquired T-Cell Deficiencies. In certain diseases of adults widespread involvement of the reticuloendothelial system with neoplasia (Hodgkin's disease) or with intracellular parasitism (lepromatous type of leprosy or disseminated leishmaniasis) or with chronic granulomas (Boeck's sarcoid) is associated with striking deficiencies in cell-mediated immunity and preservation of Ab-forming ability. Affected individuals do not give delayed-type skin reactions to any Ags and their blood lymphocytes do not respond to PHA. However, their serum Igs are normal (or even markedly elevated) and they form Abs normally in response to immunization, suggesting that some T-cell function is preserved. The reasons for their selective deficiencies are unknown. As noted above some of the deficiencies can be corrected by "transfer factor" from white blood cells of normal individuals (see above).

SOME SPECIAL ALLERGIC REACTIONS

ALLERGY TO DRUGS

Hypersensitivity reactions to drugs, particularly to penicillin, are among the more common allergic disorders in man. Most of the principles involved were noted in earlier sections of this chapter and in Chapter 19. **Sensitizing drugs, like inducers of contact skin sensitivity, must form stable covalent derivatives of proteins in vivo** (see above), which can induce Ab formation and virtually any type of hypersensitivity. In the following section both the immediate- and delayed-type responses are discussed.

Most drugs would be too toxic to be useful if they reacted rapidly with proteins under physiological conditions. If, however, the rate of reaction is sufficiently slow a drug may be tolerably nontoxic and yet may form effective hapten-protein immunogens. For most drugs that cause allergic reaction, however, it is likely that reactive contaminants, or reactive meta-

bolic derivatives formed in vivo, are solely (or additionally) responsible for the formation of immunogenic conjugates. The mechanisms involved are well illustrated with penicillins, which are models for drug allergies in general.

PENICILLIN ALLERGY

Penicillin is probably the least toxic drug in use: 20 gm per day can be given safely for prolonged periods. Nevertheless, up to 10% of persons given penicillin repeatedly can become so sensitized that an injection of 1 mg may elicit fatal anaphylactic shock.*

Immediate-type Hypersensitivity. Penicillin is unstable, and most of its solutions contain at least small amounts of **penicillenate**, a highly reactive

---

* Oral administration is less hazardous because the drug is absorbed more slowly, but it can also lead to severe reactions, such as the serum sickness syndrome (Ch. 19).

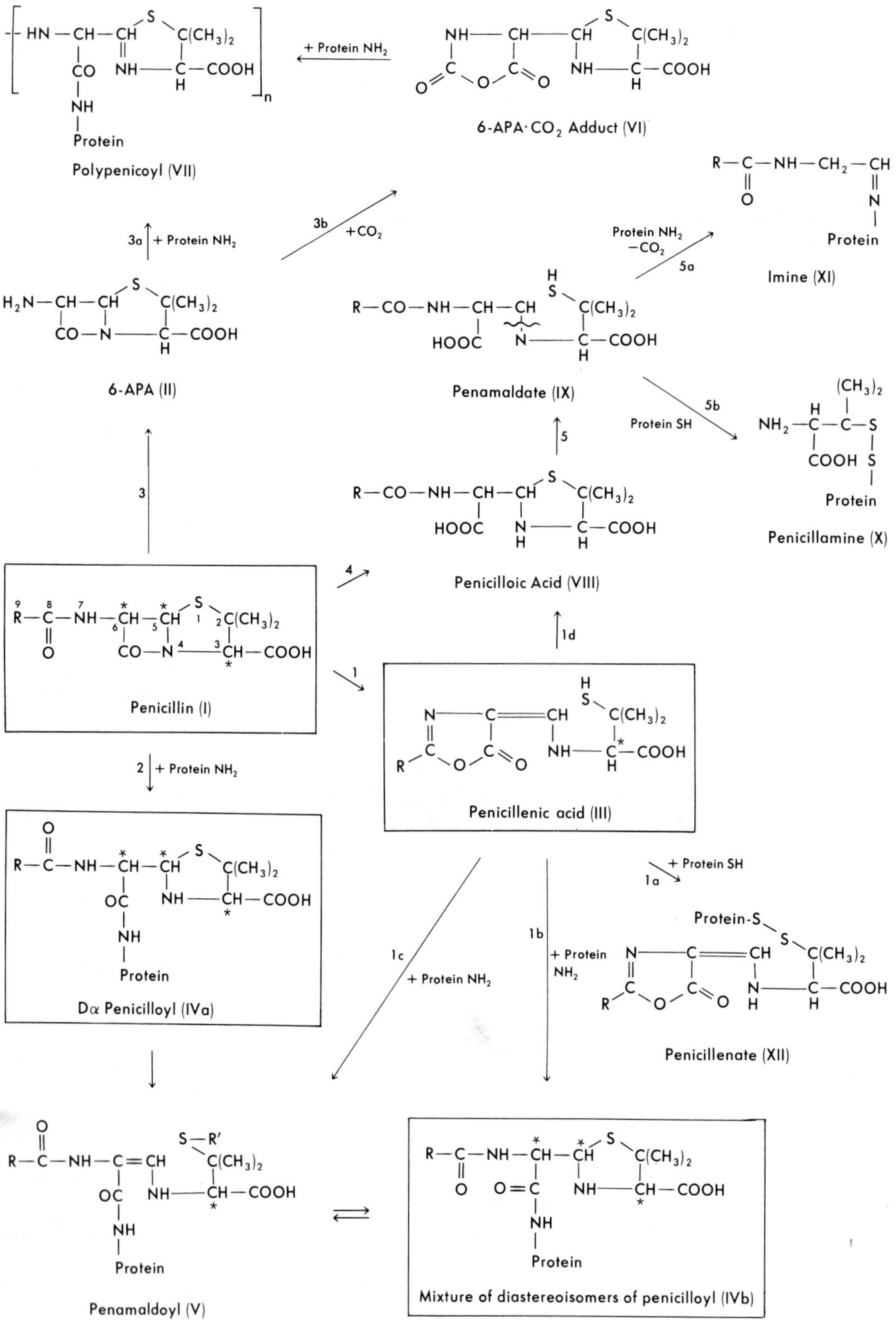
Polypenicoyl (VII)
+ Protein NH2
6-APA·CO2 Adduct (VI)
Imine (XI)
3a + Protein NH2
3b +CO2
Protein NH2 −CO2 5a
6-APA (II)
Penamaldate (IX)
5b Protein SH
Penicillamine (X)
3
5
Penicilloic Acid (VIII)
4
Penicillin (I)
1
1d
Penicillenic acid (III)
2 + Protein NH2
Dα Penicilloyl (IVa)
1a + Protein SH
1b + Protein NH2
1c + Protein NH2
Penicillenate (XII)
Penamaldoyl (V)
Mixture of diastereoisomers of penicilloyl (IVb)

derivative that forms **penicilloyl** and other substituents of amino and sulfhydryl groups of proteins (Fig. 20-13). Through its strained β-lactam ring penicillin itself can be directly attacked by nucleophilic groups (e.g., ε-NH_2 of lysyl residues), leading also to formation of penicilloyl-protein conjugates (though inefficiently at physiological pH). Penicilloic acid, formed from penicillenic acid, also forms a variety of minor determinant groups (Fig. 20-13). Conjugates with different haptenic moieties stimulate the formation of specific non-crossreacting Abs (Fig. 20-13).

Intradermal injection of small amounts of the protein conjugates (e.g., 0.01 μg) could provide diagnostic test for allergy to penicillin.* However, even small amounts of the conjugates are potentially immunogenic. A safer reagent has been prepared by introducing penicilloyl substituents into poly-D-lysine, with an average of 20 residues per molecule, to form a ligand that is multivalent but not detectably immunogenic. This reagent elicits specific wheal-and-erythema responses as effectively as penicilloyl-proteins, and its specificity can be demonstrated by inhibition with univalent ligands, e.g., ε-penicilloyl-aminocaproate:

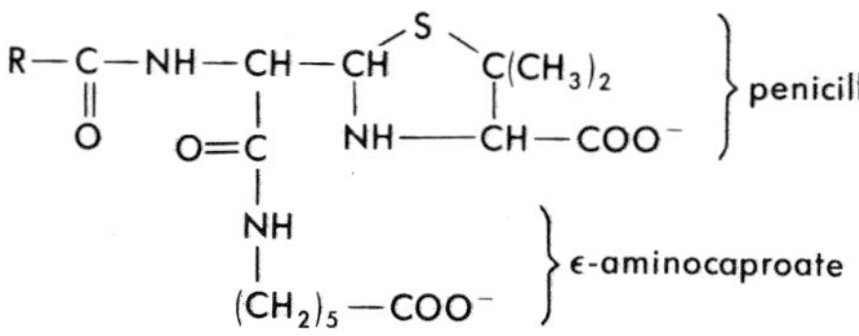

High-molecular-weight contaminants in solutions of penicillin can sometimes also cause anaphylactic reactions. The most significant are **penicilloyl proteins** in which the proteins are probably acquired,

---

† Pencillin itself only infrequently yields wheal-and-erythema responses, even in highly sensitive persons. Positive reactions, when they occur, are probably due to high-molecular-weight contaminants (see below). The unconjugated drug is univalent: if bound by Abs it should inhibit rather than elicit allergic reactions (Ch. 19).

during manufacture, from the fungus (*Penicillium*) or from the *E. coli* amidases that are sometimes added to cleave R-CO side chains in the preparation of 6-aminopenicillanic acid (6-APA) for production of semisynthetic penicillins (Fig. 20-13; also Ch. 7). Removal of the protein (e.g., by proteolysis with enzymes attached covalently to solid Sepharose beads, to avoid introducing another immunogenic impurity) reduces the frequency of reactions to penicillin. However, reactions can still be elicited with other high-molecular-weight contaminants (polymers of 6-APA or of penicillins).

Ligand and Antibody Competition. Many persons with reaginic (IgE) Abs to penicilloyl do not suffer anaphylactic reactions after injections of penicillin, even when the solutions contain penicillenate, a major source of penicilloyl conjugates. One probable reason is that the penicillin molecule itself, and the penicilloic acid formed as its major degradation product (Fig. 20-13), are univalent for antipenicilloyl Abs. Though these cross-reacting ligands are probably bound only weakly, they are present initially in great excess over the penicilloyl proteins that form in vivo, and they are thus likely to act as specific inhibitors of anaphylaxis. However, the univalent small molecules are excreted fairly rapidly, and so they are unlikely to influence the later, serum sickness-like reactions (e.g., rash, fever, joint pains) that often occur 3 to 14 days or more after penicillin is injected into persons with high antipenicilloyl Ab titers. Another reason for the infrequency of anaphylactic reactions is that persons with reaginic antipenicilloyl Abs also usually have non-reaginic Abs (IgGs, IgM) of the same specificity, which probably act as blocking Abs (Ch. 19; Table 20-6).

Hemolytic anemia due to penicillin allergy sometimes occurs in those receiving high doses of peni-

---

Fig. 20-13. Haptenic substituents derived from reactions of penicillin and its degradation products. R differs in different penicillins. (In penicillin G, the most widely used, it is benzyl ⬡—CH_2—...) Asterisks designate asymmetrical carbons.

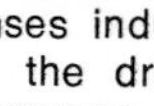

The Abs most often identified in penicillin-treated persons are specific for penicilloyl (IVa,b). Penicilloyl groups formed from penicillenic acid (III) are a mixture of diastereoisomers (IVb); those formed by direct reaction in vitro with penicillin at high pH largely retain the D-α configuration of penicillin itself (IVa). Some human antipenicilloyl Abs react better with D-α-penicilloyl than with the diastereoisomeric mixture. Penicillenate (III) is much more reactive than penicillin at physiological pH values, and it is probably the usual source of the penicilloyl groups formed in vivo. The immune responses induced by penicillin are sometimes specific for other, **"minor-determinant"** groups derived from the drug. 6-APA (II) is 6-aminopenicillanic acid, the intermediate to which many different acyl (R) groups may be attached synthetically to form a variety of penicillins (see Ch. 7). The structures of particular importance (I, III, IVa, and IVb) are enclosed. (From Parker, C. W. in *Immunological Diseases*. M. Samter, ed. Little, Brown, Boston, 1965).

TABLE 20-6.   Antibody-Mediated Reactions to Penicillin

Time of onset after penicillin administration	Clinical findings	Antibodies		Comments
		Class	Specificity	
2–30 min	Diffuse urticaria, hypotension, shock, respiratory obstruction	IgE	Penicilloyl and minor determinants	
3–72 hr	Diffuse urticaria, pruritus; rarely respiratory symptoms	IgE	Penicilloyl	IgG antipenicilloyl rises to high titer and probably acts as blocking Ab, leading to spontaneous cessation of the reaction
		IgM	Penicilloyl	
3 days to several weeks	Urticaria (sometimes recurrent), arthralgias, erythematous eruptions	IgE	Penicilloyl and minor determinants	
		IgM	Penicilloyl	

Derived from Levine, Bernard B. Immunochemical mechanisms of drug allergy in *Textbook of Immunopathology* [P. A. Miescher and H. J. Mueller-Eberhard, eds.], Vol. 1, Grune and Stratton, N.Y., 1968.

cillin for several weeks (as in treatment of subacute bacterial endocarditis): antipenicillin Abs react with penicillin adsorbed on red cells, causing excessive cell destruction and anemia. (Similar events with other, unrecognized exogenous Ags could simulate autoimmune hemolytic anemia; see chronic viral infection and autoimmune disease, below.)

Delayed-type hypersensitivity to penicillin is also common, as allergic contact dermatitis, particularly among handlers of penicillin in bulk (e.g., nurses and personnel in the pharmaceutical industry). One of the determinants that specify these reactions involves D-penicillamine, which elicits patch test reactions as effectively as penicillin in some persons with contact skin sensitivity to the drug. This compound forms stable mixed disulfides with cysteine in vitro, and probably acts in vivo by combining with protein sulfhydryl groups (X in Fig. 20-13).

Diagnosis of Immediate- and Delayed-type Penicillin Allergy. An important difference between immediate-type and delayed-type drug hypersensitivity is brought out by the diagnostic procedures used to detect penicillin allergy. The intradermal injection of penicillin itself is often not reliable for detecting immediate-type sensitivity; and even the available synthetic multivalent ligands are not effective in all sensitive individuals. In contrast, patch tests with penicillin itself are almost infallible for identifying delayed-type allergy to the drug. The differences can probably be explained by the following considerations. 1)

Intradermally injected penicillin diffuses away too rapidly to form many local protein conjugates, whereas penicillin from a patch test percolates into the skin slowly and has more time to form various derivatives that become conjugated with skin proteins in situ. 2) The pronounced carrier specificity of the cell-mediated response precludes competitive inhibition by penicillin and its low-molecular-weight derivatives.

The diversity of haptenic groups introduced into proteins by penicillin is unusual, but the principles are undoubtedly the same for all allergenic drugs. Perhaps the most important are 1) **an allergic reaction to a drug is specific for the haptenic group(s) introduced by the drug, or by its derivatives, into proteins in vivo, rather than for the drug itself;** and 2) **the haptenic derivatives may differ greatly in structure and in chemical properties from the drug itself** (Fig. 20-13).

Variations among Individuals. A striking feature of drug allergies is the extreme range in susceptibility of different individuals. Though an adequate explanation is not available, several possibilities are apparent. 1) Genetic differences could be important if enzymatic reactions are involved in converting a drug into metabolic derivatives that introduce haptenic groups into proteins; 2) the levels of Abs formed to any immunogen vary widely among different individuals, sometimes because of genetic differences (Ch. 17); 3) the tendency to form reaginic Abs is also variable, and is especially pronounced in atopic individuals (Ch. 19). In addition, certain infections could influence the response to concomitantly administered drugs; for example, killed *Bordetella pertussis* (a commonly used adjuvant in mice and rats) seems to selectively favor formation of reaginic Abs, and mycobacterial mycosides and endotoxins of gram-negative bacteria also enhance the immunogenicity of most Ags.

SPECIAL TISSUES

Most simple sensitizers react with proteins indiscriminately. Allergy to certain drugs, however, involves special tissue elements, which implies selective reactions with certain proteins. Some examples are the hemorrhagic manifestations of allergy to quinidine and to Sedormid (2-isopropyl-4-pentenoyl urea). The administration of these drugs to sensitive persons causes **thrombocytopenia,** resulting in bleeding in various tissues, including the skin (purpura).

In vitro, in the presence of the appropriate drug, the serum of a sensitive person can agglutinate platelets, his own or a normal person's, and if C is added the platelets are lysed; but platelet lysis occurs at much lower concentrations of free quinidine in vivo than in vitro. It is possible that the drug, or one of its metabolic derivatives, reacts selectively under physiological conditions with proteins on the platelet surface to form effective haptenic groups.

AUTOIMMUNE RESPONSES

Clinical and experimental observations show that individuals can sometimes respond immunologically to certain of their self-Ags. These important exceptions to the principle of self-tolerance help analyze its fundamental mechanisms, and they are frequently associated with disease. It is often not clear, however, whether these anomalous responses cause, or are the result of, disease (see below); hence it is necessary to emphasize the distinction between an **autoimmune response,** in which an individual makes Abs or becomes allergic to a self-Ag, and an **autoimmune disease,** which is a pathological condition arising from an autoimmune response. **Autoimmune reactions can be both Ab- and cell-mediated.**

MECHANISMS

Autoimmunity could arise, in principle, from the following mechanisms: 1) a change in the distribution of a self-component, allowing access to lymphoid cells that never encountered it previously; 2) a change in the structure of a self-component or introduction of a cross-reacting Ag, either of which could lead to the formation of Abs and appearance of lymphocytes that react (or cross-react) with the native self-component; and 3) emergence of abnormal ("forbidden") clones of lymphocytes. In addition, immune responses to persistent and unrecognized extrinsic Ags (such as those of certain chronic virus infections, see below) can generate chronic allergic disorders that are difficult to distinguish from those due to anti-self immune reactions.

Altered Distribution of Self-Antigens. Many self-Ags (e.g., from eye lens, spermatozoa, brain tissue) have little or no opportunity to establish tolerance because they are normally confined anatomically to sites that prevent their access to lymphoid cells. Abs to such an Ag are readily produced experimentally by removing the Ag and injecting it back into the same animal as though it were a conventional foreign Ag.

Clinical incidents that release such Ags have the same effect: thus Abs to heart muscle appear after myocardial infarction, and Abs to thyroid after the trauma of partial thyroidectomy. In these instances disease gives rise to the autoimmune response, rather than the reverse. Nonetheless, such responses can be visualized as self-perpetuating: once the response is initiated the resulting allergic inflammation in the target organ probably leads to contact of Ag with infiltrating lymphoid cells; hence resulting in further sensitization.

Altered Forms of Self-Antigens. Few self-Ags are totally isolated from lymphoid cells: for example, thyroglobulin (Tg), once thought to be completely confined to thyroid nodules, evidently leaks into lymphatics, for sensitive assays reveal its presence in serum at concentrations (ca. $0.01 \ \mu g/ml$) that could easily establish T-cell tolerance. Hence modified Tg molecules, altered by introducing or exposing new groups with "carrier" function, could engage the corresponding T cells and help stimulate persistent (not tolerized) B cells to produce Abs that react with determinants on native Tg. Thus rabbits immunized with chemically modified rabbit Tg or with cross-reacting hog Tg develop thyroiditis, associated with Abs that react with native rabbit Tg.* A clinical parallel is seen in the encephalitis that occasionally develops in people injected with rabies vaccine, which is a suspension of infected rabbit brain (Allergic encephalomyelitis, below; see Ch. 17, discussion of T and B cells in Immunological tolerance).

Some bacteria carry antigenic determinants that resemble those of the host; e.g., in rheumatic fever some of the Abs produced against group A streptococci seem to cross-react with human heart. Bacterial infections might also facilitate autoimmune responses through the adjuvant effects of certain products (e.g., mycosides, endotoxins).

Forbidden Clones. In developing the clonal selection hypothesis Burnet assumed that lymphocyte clones are somehow eliminated as they arise if they are specific for self-Ags. A breakdown in the hypothetical elimination mechanism, or the appearance of mutant lymphocytes that are resistant to this mechanism, could lead to the emergence of autoreactive "forbidden clones." There is no firm evidence in support of this possibility, but a hint of its validity is provided by clinical findings: when an individual who suffers from one autoimmune disorder is examined closely, signs of other autoimmune responses are likely to be disclosed.

Chronic Virus Infection. Mice infected at birth with certain temperate viruses (e.g., lymphocytic choriomeningitis virus, lactic dehydrogenase virus, and others that also seem not to injure infected cells) become life-long carriers, producing Abs that form virus:Ab complexes without neutralizing the virus' infectivity (see Ch. 19, discussion of Viral complexes under Immune-complex disease). Budding virions on infected cells, or viral Ags adsorbed on erythrocytes or other cells, simulate self-Ags: their combination with antiviral Abs (or perhaps with specific T cells) can give rise to chronic disorders, such as hemolytic anemia, that resemble autoimmune diseases. These circumstances in model animal systems suggest that some of the ostensibly autoimmune human diseases might also be due to unrecognized chronic viral infections (for an anal-

---

* Similar lesions and Abs can even appear when rabbit Tg itself is incorporated into Freund's adjuvant and injected back into rabbits: denaturation during preparation could expose new carrier-like groups.

ogous situation, see Hemolytic anemia due to penicillin, above).

CHARACTERISTICS OF AUTOIMMUNE DISEASES

Antibody- vs. Cell-mediated Reactions. All the mechanisms that cause allergic reactions to foreign Ags can participate in autoimmune diseases (Table 20-7). 1) Various **autoantibodies** (with or without C) can act directly on cells, e.g., lysing erythrocytes or platelets, or injuring cells of the thyroid gland (thyroiditis). 2) **Autoimmune Ab·Ag aggregates** are illustrated by systemic lupus erythematosus, in which some complexes formed from DNA, anti-DNA, and C become lodged in kidney glomeruli and lead eventually to progressive glomerulonephritis and renal failure (Ch. 19, Immune-complex diseases). Similarly, IgGs that function as autoantigens combine with certain IgM (or IgG) molecules that serve as autoantibodies (rheumatoid factors), forming aggregates that localize around synovial membranes and probably contribute to the joint inflammation of rheumatoid arthritis (Ch. 19). 3) **Autosensitized lymphocytes** have not been shown to cause human disease, but hints are provided by the striking mononuclear infiltrates in many autoimmune disorders (atrophic gastritis in pernicious anemia, thyroiditis, allergic encephalomyelitis, etc.).

Stronger support for cell-mediated mechanisms is provided by much experimental work in which bits of tissue (from thyroid, brain, adrenal, etc.) are removed surgically, emulsified in Freund's adjuvant, and injected back into the same animal. After 1 to 2 weeks the recipient develops both serum Abs and lesions infiltrated with mononuclear cells in the corresponding organ. Moreover, viable lymphocytes from the affected animal, but not serum, will usually transfer the disease to a normal recipient.

Failure to transfer the disorder with serum should not, however, be unduly stressed. Autoantibodies, like other Abs, are likely to be heterogeneous; and with the continuous presence of the target self-antigen those Abs with highest affinity are probably removed preferentially, leaving as free autoantibodies in serum the relatively ineffectual low-affinity molecules.

Localized vs. Disseminated Disease. Autoimmunity can affect almost every part of the

TABLE 20-7. Some Autoimmune Disorders in Man

Organ or tissue	Disease	Antigen	Detection of antibody*
Thyroid	Hashimoto's thyroiditis (hypothyroidism)	Thyroglobulin	Precipitin; passive hemagglutination; IF on thyroid tissue
		Thyroid cell surface and cytoplasm	IF on thyroid tissue
	Thyrotoxicosis (hyperthyroidism)	Thyroid cell surface	Stimulates mouse thyroid (bioassay)
Gastric mucosa	Pernicious anemia (vitamin B_{12} deficiency)	Intrinsic factor (I)	Blocks I binding of B_{12} or binds to I:B_{12} complex
		Parietal cells	IF on unfixed gastric mucosa; CF with mucosal homogenate
Adrenals	Addison's disease (adrenal insufficiency)	Adrenal cell	IF on unfixed adrenals CF
Skin	Pemphigus vulgaris	Epidermal cells	IF on skin sections
	Pemphigoid	Basement membrane between epidermis-dermis	IF on skin sections
Eye	Sympathetic ophthalmia	Uvea	Delayed-type hypersensitive skin reaction to uveal extract
Kidney glomeruli plus lung	Goodpasture's syndrome	Basement membrane	IF on kidney tissue; linear staining of glomeruli (see Ch. 19, Fig. 19-19B)
Red cells	Autoimmune hemolytic anemia	Red cell surface	Coombs' antiglobulin test
Platelets	Idiopathic thrombocytopenic purpura	Platelet surface	Platelet survival
Skeletal and heart muscle	Myasthenia gravis	Muscle cells and thymus "myoid" cells	IF on muscle biopsies
Brain	? Multiple sclerosis	Brain tissue	Cytotoxicity on cultured cerebellar cells
Spermatozoa	Male infertility (rarely)	Sperm	Agglutination of sperm
Liver (biliary tract)	Primary biliary cirrhosis	Mitochondria (mainly)	IF on diverse cells with abundant mitochondria (e.g., distal tubules of kidney)
Salivary and lacrimal glands	Sjögren's disease	Many: secretory ducts, mitochondria, nuclei, IgG	IF on tissue
Synovial membranes, etc.	Rheumatoid arthritis	Fc domain of IgG	Antiglobulin tests: agglutination of latex particles coated with IgGs, etc.
	Systemic lupus erythematosus (SLE)	Many: DNA, DNA-protein, cardiolipin, IgG, microsomes, etc.	Precipitins, IF, CF, LE cells (see text)

* IF = immunofluorescence staining, usually with fluorescent antihuman Igs (see Ch. 14).
CF = complement fixation (Ch. 18).
Based on Roitt, I. *Essential Immunology.* Blackwell, Oxford, 1971.

body (Table 20-7). Some responses are directed to **organ-specific** Ags and may even be limited to a particular cell type (e.g., parietal cells of gastric mucosa in pernicious anemia). Other responses are directed to widely distributed Ags and are associated with **disseminated** disease (e.g., antinuclear Abs in systemic lupus erythematosus). In still other diseases the responses are **intermediate** between these extremes: for instance, in Goodpasture's disease, characterized by chronic glomerulonephritis and pulmonary hemorrhages, Abs are deposited on basement membrane of kidney glomeruli and lung parenchyma, in accord with a strong cross-reaction between these particular basement membranes, shown by localization in vivo of ^{125}I-labeled heteroantisera (e.g., rabbit antirat glomeruli).

Multiplicity of Responses. An individual who makes one autoimmune response is likely to make others. For instance 10% of persons with autoimmune thyroiditis have pernicious anemia, which is present in only 0.2% of the population at large (of the same age and sex distribution). Thyroid disease is similarly found with excessive frequency in those who suffer from pernicious anemia. Serological evidence for multiple reactions is even more frequent: 30% of those with autoimmune thyroiditis have Abs to parietal cells of gastric mucosa (involved in pernicious anemia), and 50% of those with pernicious anemia have Abs to thyroid, though the two kinds of Abs are entirely non-cross-reacting. Similar associations are found among the disseminated group of autoimmune diseases: persons with systemic lupus erythematosus often have evidence of rheumatoid arthritis, autoimmune hemolytic anemia, or thrombocytopenia.

Genetic Factors. Relatives of patients with autoimmune thyroiditis commonly have antithyroid Abs, and relatives of those with pernicious anemia have a high incidence of Abs to gastric parietal cells. Moreover, some inbred animal strains suffer from a high frequency of autoimmune disorders: all mice of the NZB strain (New Zealand Black) eventually develop autoimmune hemolytic anemia, and most of the hybrids (B×W) made by crossing NZB with another inbred strain (New Zealand White, NZW) develop a syndrome

that is strikingly similar to systemic lupus erythematosus in man.

The genetic factors and the multiplicity of autoimmune disorders in some individuals suggest that the key to autoimmunity may reside in a breakdown of the still unknown central mechanisms that are responsible for self-tolerance (Forbidden clones, above).

Age and Sex. Autoimmune responses are improbable events; their frequency increases with age (Fig. 20-14). They are also more frequent in women than in men, perhaps because different cells in females express different X chromosomes (Lyon effect): the resulting cellular mosaicism might increase opportunities for a breakdown in self-tolerance (see tetraparental mice under Tolerance, above, and Allelic exclusion, footnote p. 470).

SOME REPRESENTATIVE AUTOIMMUNE DISEASES

Acquired Hemolytic Anemia. In this disorder a person forms Abs that react with his own red blood cells. Such Abs are sometimes found in persons with other diseases that might alter self-antigens or introduce cross-reacting ones: e.g., malignant neoplasms of lymphoid tissue, syphilis, mycoplasma

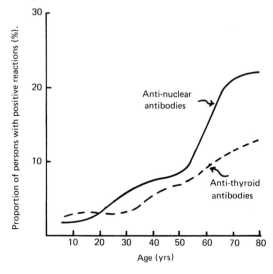

Fig. 20-14. Increasing incidence of autoantibodies with age in general population. Antinuclear Abs were detected by immunofluorescence (e.g., Fig. 20-17) and antithyroid by passive hemagglutination with thyroglobulin on tanned red cells. (From Roitt, I. *Essential Immunology.* Blackwell, Oxford, 1971).

pneumonia, infectious mononucleosis. More often, however, this disorder is idiopathic (i.e., it is unassociated with other diseases or with known exposure to agents toxic to red cells).

Abs to the patient's red cells are demonstrated by two procedures. 1) In the **direct antiglobulin (Coombs) test** the patient's washed red cells are agglutinated by rabbit antiserum to human Igs (Ch. 15). 2) In the **indirect test,** red cells from another person are incubated with the patient's serum, washed, and examined for clumping by the rabbit antiserum.

The anti-red cell Abs have no hemolytic activity in vitro, but they accelerate destruction of red cells in vivo. Thus, transfused normal red cells have a shortened survival in affected patients only if the injected cells have the particular surface Ag that binds the patient's autoantibody, indicating that red cell breakdown is due to the bound Abs. The Ab-coated (opsonized) cells are phagocytized by macrophages and their breakdown occurs especially in the spleen. Therapy includes nonspecific immunosuppressants (Ch. 17) and splenectomy.

Mice of the inbred NZB strain almost invariably develop hemolytic anemia as they age, and viable lymphoid cells (including Ab-forming clones) from older (affected) animals transfer the disease efficiently to young, unaffected mice of the same strain. These mice are chronically infected from birth with C-type viruses (resembling murine leukemia virus; see Ch. 63), and it is possible that what looks like autoimmune disease is really due to a conventional immune reaction to viral Ags absorbed on red cells or present on budding virons of infected cells.

Thrombocytopenic Purpura. In this disease platelets can decline to ca. 1/10 the normal level and bleeding occurs in many organs, including the skin, causing petechial rash and purpura. In the dramatic experiment that first provided evidence of the immune nature of this disease, a human volunteer injected with a patient's plasma suffered a precipitous fall in platelets and extensive bleeding into internal organs and skin (Fig. 20-15). A patient's serum can cause clumping of normal platelets, and lysis if C is present. Infants born to mothers with the disease may have transient thrombocytopenia and bleeding, owing to placental transmission of the maternal Abs.

Allergic Encephalomyelitis. When laboratory animals (e.g., rat, guinea pig, monkey) are injected with suspensions of central nervous system tissue from individuals of the same or other species they develop patchy areas of vasculitis and demyelination in the brain and spinal cord (Fig. 20-16). This response is readily evoked with a single injection of a small amount of brain or spinal cord tissue, even from the same animal, in Freund's adjuvant.

The immune nature of the disease is indicated by

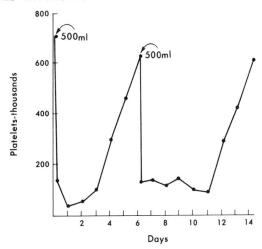

Fig. 20-15. Passive transfer of thrombocytopenic purpura. The drop in platelet count of a normal human volunteer following transfusion (arrows) of blood from a patient with idiopathic thrombocytopenic purpura. Similar results were obtained with Ig fractions from other donors with the disease. Some of the recipients suffered bleeding in internal organs simulating the natural course of the disease. [From Harrington, W. J., Minnich, V., Hollingsworth, J. W., and Moore, C. V. *J Lab Clin Med 38*:1 (1951).]

the following. 1) Lesions appear 9 days or more after the primary injection, but the onset is more rapid in animals that have recovered and are then reinjected (secondary response). 2) The lesions are specific: they follow inoculation only of myelin-containing tissues, and appear only in myelinated tissue, especially white matter of brain. 3) Abs that react with brain tissue can be demonstrated in serum, and lymphoid cells from inoculated animals produce cytopathic effects on myelinated brain tissue and glial cells in culture. 4) The lymphoid cells can also cause specific neural lesions in nonsensitized syngeneic recipients. 5) Intradermal injection of myelinated tissue evokes a delayed skin response in affected animals. Though serum Abs are present they do not seem to play a major role in the disease: the intensity of the lesions does not parallel their levels and serum, unlike lymphoid cells, fails to cause lesions in recipient animals.

The responsible self-antigen is a basic protein, extractable at low pH from myelinated nervous tissue and localized by immunofluorescence in myelinated nerve fibers. It is heterogenetic (i.e., distributed in many species) and organ-specific, being confined to the central nervous system.

The experimental background clarifies the post-vaccination encephalitis that often occurs in humans after vaccination with the standard rabiesvirus, which is a suspension of infected rabbit brain.

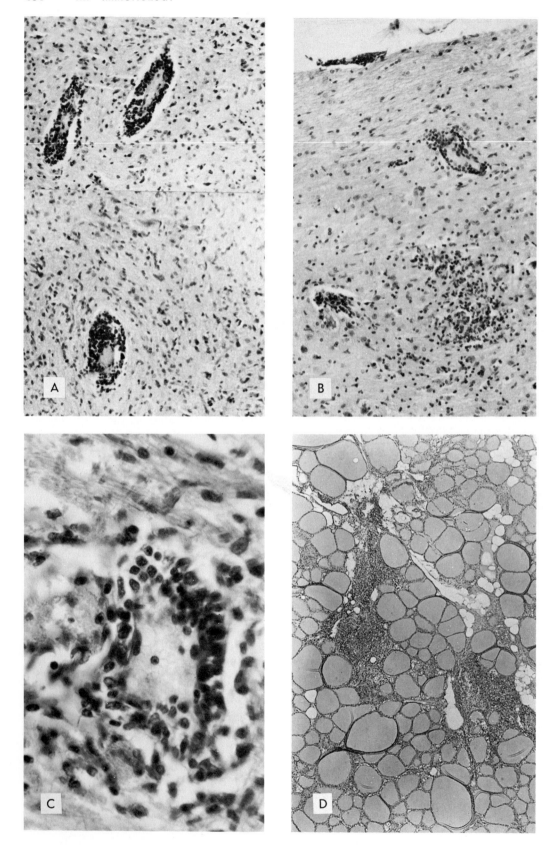

Rabies vaccine from virus grown in tissue culture or in duck embryo tissues that lack myelin (Ch. 58) is now preferred. The demyelinating encephalitides that occasionally follow measles and vaccinia could arise because infection of the nervous system brings the encephalitogenic Ag into contact with inflammatory (lymphoid) cells. A similar mechanism is suspected for multiple sclerosis, a common disabling neurological disorder of unknown etiology with characteristic focal demyelinating lesions.

Thyroiditis. Patients with chronic inflammation of the thyroid (Hashimoto's disease) suffer destruction of secretory cells and loss of thyroid function. Their sera contain some Abs that react in high titer with thyroglobulin (Tg), and others that react with Tg-free particulate fractions of thyroid (? cell membranes; e.g., in immunofluorescence assays as illustrated in Fig. 20-17). The possibility that these Abs cause the disease is supported by observations on an inbred strain of chickens that spontaneously develops antithyroid Abs and thyroiditis (and finally hypothyroidism and obesity): the Abs appear to be causal, since neonatal bursectomy, but not thymectomy, prevents the anomalies. However, experimental thyroiditis induced in mice, rats, etc, is very similar in pattern to experimental allergic encephalomyelitis (above). The suspicion therefore remains that cell-mediated rather than (or in addition to) humoral autoimmunity is involved in the lesions of the human disease.

The interaction of Abs with Ags on cells sometimes causes cell proliferation and differentiation rather than destruction—e.g., when anti-Igs react with B lymphocytes (blast transformation, Ch. 17), or when appropriate Abs react with sea urchin eggs. Similar mechanisms appear to be involved in some patients with hyperplastic and hyperfunctional thyroid glands, who have antoantibodies to the thyroid. If present during pregnancy, these autoimmune Abs (also called **long-acting thyroid stimulators**) can cross the placenta and cause neonatal hyperthyroidism, which subsides within a few weeks of birth (as the maternal IgG is degraded; see Ch. 17, Ontogeny). The autoantibody might bind specifically to the same cell surface receptors as thyroid-stimulating hormone, for the actions of both are potentiated by theophylline, indicating that they act through the adenyl cyclase system (see Ch. 19, Fig. 19-13).

Pernicious Anemia. Defective red cell maturation in this disease is due to lack of vitamin B_{12}, caused by faulty absorption of the ingested vitamin. Affected persons have an atrophic gastritis, and their poor absorption of vitamin B_{12} is due to lack of intrinsic factor (IF), a protein that is necessary for this absorption and is secreted into the stomach by special (parietal) cells of the gastric mucosa. Most patients with the disease have Abs to parietal cells (revealed by immunofluorescence of gastric biopsies) and cell-mediated immunity to these cells could also be present. In addition, autoantibodies to IF itself are also involved, for large amounts of oral B_{12} (which ordinarily cure the anemia) are ineffective if given together with serum from many patients, and the active sera contain Abs to IF. Evidently the inhibitory effect of anti-IF is exercised within the stomach, for absorption of the fed vitamin remains normal in immunized human volunteers even when they develop a high serum titer of these Abs, or intense delayed-type hypersensitivity to IF. The gastric Abs, produced by plasma cells in the gastric lesions, are able to function within the stomach (normally extremely acidic) because loss of cells from the affected mucosa reduces secretion of HCl. Thus, by decreasing production of IF and of HCl, and by secreting Abs to IF the autoimmune atrophic gastritis contributes to (and may even cause) B_{12} deficiency and pernicious anemia.

Systemic Lupus Erythematosus. At various stages in this complex disease patients produce several of an immense variety of autoantibodies to various blood cells, clotting factors, and intracellular components (e.g., mitochondria, nuclear components; Fig. 20-17). The resulting difficulties include hemolytic anemia, leukopenia, thrombocytopenic purpura, and bleeding tendencies. The Abs to some cell com-

Fig. 20-16. Autoimmune allergic reactions. **A–C.** Allergic encephalomyelitis in a rat sensitized adoptively with viable lymph node cells from a donor rat that had been immunized with rat spinal cord (injected in complete Freund's adjuvant). The recipient animal, which had severe ataxia and hind-leg paralysis 5 days after receiving the donor's lymphoid cells, was sacrificed at 7 days. Sections of brain show a focal inflammation with perivascular infiltration by mononuclear cells. H & E stain. **A and B,** ×130 (reduced); **C,** ×500 (reduced). **D.** Thyroiditis in a rabbit that had been immunized repeatedly with hog thyroglobulin. A small proportion of the rabbit's Ab (to the hog protein) reacted also with rabbit thyroglobulin. Note intense focal infiltration of the immunized rabbit's thyroid with mononuclear cells. ×60 (reduced). Similar lesions appear in animals injected with their own thyroglobulin or with homogenates of a bit of their own thyroid tissue. [**A–C** from Patterson, P. Y. *J Exp Med 111*:119 (1960). **D** from Witebsky, E., and Rose, N. R. *J Immunol 83*:41 (1959).]

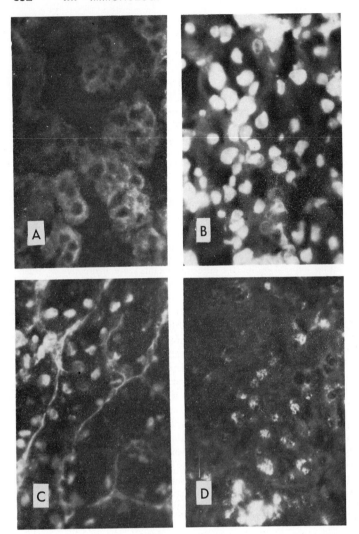

Fig. 20-17. Variety of antitissue Abs in sera of different patients with systemic lupus erythematosus. Mouse kidney sections were incubated with the sera and, after washing, were stained with fluorescein-labeled rabbit antiserum to human 7S Igs. Similar reactions occur with human tissues. **A.** Normal human serum control. **B.** Abs in a lupus serum react uniformly with all nuclei, giving homogeneous nuclear staining. **C.** Abs react with nuclei and with basement membrane of renal tubules. **D.** Abs react with selected parts of nuclei, giving speckled staining. All ×250. (Courtesy of Drs. E. Tan and H. Kunkel.)

ponents (e.g., to DNA) seem to cause difficulty mainly through deposition of Ab · Ag · C complexes in walls of small blood vessels leading to widespread vasculitis (Arthus lesions); deposits in capillaries of renal glomeruli are especially threatening, for they can lead to glomerulonephritis and renal failure (Ch. 19). The production of so many autoantibodies is accompanied by elevated serum Ig levels, and

during the active phases of the disease serum C falls to low levels as Ab · Ag aggregates bind these proteins.

The multiplicity of Abs to self-Ags and the appearance of "lupus erythematosus" (LE) cells are diagnostic. These cells appear simply on incubation of blood or bone marrow: the breakdown of some cells evidently releases DNA which combines with serum anti-DNA, and the resulting Ab · Ag aggregates are taken up by granulocytes, which acquire a characteristic appearance (a large amorphous mass in the center of the cell, with the surrounding multilobed nucleus pushed to the periphery).

PATHOLOGICAL CONSEQUENCES OF AUTOIMMUNE REACTIONS

When autoantibodies were first discussed, at the turn of the century, they were imagined to occur either not at all or with disastrous consequences. Now, with the development of increasingly sensitive and reliable assays for Abs and for hypersensitivity, it is clear that autoimmune responses are not so uncommon. However, their pathological effects are often conjectural, with three possibilities to be considered. 1) The response can be innocuous. For example, though anticardiolipin (i.e., Wasserman Abs) in a person with syphilis (Ch. 37) can react with cardiolipin extracted from his own tissues, these Abs do not appear to be pathogenetic: they may be present at high titer in apparently healthy persons. Presumably cardiolipin is buried within membranes and is thus inaccessible. 2) The response can be secondary to another disease (e.g., antithyroglobulin Abs following the trauma of partial thyroidectomy); but it may then be responsible for continuing disease (i.e., inflammation in the affected organ introduces new lymphoid cells that increase autosensitivity). 3) The response can be the main causal factor in disease, e.g., in autoimmune hemolytic anemia or thrombocytopenic purpura.

Witebsky's Criteria. The spectrum of allergic effects is so wide—from hemolysis to demyelinating inflammatory lesions—that autoimmune processes are now commonly invoked for many diseases of unknown etiology; and highly sensitive assays often reveal autoantibodies. In an effort to provide guidelines for interpretation Witebsky suggested the following criteria (reminiscent of Koch's postulates for bacterial etiology): an autoimmune response should be considered the cause of a human disease if 1) it is regularly associated with that disease 2) immunization of an experimental animal with Ag from the appropriate tissue causes it to make an immune response, 3) the responding animal develops pathological changes similar to those of the human disease, and 4) the experimental disease can be transferred to a nonimmunized animal by serum or by lymphoid cells.

ALLERGY AND IMMUNITY

Many of the allergic reactions described in this and in the preceding chapter can be elicited with microbial Ags in persons who are suffering, or have recovered, from the associated infectious disease. Two questions arise: 1) Do allergic responses occur naturally during the infectious disease? 2) If they occur, do they enhance or diminish the host defenses?* Broadly speaking, the answers seem to depend on 1) the mass and distribution of microbial Ags, 2) the concentration and types of Abs present, and 3) the intensity and localization of cell-mediated responses. The range of possibilities is large, as is illustrated by the following examples.

1) **No detectable allergic reactions.** In some infectious diseases allergic reactions are

---

* These questions are also considered elsewhere from different viewpoints (see Ch. 22, and also chapters dealing with particular microorganisms).

not likely to occur, or to be significant if they do. For example, in diseases caused primarily by exotoxins, such as diphtheria and tetanus, the quantities of toxin involved are too small to elicit an obvious allergic response even if the host were hypersensitive. Moreover, only a minority of persons successfully immunized with the corresponding toxoids exhibit allergic responses to intradermal tests with these proteins.

2) **Coincidental allergic reactions.** In the course of many infections various sterile skin eruptions appear and are probably due to allergic reactions to microbial Ags. For example, transient erythematous rashes and urticaria, resembling cutaneous anaphylaxis, often occur in group A streptococcus infections; erythematous skin nodules (erythema nodosum), resembling the Arthus reaction, occur sometimes in the course of tuberculosis, coccidioidomycosis, and many other infectious diseases;

and vesicular lesions ("ids"), resembling delayed-type reactions, occur often in fungal infections (dermatophytosis and candidiasis; Ch. 43). Though these reactions are useful for clinical diagnosis there is no evidence that they affect the host's resistance.

3) **Significant allergic reactions.** Mycobacterial diseases regularly produce delayed-type allergy to the bacillary proteins, and the mass of bacteria in tissues is unusually large. Hence it is probable that intense allergic reactions occur regularly at infected foci in these diseases and account for much of the observed inflammatory reaction and tissue necrosis. As noted elsewhere (Chs. 22 and 35), the consequences at these severe reactions depend on their localization: if the reaction occurs in the skin and causes ulceration it can lead to the drainage of virulent microbes from the body, but if it takes place on the surface of the brain or in a bronchus the same response can lead to fatal meningitis or to a spreading pulmonary infection.

The sterile cardiac lesions that sometimes develop after streptococcal infections can also cause severe disease (e.g., rheumatic fever), and seem to be allergic in origin (Ch. 26). Thus the Abs to a cell wall Ag of β-hemolytic streptococci cross-react with an Ag from human cardiac muscle, suggesting that rheumatic carditis may be an autoimmune disease. A similar mechanism may contribute to the glomerulonephritis that frequently follows recovery from infection with the type 12 group A streptococcus (Ch. 26).

The following considerations suggest, however, that allergic responses to microbial Ags generally favor host defenses. 1) A given microbe contains many Ags (probably hundreds with bacteria and fungi), of which only a few are directly concerned with virulence. Thus very few Ab-Ag reactions that occur during an infectious disease are likely to result in specific neutralization of substances that cause toxicity and virulence. Nevertheless, many of the other reactions could well contribute indirectly to the host's resistance by provoking localized allergic responses around the microbial agents, leading to the accumulation of granulocytes, lymphocytes, macrophages, and serum proteins, including Abs and C. 2) Delayed-type responses are associated with "activated" macrophages, which can destroy those bacteria (such as *M. tuberculosis*) that normally proliferate within phagocytic cells (Chs. 22 and 35).

Delayed-type (T-lymphocyte) reactions with cell surface Ags also seem to be more effective than the Ab-C system in destroying target animal cells: such reactions with infected cells that have budding virions on the surface may be a particular effective means for eliminating infectious centers in many virus diseases. Thus children who are unable to produce Abs but who have an intact cell-mediated immunity system recover normally from mumps, measles, and other common childhood viral infections (Ch. 17, Infantile X-linked agammaglobulinemia). The same effect, functioning as a surveillance mechanism, seems to be important in aborting incipient cancer clones via attack on cell surface tumor-specific Ags (see also Ch. 21). The Ag-binding receptors on T lymphocytes might have high affinity for Ag, related perhaps to the large determinant recognized, and this could provide for early elimination of small numbers of target cells. On balance therefore, allergic responses are likely to benefit the host. Perhaps it is for this reason that allergic reactivity has persisted through evolution, being represented in all species of vertebrates, along with Ab formation, from primitive cyclostomes up.

SELECTED REFERENCES

Books and Review Articles

BLOOM, B. R. In vitro approaches to the mechanisms of cell-mediated immune reactions. *Adv Immunol* 13:101 (1971).

BLOOM, B. R., and GLADE, P. (eds.). *In Vitro Methods in Cell-Mediated Immunity*. Academic Press, New York, 1971.

Cell-mediated immune responses. *WHO Tech Rep Ser* No. 423, 1969.

DAVID, J. R. Mediators produced by sensitized lymphocytes. *Fed Proc* 30:1730 (1971).

LAWRENCE, H. S. Transfer factor. *Adv Immunol* 11:195 (1969).

LAWRENCE, H. S., and LANDY, M. (eds.). *Mediators of*

Cellular Immunity. Academic Press, New York, 1970.

MACKANESS, G. B., and BLANDEN, R. V. Cellular immunity. *Progr Allergy 11*:89 (1967).

PERLMANN, P., and HOLM, G. Cytotoxic effects of lymphoid cells in vitro. *Adv Immunol 11*:117 (1969).

Proceedings of Conference on Antilymphocyte Serum. *Fed Proc 29*:101 (1970).

ROITT, I. M., GREAVES, M. F., TORRIGIANI, G., BROSTOFF, J., and PLAYFAIR, J. H. L. The cellular basis of immunological responses (an occasional survey). *Lancet 2*:367 (1969).

SIMONSEN, M. Graft-vs.-host reactions. *Progr Allergy 6*:349 (1962).

SMITH, R. T., and LANDY, M. (eds.). *Immunologic Surveillance*. Academic Press, New York, 1971.

TURK, J. L. *Delayed Hypersensitivity*. North Holland, New York, 1967.

WAKSMAN, B. H. *Atlas of Experimental Immunobiology and Immunopathology*. Yale Univ. Press, New Haven, 1970.

Specific Articles

ALLISON, A. C. New antigens induced by viruses and their biological significance. *Proc R Soc Lond (Biol) 177*:23 (1971).

BLANDEN, R. V., LEFFORD, M. J. and MACKANESS, G. B. Host response to Calmette-Guerin Bacillus (BCG) infection in mice. *J Exp Med 129*:1079 (1969).

BRUNNER, K. T., MAVEL, J., CEROTTINI, J. C., and CHAPUIS, B. Quantitative assay of the lytic action of immune lymphoid cells on ^{51}Cr-labeled allo-geneic target cells in vitro. *Immunology 14*:181 (1968).

DAVIE, J. M., and PAUL, W. E. Receptors on immuno-specific cells: Receptor specificity of cells participating in cellular immune responses. *Cell Immunol 1*:104 (1970).

DVORAK, H. F., DVORAK, A. M., SIMPSON, B. A., RICHERSON, H. B., LESKOWITZ, S., and KARNOVSKY, M. J. Cutaneous basophil hypersensitivity: A light and electron microscopic description. *J Exp Med 132*: 558 (1970).

GINSBURG, H. Graft-vs-host reaction in tissue culture: Lysis of monolayers of embryo mouse cells from different strains differing in H-2 histocompatibility locus by rat lymphocytes sensitized in vitro. *Immunology 14*:621 (1968).

GOLDSTEIN, P., WIGZELL, H., BLOMGREN, H., and SVEDMYR, E. Cells mediating specific in vitro cytotoxicity: Probable autonomy of thymus-processed lymphocytes (T cells) for the killing of allogeneic target cells.

MCCLUSKEY, R. T., BENACERRAF, B., and MCCLUSKEY, J. W. Studies on specificity of the cellular infiltrate in delayed hypersensitive reactions. *J Immunol 90*:466 (1963).

RUDDLE, N. H., and WAKSMAN, B. H. Cytotoxicity mediated by soluble antigen and lymphocytes in delayed type hypersensitivity. *J Exp Med 128*: 1267 (1968).

WAKSMAN, B. H., ARNASON, B. G., and JACKOVIC, B. D. Role of thymus in immune reaction in rats. III. Changes in lymphoid organs of thymectomized rats. *J Exp Med 116*:187 (1962).

WARD, P. A., OFFEN, C. D., and MONTGOMERY, J. R. Chemoattractants of leukocytes with special reference to lymphocytes. *Fed Proc 30*:1721 (1971).

chapter 21

ALLOANTIGENS ON CELL SURFACES: BLOOD GROUP SUBSTANCES AND HISTOCOMPATIBILITY ANTIGENS

This chapter deals with the immunology of blood group substances, which are of practical importance in the transfusion of blood, and with histocompatibility antigens (Ags) on diverse cells, which are responsible for the reactions that limit the survival of transplanted organs and tissues. The characteristic immunological effects of all these Ags derive mainly from their position on cell surface membranes. Similar effects are elicited by certain distinctive tumor-specific Ags on surface membranes of tumor cells, which are therefore also considered in this chapter.

The blood group and transplantation Ags are **alloantigens** (Gr. *allo* = other), which are identified operationally as substances from certain individuals that are immunogenic in some other members of the same species, but not in the donor. They may be defined formally as Ags that segregate genetically within a species: they are present in some individuals and absent in others.

An older synonym, isoantigen (Gr. *iso* = same), emphasizes that the variations occur among diverse individuals of the **same** species; this term is still widely applied to blood group substances, while alloantigen is the synonym commonly applied to histocompatibility Ags. We shall use alloantigen for both not only for consistency but because it is the differences among these Ags that should be emphasized, rather than the sameness of the species.

Alloantigens were first recognized on erythrocytes over 60 years ago (see below), and those on nucleated cells were later shown to account for the general observation that tissues transplanted from one individual to another are ultimately rejected, unless donor and recipient are genetically identical (**syngeneic**, see p. 610). Though Ags of this type were thought for many years to be limited to cells, several soluble proteins have recently also been recognized as alloantigens (e.g., haptoglobins, transferrins, and some β-lipoproteins). The alloantigenic forms of immunoglobulins (Igs), known as allotypes, have been exploited to great advantage in clarifying the genetics and structure of antibody (Ab) molecules (Ch. 16).

BLOOD GROUP SUBSTANCES

THE ABO SYSTEM

Following Harvey's discovery of the circulation, repeated attempts were made to transfuse blood from one individual to another. Disastrous reactions in the recipients were frequent, however, and were not understood until Landsteiner discovered the alloantigens of human red blood cells in 1900.

Stimulated by observations in the 1890s that animal species could be distinguished by the reactions of their red cells and serum proteins with specific antisera, Landsteiner sought to determine whether individuals of the **same species** could be distinguished in the same way. When individual samples of serum and erythrocytes from 22 human subjects were mixed in all possible combinations the red cells of some persons were found to be clumped by the sera of certain other indi-

TABLE 21-1. Division of Human Populations into Four Blood Groups on the Basis of Red Cell Agglutination by Normal Human Sera

Serum from group	Red cells from group			
	A	B	O	AB
A	0	+	0	+
B	+	0	0	+
O	+	+	0	+
AB	0	0	0	0

+ = clumping; 0 = no clumping.

viduals. On the basis of these reactions the subjects could be classified into three groups, A, B, and O; and within 1 year a less common fourth group, AB, was also recognized (Table 21-1).

From these results Landsteiner concluded that 1) two different Ags or blood group substances, A and B, are associated with human red cells and one, both, or neither may be present in any given individual's cells; 2) Abs for these alloantigens (called **alloantibodies** or isoantibodies) are regularly present in the sera of those individuals who lack the corresponding alloantigen, and never present in the sera of those who possess it. These observations, later confirmed in vast numbers of humans, contributed greatly to the early acceptance of the doctrine of self-tolerance (Ch. 17).

The **blood groups** or types in human populations are named for the red cell Ags: group A has the A alloantigen, group B has the B alloantigen, group O has neither, and in group AB **each** red cell has both A and B. The corresponding serum alloantibodies are anti-A in group B persons and anti-B in group A; group O has both anti-A and anti-B; group AB has neither.

When anti-A sera are adsorbed with cells from certain A persons (A_2), making up about 20% of the A population, they lose their ability to clump these cells but retain their ability to clump A cells from the remaining 80% (A_1). On the other hand, adsorption of these sera with A_1 cells abolishes their capacity to agglutinate all A cells. Thus there are two kinds of A: A_1 adsorbs anti-A completely, and A_2 adsorbs only some of the anti-A. Correspondingly, there are two types of AB cells: A_1B and A_2B.

GENETIC DETERMINATION OF THE ALLOANTIGENS

Family studies established the heritability of blood cell alloantigens. Analysis of large populations led Bernstein to propose that the *ABO* gene has three alleles—*A, B,* and *O,* with *A* and *B* dominant over *O.* Since man is diploid, the two alleles per individual provide the six genotypes and four phenotypes shown in Table 21-2.

Since each allele has the same probability of being inherited, the Bernstein theory accounts for the distribution of blood groups within families. For example, children of an O and an AB parent (*OO × AB*) average 50% A (genotype *AO*) and 50% B (genotype *BO*); none are AB or O. The large number of families examined are consistent with the foregoing scheme; the small proportion of inconsistent results (less than 1%) are reasonably ascribed to illegitimacy, technical errors in typing (or possibly very rare mutations).

H Antigen. Though the *A* gene controls the formation of the A substance, and the *B* gene the B substance, the *O* gene is an "amorph," i.e., it does not specify a particular red cell alloantigen. Nevertheless, O cells have a distinctive Ag that has been recognized from their agglutination by some normal animal sera (from eels and cattle), antisera (goat anti-*Shigella*), or plant proteins (extracted from the seeds of *Ulex europeus*). This Ag (as well as the A and B alloantigens) is lacking in the red cells of certain rare humans, first recognized in Bombay; and such **Bombay-type individuals** can form Abs in high titer to the characteristic Ag of O cells, either spontaneously or in response to injec-

TABLE 21-2. Genotypes and Phenotypes in the ABO Blood Group System

Genotype	Phenotype
AA ⎱ AO ⎰	A
BB ⎱ BO ⎰	B
OO	O
AB	AB

tions of O cells. The O cell Ag is present not only in man, but also in a variety of other species; i.e., it is **heterogenetic*** and is therefore called **H substance.** This Ag cannot, however, be considered the product of the *O* gene since it is also detectable, with anti-H sera, on the red cells of persons who **lack** the *O* gene, such as A_2B or homozygous A_2 individuals.

As we shall see below there are good reasons for believing that 1) the gene for H substance is independent of the *ABO* gene, and 2) the H substance provides an obligatory precursor to which the A and B groups are attached. **In O individuals the H substance is exposed and fully expressed.** Partial expression in red cells of other types is revealed by reaction with monospecific anti-H sera, the order of reactivity being $O >> A_2 > A_2B > B$; the sera react weakly with some A_1 and A_1B cells, and, as noted above, not at all with Bombay-type. In Bombay-type persons a defective (or absent) *H* gene apparently leads to the absence of H substance, and thereby of A and B determinants as well (see below).

Another pair of blood group activities, called Lewis a and b (Le^a and Le^b), are associated with the A, B, H substances. The Le^a activity is specified by another gene, *Le,* that segregates from the *ABO* and *H* genes. The Le^b activity is not due to a separate allele, but represents instead a novel specificity formed by the combined presence of the individual structures that, by themselves, determine the Le^a and H activities (see below).

---

* An Ag is called heterogenetic when it is formed by a variety of phylogenetically unrelated species. The best known examples are the **Forssman Ags,** one of which is of clinical importance in the diagnosis of infectious mononucleosis (Ch. 61). These Ags, defined by their ability to induce rabbits to form hemolytic Abs to sheep red blood cells (sheep hemolysins), are found in many animal and some bacterial species, e.g., in tissues of guinea pig, horse, cat, and chicken, but not rat or rabbit. The anti-Forssman Abs, sometimes called **heterophile** Abs, are of two types, differing in their ability to distinguish human A and AB from O and B cells. Actually, A and B substances are probably also heterogenetic; similar substances are found in a variety of animal and bacterial species.

DISTRIBUTION OF ALLOANTIGENS: SECRETORS AND NONSECRETORS

The A, B, H, and Le^a substances are not confined to the red cell membrane. Though absent on connective tissue and muscle cells, they are present as surface components of many epithelial and virtually all endothelial cells (Fig. 21-1), and they are also abundant (in some persons) in many secretions: saliva, gastric juice, pancreatic secretions, sweat, meconium, ovarian cyst mucin, etc.

The presence of A, B, and H in secretions is controlled by alleles *Se* and *se* at a separate genetic locus. About 80% of the all persons are **secretors** (*Se/Se* or *Se/se*): depending on their blood type, their secretions contain water-soluble glycopeptides with A, B, or H activity. The other 20% are **nonsecretors** (*se/se*): their secretions lack A, B, and H, but contain instead a similar glycopeptide with Le^a activity. In about 1% of all persons the secretions lack all these activities but contain a related glycopeptide that corresponds to the "core" of the blood group glycopeptides (see below).

Because of their abundance and solubility, blood group substances in secretions have been invaluable for chemical and antigenic analyses. They are serologically indistinguishable from the blood group substances that are isolable in trace amounts, and with great difficulty, from red cell membranes; the few chemical differences are not relevant for their antigenic properties. The purified substances from secretions are glycopeptides, whereas those from red cells are glycopeptides plus glycolipids, with the same oligosaccharides.

A, B, and H antigens when present in saliva are all found to be determinants on the same macromolecule, for all are coprecipitated by a monospecific antiserum to any one.

CHEMISTRY OF THE A, B, H, AND LE ALLOANTIGENS

Regardless of their A, B, H, or Le^a activity, the purified water-soluble glycopeptides have a similar over-all structure: they are polydisperse macromolecules (MW 200,000 to 1,000,000) of similar composition (75 to 80% carbohydrate, 15 to 20% protein);

Fig. 21-1. Localization of A and B alloantigens in human tissue by immuno-fluorescence. The A substance is shown in lymph node (**A**), epidermis (concentrated in stratum corneum) (**B**), Hassall's corpuscle of the thymus (**D**), and the goblet cells of a villus in the small intestine (**F**). The B substance is shown in squamous epithelium of the tongue (**C**) and in transitional epithelium of renal calyces (**E**). [From Szulman, A. E. *J Exp Med 111*:789 (1960).]

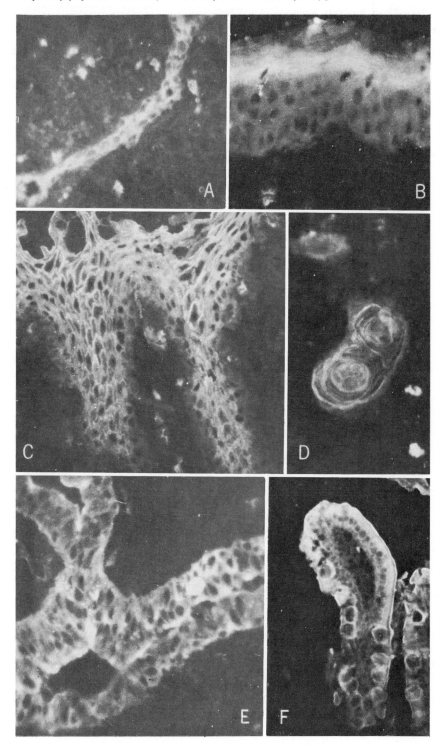

they all consist of multiple heterosaccharide branches attached by glycosidic linkage at their internal, reducing ends to serine or threonine of the polypeptide backbone (see Fig. 21-3, below).

Degradation Products. Stepwise enzymatic removal of sugars from the free, nonreducing ends of branches eliminates some determinant groups and exposes others that were previously detected only feebly or not at all (Fig. 21-2). Thus, when purified A substance is digested with a crude enzyme preparation (from clostridia) the A activity is lost, and H activity increases. Similarly, when B substance is digested with another enzyme (an α-glycosidase from coffee) the B activity is lost and H activity appears. Furthermore, when the H-active glycopeptides derived from these procedures (or isolated directly from O individuals) are treated with still another enzyme preparation, the H activity disappears and the capacity to react with Abs to the Le^a determinant appears. Finally, with further degradation Le^a activity is lost; the remaining glycopeptide cross-reacts with type 14 pneumococcal polysaccharide (Fig. 21-2).

These relations led Watkins and Morgan, and Ceppellini, to postulate that the blood group macromolecule of the ABO and Lewis systems is built from a single large glycopeptide, on which the various sugars that correspond to the Le^a, H, A, and B specificities are added sequentially by enzymes that are specified by the corresponding genes (*A, B, H, Le*). As each sugar is added it introduces a new antigenic specificity, masking the previous one.

This hypothesis has been thoroughly substantiated. Fragmentation of purified blood group glycopeptides (by periodate oxidation,

alkaline borohydride reduction, partial acid hydrolysis) has yielded a large variety of small oligosaccharides from whose properties the structure shown in Figure 21-3 was gradually deduced. Since many of these fragments specifically inhibit various alloantibodies (e.g., in hemagglutination or precipitin assays) specificities can be assigned to particular saccharides. For instance with fucose residues attached ($\alpha 1 \rightarrow 2$) at residues ② and ④ of Figure 21-3 the heterosaccharide has H activity; but if N-acetyl galactosamine is also present ($\alpha 1 \rightarrow 3$) on both ② and ④, A$_1$ activity is established and H activity is negligible, even though fucose is still present on ② and on ④. If galactose ($\alpha 1 \rightarrow 3$) is the additional residue at ② and at ④ the substance has B activity, rather than A, and H activity is also masked.

Structural analysis also accounts for the antigenic difference between A$_1$ and A$_2$. In A$_2$, N-acetyl galactosamine is present only on ④ (branch II), and branch I lacks a terminal substituent on ②; hence A$_2$ also has a good deal of H activity.

Thus the antigenic difference between A and B determinants, of vast clinical importance for blood transfusions, is determined by the presence or absence of acetylated amino groups in the terminal sugars of complex, branched glycopeptides. While these few atoms are the crucial elements, the actual A and B determinants are probably as large as the terminal tetra- or pentasaccharides shown in Figure 21-3.

The Watkins-Morgan hypothesis postulates that the direct products of the *A, B, H,* and *Le* genes are enzymes (glycosyltransferases) that carry out the additions of particular sugars in the biosynthesis of the heterosaccharides, rather than the antigenic sugars themselves.

In support of this idea Ginsburg *et al.* identified in human milk the four postulated enzymes: they transfer the appropriate sugar moieties from nucleotide-activated substrates to a milk tetrasaccharide that resembles the termini of branches I and II of the core heterosaccharide in the blood group glycopeptide (Fig. 21-3). The presence or absence of these glycosyltransferases in different individuals coincides with their A, B, O, Le blood type (Fig. 21-4)

The A and B glycosyltransferases can function only if the core heterosaccharide has

Fig. 21-2. Antigenic determinants of blood group mucopeptides revealed by sequential enzymatic removal of terminal sugar residues from A and B substances. [From Watkins, W. M. *Science* 152:172 (1966).]

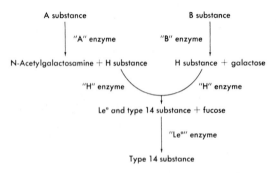

A substance   B substance

"A" enzyme   "B" enzyme

N-Acetylgalactosamine + H substance   H substance + galactose

"H" enzyme   "H" enzyme

Le^a and type 14 substance + fucose

"Le^a" enzyme

Type 14 substance

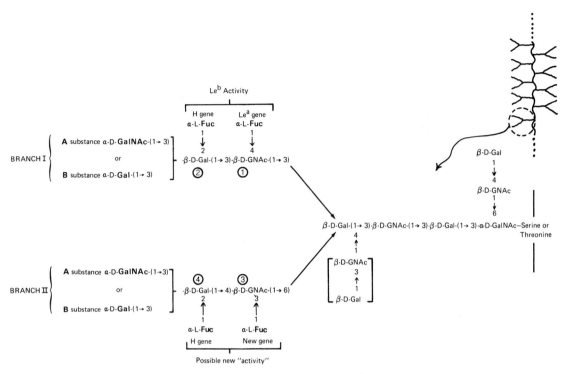

Fig. 21-3. Proposed structure of the ABO megalosaccharide. Branched heterosaccharides project from a polypeptide backbone in secreted water-soluble substances, or are associated with lipid in cell membrane glycolipids. A representative branched structure (enclosed in dotted line) is shown in detail. The residues responsible for A, B, H, Le^a, Le^b activities are in heavy type; they are added by glycosyltransferases to the "core"structure, whose residues are in light type. The core, devoid of the heavy substituents, reacts with antisera to type 14 pneumococcal capsular polysaccharide; a fragment of the core (branch II) reacts with certain monoclonal human Abs ("cold agglutinins" called anti-I). [Modified from Lloyd, K. O., and Kabat, E. A., *Proc Natl Acad Sci USA 61*:1470 (1968), and Lloyd, K. O., Kabat, E. A., and Liverio, E., *Biochemistry 9*:3414 (1970).]

terminal fucose residues, corresponding to H activity. In the Bombay-type blood mentioned earlier the absence of these fucose residues— owing to an absent or defective *H* gene— prevents addition of the terminal hexoses; the resulting glycopeptide in these persons lack A and B as well as H determinants. The *O* allele evidently produces an inactive enzyme or no protein at all.

From the foregoing results it is clear that both allelic (*A, B*) and nonallelic (*H, Le*) genes cooperate in sequential additions of different sugar determinants on a complex heteropolymer. The process resembles other complex interactions of genes that determine the numerous different specificities of the cell wall antigens (O polysaccharides) in the salmonellae (Ch. 29) and other bacteria.

THE AB ALLOANTIBODIES

The anti-A and anti-B alloantibodies are natural Abs (Ch. 14), probably formed in response to ubiquitous A- and B-like polysaccharides of many intestinal bacteria and of some foods. Additional inconspicuous immunogenic stimulation probably comes from inapparent infections. Because of self-tolerance (Ch. 17), an individual would form only those natural Abs that are specific for the alloantigens he lacks; for example, a person of type A forms anti-B, not anti-A. [Chickens have blood groups, including alloantibodies, that resemble the human AB system; when raised under germ-free conditions chicks form alloAgs (A, B, etc.) but not anti-A and anti-B.]

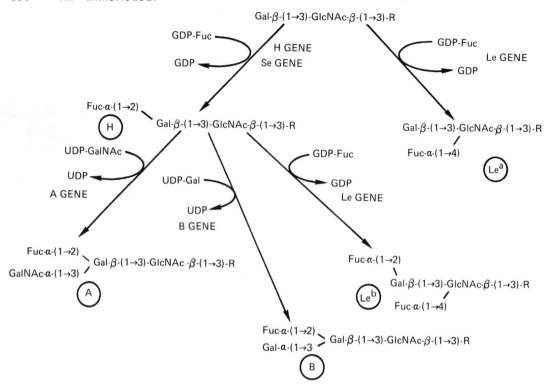

Fig. 21-4. Glycosyltransferases in the synthesis of A, B, H, and Le antigenic specificities. Enzymes speci-fied by *A, B, H,* and *Le* genes transfer hexoses from activated precursors (uridine or guanosine diphos-phosugars) to a tetrasaccharide (from human milk) that correponds to branch I of the core heterosac-charide of Figure 21-3. R is lactose. [From Kobata, A., Grollman, E. F., and Ginsburg, V. *Biochem Biophys Res Commun* 32:272 (1968).]

Classes of Immunoglobulin. Natural anti-A and anti-B are predominantly IgM molecules in persons of groups B and A, but they are both IgM and IgG in those of group O. The Abs formed in response to intensive antigenic stimulation by injections of A and B substance are largely of the IgG class.*

Evolution. It has been suggested that some severe infectious diseases could have served as selective agents in the evolution of blood group substances and accounted for the different frequencies of A, B, O blood types in different ethnic groups (Table 21-3). If, for instance, a particular blood group substance were the same as a surface Ag of a microbial pathogen, persons with that alloantigen would be immunologically unresponsive to it and might be more susceptible to infection (Ch. 17, Tolerance), assuming that the corresponding Abs (if formed) would be protective. So far the lack of

correlation between blood type and incidence or severity of certain infectious diseases (e.g., smallpox, whose virion has been thought to contain an A-like substance) does not support this idea, but it never-theless remains an attractive possibility.

That pathogens might operate as selective agents in another way is suggested by evidence that a blood group Ag of chicken red cells serves as specific receptor for an avian leukosis-sarcoma virus. Sim-ilarly, the MN blood group substances (see below) resemble cell surface receptors for influenza virus: isolated MN blocks agglutination of human red cells by the virus (Ch. 56, Influenza virus hemag-glutinin).

OTHER RED CELL ALLOANTIGENS

The discovery of the ABO system was fa-cilitated by the presence of anti-A and anti-B Abs in most normal human sera. Since then many other red cell alloantigens have been

---

* Purified A and B substances are sometimes in-jected deliberately to raise the Ab titer, as in the preparation of typing sera.

TABLE 21-3. Frequency of ABO Blood Types in Various Ethnic Groups

Population	Phenotypes (%)			
	O	A	B	AB
Scotland (Stornoway)	50	32	15	3
Sweden (Uppsala)	37	48	10	6
Switzerland (Berne)	40	47	9	4
Pakistan (N.W. frontier province)	25	33	36	5
India (Hindus in Bombay)	32	29	28	11
United States (Chippewa Indians)	88	12	0	0
Eskimos (Hudson Bay)	54	43	1.5	1.5

Based on Mourant, A. E. *The Distribution of the Human Blood Groups.* Thomas, Springfield, Ill., 1954.

recognized, but different means were required for their detection, because the corresponding natural Abs are not found in normal human sera. One approach involves skillfully adsorbed animal antisera to human red cells. Another depends on the appearance of alloantibodies in persons who have received multiple blood transfusions, and in women who have had multiple pregnancies; for a fetal alloantigen, inherited from the father and absent from the mother, can stimulate maternal Ab formation if it enters the maternal circulation. These several approaches are illustrated with selected blood group systems described below.

MNSs BLOOD GROUPS

MN Antigens. About 25 years after the ABO system was recognized Landsteiner and Levine found that occasional rabbit antisera to human blood would, after adsorption with red cells from certain persons, agglutinate many but not all human erythrocytes, regardless of their ABO type. The adsorbed antisera were thus specific for an additional red cell alloantigen, which they called M. Rabbit antisera subsequently elicited with various samples of M+ cells revealed still another red cell alloantigen, which was called N. All human red cells react with either anti-M or anti-N sera, or with both. From the distribution of the M and N Ags in many human families, it has become clear that these Ags are governed by a pair of allelic genes that segregate inde-

pendently from the ABO locus: irrespective of an individual's ABO type, his cells also have M or N, or both. The *MN* alleles are codominant; hence genotypes *MM, NN,* and *MN* correspond to phenotypes M, N, and MN.

Ss Antigens. Human sera (e.g., from a mother with Abs to her fetus' red cells) later identified another pair of alloantigens, called S and s, that are associated genetically with M and N. S and s are distributed in families as though governed by a pair of codominant allelic genes: i.e., every person has one or the other or both.

S is much more frequently found on M or MN than on N cells. This suggests that the S specificity might be due to a mutation of the *M* gene (and less frequently of *N*) that adds a determinant group (S) without modifying the original determinants: a similar basis for the s specificity would mean that there are four alleles for the *MN* locus (*MS, Ms, NS, Ns*). However, family studies are also consistent with the alternative possibility that these alloantigens represent two separate but tightly linked genes (*M,N* and *S,s*): for example, the child of homozygous MS and Ns parents (*MMSS × NNss*) would be MSNs but would contribute to each of his offspring *either MS or Ns,* as though each pair were inseparable.

It is not possible to make a firm decision between the alternative genetic possibilities. But the nonrandom association of *S* with *M* argues against linkage of separate genes; for even with tightly linked genes, and correspondingly infrequent crossover events, over a long period of evolution genetic equilibrium should have led *S* (and *s*) to be as frequently associated with *N* as with *M*, unless there are unknown selective advantages to the *M-S* combination, or unless contemporary populations resulted from relatively recent interbreeding of different racial groups that originally had considerably different frequencies of these genes.

Rh ANTIGENS

Like ABO, the Rh system was discovered as a byproduct of curiosity about alloantigens and was then found to solve an important clinical problem. In the 1930s, Landsteiner and Wiener, investigating the phylogeny of M antigen, found that rabbit antisera to *Rhesus* monkey red cells (after removal of anti-M) clumped the red cells of about 85% of all persons (Rh+) but not those of the remaining 15% (Rh−). Wiener then showed that some severe reactions to blood transfusions could be explained by Rh incompatibility: donors were Rh+ while recipients were Rh− but had anti-Rh Abs.

At about the same time Levine and Stetson described the case of a mother who, after giving birth to a baby with a hemolytic disease called erythroblastosis fetalis, suffered a severe reaction upon receiving blood from her husband, though both parents had the same ABO type. The newly discovered anti-*Rhesus* serum was subsequently found to clump the father's cells (Rh+), not the mother's (Rh−); and in similar cases erythroblastotic babies were found to be Rh+ with an Rh− mother and an Rh+ father. Evidently fetal red cells, carrying the paternal Ag, can cross the placenta and immunize the mother; maternal Abs can then enter the fetal circulation and react with fetus' red cells, causing massive breakdown of red cells.

Nonagglutinating Rh Antibodies. The foregoing explanation presented one difficulty: most sera from affected Rh− mothers did not clump red cells from the erythroblastotic Rh+ babies or from other Rh+ individuals. It was later discovered, however, that human anti-Rh Abs are often of the "incomplete" type (Ch. 15): they combine specifically with Rh+ cells without causing agglutination. Because these nonagglutinating Abs are of the IgG class, they cross the placenta; and they are ultimately responsible for destruction of the fetal red cells: they probably act as opsonins and promote phagocytosis and degradation by macrophages. The initial puzzle was complicated by the presence in some mothers of anti-Rh Abs of the IgM class: these Abs are readily recognized because they agglutinate Rh+ cells but they do not cross the placenta (Ch. 17, Ontogeny) and therefore do not affect the Rh+ fetus.

The search for anti-Rh Abs in hemolytic disease provided the main impetus for the development of a number of ingenious methods for detecting incomplete Abs (see, for example, the antiglobulin or Coombs test, Ch. 15). Though these Abs were originally considered to be univalent they almost certainly are bivalent since they can clump red cells

under special circumstances, e.g., when 1) reactions are carried out in the presence of a high protein concentration, such as 30% serum albumin, or 2) red cells are first treated with proteolytic enzymes, such as trypsin or ficin. (See Ch. 15, Monogamous binding, for other bivalent Abs that do not cross-link Ag particles.) Nonagglutinating anti-Rh Abs also played a key role in the discovery of diverse alloantigenic forms of human immunoglobulins (Ch. 16, Allotypes; Fig. 16-13).

Frequency of Hemolytic Disease in the Newborn Due to Blood Group Incompatibility. Fetal red cells probably enter the maternal circulation in small numbers in most pregnancies. However, only about 1 in 100 Rh+ babies with Rh− mothers have significant hemolytic disease. Yet the Rh factor is more immunogenic than most other alloantigens and it accounts for the vast majority of fetal deaths due to red cell incompatibilities. [On rare occasions incompatibilities in the ABO and the Duffy and Kell blood group systems (see below) also cause severe hemolytic disease of the newborn.] One reason is that entry of fetal red cells into the maternal circulation is usually slight during early pregnancy, and is only pronounced during expulsion of the placenta at parturition. Hence it is only after the immunogenic stimulus experienced at delivery of her first Rh+ baby that the Rh− mother can make a substantial anamnestic response to the small numbers of Rh+ fetal cells that cross the placenta during subsequent pregnancies. Thus the first Rh+ baby is usually unaffected and the risk of hemolytic disease increases in successive pregnancies.

Prevention of Rh Disease. The incidence of Rh disease is less when mother (Rh−) and baby (Rh+) are also incompatible in ABO type (e.g., an O mother with B baby): rapid removal of fetal cells from maternal circulation by anti-B (or anti-A) evidently reduces the antigenic Rh stimulus (see discussion of Suppression of Ab formation by other Abs acting as antiimmunogens, Ch. 17). This observation led eventually to the development of a simple and effective means for reducing the incidence of erythroblastosis in the successive children born to high-risk parental combinations (Rh+ father, Rh− mother). At each delivery the mother is injected with anti-Rh Abs (γ-globulin fraction of human anti-Rh serum), causing rapid clearance of Rh+ fetal cells from maternal blood: this minimizes immunogenic priming of the mother.

Multiplicity of Rh Antigens. Analyses of many fetal–maternal incompatibilities have yielded a large variety of anti-Rh sera, of which there now seem to be about 27 distinctive types, each corresponding to a particular alloantigenic determinant or "specificity." Family studies have established that these serologically distinctive specificities are all genetically linked. However, since structural information about Rh antigens is lacking the genetic basis for their extreme polymorphism remains controversial. Before so many specificities were identified there was wide acceptance of Fisher's view that three allelic pairs of closely linked genes (*Cc, Dd, Ee*) were responsible. However, the multiplicity of specificities now known can hardly be reconciled with this scheme, but they can be accommodated by Wiener's view that all Rh specificities are due to a single Rh locus with many alleles. Various terminologies for the Rh Ags are still widely used (Table 21-4).

Antigen D. Despite the large number and complexity of the genetically linked Rh Ags their clinical utility is simplified by the outstanding importance of one of them, the factor called D. This alloantigen was responsible for the first case recognized by Levine and Stetson; it accounts for over 90% of all cases of erythroblastosis fetalis. Hence anti-D sera, from transplacentally immunized women, are used routinely to establish Rh type.* A person who is D− is commonly referred to as being Rh−; he will, however, usually possess some of the other antigenic determinants of the Rh locus.

---

* Guinea pig and rabbit antisera to *Rhesus* red cells do not distinguish consistently between D+ and D− red cells in umbilical cord blood, and so they are not used for typing purposes.

TABLE 21-4. Notations for Rh Alloantigens and Genes*

Some Rh alloantigens		Some genes or gene combinations		
Fisher-Race	Wiener	Fisher-Race	Wiener	Commonly used
D	Rh_0	cDe	Rh_0	R_0
C	rh'	CDe	Rh_1	R_1
E	rh''	cDE	Rh_2	R_2
c	hr'	CDE	Rh_z	R_z
e	hr''	cde	rh	r
		Cde	rh'	R'
		cdE	rh''	R''
		CdE	rh_y	R_y

* If a person's red cells react only with anti-C, anti-D, and anti-e sera, the cells are called CDe in the Fisher-Race terminology, and the genotype is assumed to be *CDe/CDe*. In the Wiener terminology the same antisera are called anti-rh', anti-Rh_0, and anti-hr'', and the red cells that react with all three are called Rh_1, as though a large antigen, Rh_1, is composed of three distinguishable antigenic determinants (rh$_1$, Rh$_0$, hr''). The more recent terminology of Rosenfield, Allen, Swisher, and Kochwa (*Transfusion 2*:287, 1962) is purely descriptive: the antisera are numbered and the red cells' antigenic structure is given by listing the sera with which they have been tested, with a minus sign before the number meaning that no reaction was observed. Thus, anti-Rhl = anti-D; anti-Rh2 = anti-C; anti-Rh3 = anti-E; anti-Rh4 = anti-c; anti-Rh5 = anti-e; anti-Rh6 = anti-ce or anti-f, etc. The CDe (Rh$_1$) cells receive the following designation: Rh: 1, 2, -3, -4, 5, -6.

THE KELL AND DUFFY BLOOD GROUPS

Besides ABO and Rh, several other Ag systems are important causes of severe transfusion reactions (and rarely of hemolytic disease in the newborn). The most common Ags of the Kell system are called K and k. K, present in about 10% of the population (Table 21-5), is a potent immunogen. Abs to K, formed as a result of pregnancy or transfusion, are usually incomplete and are detected by the Coombs antiglobulin test (Ch. 15). Unlike the red cells coated with Abs to most of the other blood group Ags, cells coated with anti-K are lysed by complement (C; see below).

The most common Ags of the Duffy system are termed Fy^a and Fy^b. Abs to Fy^b, formed as a result of transfusion or pregnancy, are being detected with increasing frequency in transfusion reactions and usually also require the Coombs antiglobulin test for their detection.

TABLE 21-5. Incidence of Some Red Blood Cell Phenotypes in the United States*

Blood group system	Phenotype	Frequency (%)	
ABO	O	44	
	A ($A_1 + A_2$)	42	
	B	10	
	AB ($A_1B + A_2B$)	4	
MN	M	27	
	N	24	
	MN	50	
Ss†	S	11	
	s	45	
	Ss	44	
P	P_1	80	
	P_2	14	
	p	rare	
Rh‡	DCe (Rh_1, R_1)	54	⎫
	DCE (Rh_z, R_z)	15	⎬ 85% react with anti-D
	DcE (Rh_2, R_2)	14	⎪ (= "Rh-positive")
	Dce (Rh_0, R_0)	2	⎭
	dce (rh, r)	13	⎫
	dCe (rh', R')	1.5	⎬ 15% do not react with anti-D
	dcE (rh", R")	0.5	⎪ (= "Rh-negative")
	dCE (rh_y, R_y)	rare	⎭
Lutheran	Lu^a	6	
	Lu^b	94	
Kell	K+	6	
	K−	94	
Lewis	Le^a	22	
	Le^b	78	
Duffy	Fy^a	38	
	Fy^b	28	
Kidd	Jk^a	83	
	Jk^b	17	

* Based on *Zinsser's Microbiology,* 13th ed. (D. T. Smith, N. F. Conant, and J. R. Overman, eds.), Appleton, New York, 1964.

† The incidence of S, s, and Ss is from Race, R. and Sanger, R. *Blood Groups in Man,* 2nd ed., Blackwell, Oxford, 1954. Anti-S sera agglutinate 73% of M, 54% of MN, and 32% of N cells.

‡ From Levine, P., Stroup, M. and Pollack, W. In *Bacterial and Mycotic Infections of Man,* 3rd ed. (R. J. Dubos, ed.), Lippincott, Philadelphia, 1958.

BLOOD TYPING

The identification of red cell alloantigens, called blood typing or grouping, is required for blood transfusions. In addition, it is commonly used for genetic analysis in cases of disputed paternity, and for anthropological surveys of human populations. It has even been used in archeological work, since the red cell Ags are extraordinarily stable: they have apparently been identified (by specific inhibi-

tion of hemagglutination reactions) in Egyptian mummies thousands of years old. King Tutankhamen, for instance, has been typed A_2MN.*

Blood typing is performed by agglutination

* Blood typing and other serological procedures are widely used in forensic medicine: to distinguish human from animal blood; to identify human blood types in blood stains, semen, or saliva; to distinguish horse meat from beef; etc.

reactions; unknown red cells are typed with known antisera and unknown alloantibodies with red cells of known type. The C-fixation test is not used; red cells coated by Abs to most alloantigens are not lysed by C. This might be due to a peculiar distribution of most alloantigens on the red cell surface, or blood group Abs might often belong to classes of immunoglobulins that do not react effectively with the first component of C (Ch. 18).

Transfusion Reactions. Blood transfusion can lead to serious reactions if massive intravascular clumping and hemolysis of red cells take place.* Such reactions are usually the result of an attack on the donor's red cells by the recipient's alloantibodies. Rarely is the reverse reaction serious, between the donor's Abs and the recipient's cells, since 1) the alloantibody titer in most normal individuals (as donors are supposed to be) is usually low to begin with, and 2) the dilution of donor blood in the recipient (usually about 10-fold) is generally sufficient to lower the titer to an innocuous level. Nevertheless, each lot of blood drawn from a prospective donor is screened against standard samples of red cells with 8 to 10 of the Ags that are most often responsible for transfusion reactions; bloods with a high titer of either agglutinating or incomplete Abs are used for other purposes (for example, the washed red cells might be injected).

The blood considered for a particular transfusion must, of course, have the same major red cell Ags as those in the prospective recipient's blood. In addition, "major" cross-matching must be performed routinely, with the prospective donor's red cells and the recipient's serum; if no agglutination is observed the cells must be washed and tested for adsorbed incomplete Abs by addition of rabbit antiserum to human γ-globulins (Ch. 15, Coombs' test). As a further precaution "minor" cross-matching is similarly carried out, i.e., with the prospective donor's serum and the recipient's red cells.

Universal Donors and Recipients. Under emergency conditions certain persons can donate blood to any recipient, and certain others can accept blood from any donor. The "universal donors" are type O; their red cells cannot react with either anti-A or anti-B in the recipient. However, type O donors are avoided if they have unusually high titers of anti-A and anti-B. The "universal recipients" are type AB; they lack both anti-A and anti-B. As an additional precaution under such circumstances, soluble A and B substances are often added to the transfused blood as specific inhibitors to minimize the possibility of AB alloimmune reactions.†

Uniqueness of the Individual's Red Cell Alloantigen Pattern. The foregoing precautions are not always reliable, however, since there are other red cell alloantigens that can cause serious incompatibilities (Table 21-5). In fact, so many different blood group alloantigens have now been identified (at least 60) that no two individuals are likely to be found with identical combinations, except for monozygotic twins.

In spite of this extreme diversity blood transfusions are extraordinarily successful, even when recipients undergo multiple transfusions from many different donors. Aside from the care exercised in the selection of prospective donors, through scrupulous typing procedures, the infrequency of transfusion reactions appears to be due to the fortunate fact that most red cell alloantigens are only feebly immunogenic. Moreover, transfused red cells survive for only a limited time (an average of perhaps about 3 to 4 weeks), so that even if Ab formation should be stimulated in the recipient the transfused cells are

---

* After multiple transfusions or multiple pregnancies alloantibodies are also sometimes formed to diverse alloantigens on white blood cells and on platelets (HL-A transplantation antigens, below). These Abs sometimes also cause serious transfusion reactions, which are characterized by high fever when leukocytes are involved, or by thrombocytopenic purpura when platelets are involved (Ch. 20; Fig. 20-15). Alloantibodies to Am allotypes of IgA-2 Igs (Ch. 16) can also cause transfusion reactions.

---

† Except for life-saving circumstances, A and B substances are not added to blood that is to be transfused into women of reproductive age; any enhancement of their immune response to A or B would increase the possibility that the babies they subsequently bear might have hemolytic disease due to A or B incompatibilities.

likely to be few in number by the time his al-loantibodies reach an effective level; the destruction of a small number of cells is not likely to be serious. As we shall see below, however, nature is less benevolent in the immune response to the alloantigens of transplanted tissues.

TRANSPLANTATION IMMUNITY: THE ALLOGRAFT REACTION

The immunological mechanisms underlying host reactions to transplanted tissues are difficult to decipher because of the complexity of the substances involved. But these reactions are among the most significant problems in immunology today, both because their suppression could make organ transplantation as feasible in the future as blood transfusions are at present, and because similar mechanisms are probably also involved in immune reactions against cancer cells.

DEFINITIONS

Four terms are used to describe tissue grafts.

1) **Autografts** are transplants from one region to another of the same individual.

2) **Isografts** are transplants from one individual to a genetically identical individual. These are possible only between monozygotic twins or between members of certain lines of mice and other rodents that have been so highly inbred (by brother-sister mating) as to be **syngeneic** or **isogenic,** i.e., genetically identical.*

3) **Allografts** or **homografts** are transplants from one individual to a genetically nonidentical (i.e., allogeneic) individual of the same species.

4) **Heterografts** or **xenografts** (Gr. *xenos* = foreign) are transplants from one species to another.

In these four types of grafts the donors are designated respectively as autologous, isologous, homologous, or heterologous with respect to the recipient.

---

* Syngeneic in the transplantation field refers operationally to the absence of any discernible tissue incompatibility, i.e., to genetic identity with respect to the genes controlling histocompatibility Ags. It approximates the situation in isogenic individuals, who are identical with respect to all their genes.

THE ALLOGRAFT REACTION AS AN IMMUNE RESPONSE

Among vertebrates autografts and isografts are usually enduring, but allografts (and heterografts) are regularly rejected.† Successful transfer of experimental tumors between individuals of an inbred mouse strain, but not between mice of different strains, provided the first indication that rejection of a graft was due to genetic differences between host and donor. It is now clear that grafted cells with genetically determined surface **histocompatibility or transplantation antigens** that are lacking in the recipient elicit an immune response that is directed against these Ags and leads to destruction (rejection) of the graft.

In investigating mechanisms of the allograft reaction skin grafts have been used most extensively, because of technical advantages: they are easy to prepare, their rejection is readily detected, and their median survival times provide an estimate of the intensity of the host's immune response. However, the same principles are involved in grafts of other tissues and cells.

THE SECOND-SET REACTION

When an allograft of skin is placed on a recipient animal, in a bed created by excising a slightly larger piece of skin, the graft at first becomes vascularized and its cells proliferate; but after about 10 days it quite abruptly becomes the seat of intense inflammation, withers, and is sloughed. If a second graft is then made to the same recipient, with another piece of skin from the same donor, it is rejected much more rapidly than the first graft, perhaps in 5 to 6 days. This accelerated re-

---

† Allografts are accepted by most invertebrates, which display few if any adaptive immune responses (see Chs. 17 and 20).

jection, the "second-set" reaction, is specific for a particular donor: if after the accelerated rejection another donor, antigenically different from the first, provides skin grafts to the same recipient, first- and second-set reactions to successive grafts are again seen. Thus, the capacity to reject an allograft (**transplantation immunity**) is acquired by virtue of exposure to the donor's cells; and it is specific for transplantation Ags of that donor. The shorter survival of the second graft results from persistence of the immunity acquired from the first graft or, perhaps, from an anamnestic response.

The second-set reaction to a skin graft can be induced not only by a prior skin graft, but just as well by prior inoculation of various other cells (e.g., spleen cells) from the same donor. In fact, virtually all cells induce transplantation immunity except erythrocytes; some histocompatibility Ags are present on red cells, but apparently not in immunogenic form (H-2 antigens in the mouse, below).

TRANSFER OF ALLOGRAFT IMMUNITY

Adoptive Transfer. The second-set reaction can be transferred "adoptively" from an immunized donor to a nonimmune recipient by viable lymphoid cells (T lymphocytes, Ch. 20). Thus if a mouse of strain X is immunized with a graft from a mouse of strain Y and viable lymphoid cells from the immune X animal are inoculated into a nonimmunized X mouse, the latter can respond as would the donor, giving a specific second-set reaction to a Y graft. [When the donor of sensitized lymphoid cells is syngeneic with the recipient the adoptive immunity can be enduring; when the donor is allogeneic the recipient's adoptive immunity is short-lived (1 to 2 weeks) and is terminated by an allograft reaction against the donor's lymphoid cells.]

HUMORAL VS. CELL-MEDIATED IMMUNITY

The rejection of most allografts appears to be an expression of cell-mediated hypersensitivity because the capacity for accelerated rejection is transferred by viable lymphocytes, not by serum. Moreover, in some species, such as the guinea pig, lymphocytes from a sensitized animal can elicit a delayed cutane-

ous reaction if injected into the skin of the animal to whose tissues they are sensitive. As in other cell-mediated reactions, the site of an allograft undergoing rejection is intensely infiltrated with lymphocytes and macrophages; granulocytes and plasma cells are much less conspicuous (Ch. 20).

Nevertheless, an animal that has rejected an allograft will often have serum Abs for the donor's histocompatibility Ags, some of which are also present on red blood cells; **hemagglutination reactions** have therefore provided a simple but powerful means of characterizing these Ags and for their genetic mapping (see below). However, these serum Abs seem not to be responsible for rejection of skin grafts: they generally appear late in the course of the allograft response, their levels bear no consistent relation to the intensity or rapidity of the rejection reaction, and as noted above they are generally incapable of transferring the ability to mount a typical second-set reaction.

However, some antisera from intensively immunized individuals can interfere specifically with the healing-in of a fresh graft, causing unusually rapid rejection (the "white-graft" reaction). Moreover, allogeneic lymphocytes, unlike "solid" tissue cells, are readily destroyed by Abs to histocompatibility Ags, and complement is required. Broadly speaking, therefore, rejections of allografts, like allergic reactions to most Ags, can be a manifestation of either humoral or cell-mediated immunity; but the cell-mediated reaction is primarily responsible for rejection of skin and other "solid" tissue grafts.

TOLERANCE OF ALLOGRAFTS

Under a number of exceptional circumstances allografts are not rejected.

Privileged Sites. There are a few special ("privileged") sites where allografts may flourish for prolonged periods without inducing immunity, such as the meninges of the brain and the anterior chamber of the eye. Lymphatic drainage is lacking in these sites; hence stimulation of immunologically competent cells of the host's lymphatic tissue is minimal.

Pregnancy. Histocompatibility Ags are formed early in embryonic life, and many of these Ags, inherited from the father, are alien to the mother. Hence in man and other mammals **the intrauterine fetus is actually an allograft.** Its failure to evoke an allograft reaction, even when the mother has been previously immunized deliberately to the father's histocompatibility Ags, is probably explained by the absence (or masking by mucinous secretions) of these Ags in the special fetal cell layer (trophoblast) at the placental interface between the fetus and its maternal host.

Induction of Immunological Tolerance. The induction of immunity to allografts has dose-response features that resemble those of immune responses in general. The routine success of corneal transplants in man (which are always allografts) is due to the small amount of tissue transplanted and the relative avascularity of the transplantation site. At the other extreme, large doses of allogeneic cells can establish tolerance to allografts, especially when introduced around the time of birth (see below).

Current interest in immunological tolerance in general actually began with experiments on allografts, which grew out of a crucial observation on red cell alloantigens in nonidentical cattle twins, which frequently have in utero anastomoses of their placental blood vessels. Owen observed in 1945 that each twin often had two antigenically different kinds of red cells, which persisted as the twins grew to maturity. It was inferred that hematopoietic stem cells from each twin, transferred through the common circulation in utero, had settled in the marrow of the other and then survived in the genetically foreign soil through the animal's lifetime. Each twin thus produced two kinds of red cells, with its own and with its twin's characteristic alloantigens. Such individuals, with mixtures of genetically different cells, are called **chimeras,** after the monster in Greek mythology with a lion's head, a goat's body, and a serpent's tail. (Rare blood group chimeras among nonidentical human twins have also been found.)

Surmising that such chimeras might also be generally tolerant of each other's tissues, Billingham, Brent, and Medawar then demonstrated that they accepted skin grafts from each other without an allograft reaction. By taking advantage of the fact that mice of a given inbred strain are exact genetic replicas, it was subsequently shown that mice of one strain (A) could be rendered permanently tolerant of skin allografts from another strain (CBA) if embryonic or newborn A mice were inoculated with viable cells (e.g., of spleen) from CBA animals. When the inoculated animals matured they accepted allografts permanently from CBA donors, though they rejected grafts from any other strain in a normal manner.

The newborn mouse appears to develop allograft tolerance with ease because its immune apparatus is relatively immature, and it therefore cannot reject the foreign cells by an allograft reaction. Once established, the tolerance persists, probably because the foreign cells continue to proliferate and to maintain a sufficient level of the tolerated transplantation Ags. An individual rendered tolerant in this manner is, therefore, a chimera, carrying allogeneic cells in advance of the allograft that reveals tolerance.* Since tolerance of allografts depends on an adequate level of foreign histocompatibility Ags (i.e., allogeneic cells) it seems to be fundamentally the same as the tolerance that can be established to other Ags, such as globular proteins and polysaccharides (Ch. 17). Another mechanism that might account for the persistence of allogeneic cells in a chimera is discussed below (blocking Abs in enhancement).

The immunological balance in the chimera can be readily tipped, and the tolerance abrogated, by introducing immunologically competent cells that recognize the tolerated tissue as genetically alien. Thus when a mouse of strain X, rendered tolerant as a newborn to tissues of strain Y, carries a successful and enduring Y graft, the graft can be made to undergo prompt rejection by inoculating the tolerant host with viable lymphoid cells from a strain-X animal that had previously been immunized against Y (Fig. 21-5). The rejection can also be elicited by inoculating the tolerant X animal with lymphoid cells from a normal, nonimmune animal of strain X, but

---

* The chimerism can be demonstrated by using spleen or white blood cells from such a tolerant animal (A strain tolerant of CBA) as immunogens to induce in a third strain of mice allograft sensitivity to both A and CBA.

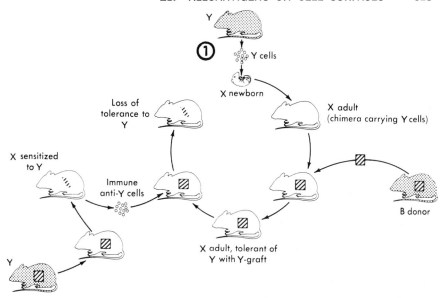

Fig. 21-5. Establishment and loss of tolerance to histocompatibility Ags. Newborn X was injected with Y cells. The subsequent injection of the tolerant X animal (shown carrying a Y skin graft) with lymphoid cells from a Y-sensitive X donor leads to adoptive immunity, with rejection of the previously tolerated graft. The risk of a graft-vs.-host reaction can be eliminated in step 1 (top) if the donor of cells to the newborn is an X × Y hybrid, rather than a purebred Y-strain mouse, as shown.

the effect requires more cells and takes longer to develop.

Adult animals have, with difficulty, also been rendered tolerant of allografts by inoculation of viable cells from prospective donors, but special measures are required: the adult is first converted temporarily to a state of immunological incompetence, resembling that of the newborn period, by intensive X-irradiation or treatment with cytotoxic drugs (Ch. 17), and multiple injections of the allogeneic cells are then usually given. Reactions of allogeneic lymphoid cells against the immunologically incompetent host creates other severe problems (Graft-vs.-host reaction, below and Ch. 20).

The genetic basis for both transplantation tolerance and transplantation immunity is evident with the hybrid offspring (AB) of a cross between inbred parental strains (AA and BB). **The AB hybrids are tolerant of grafts from either parental strain, but mice of either parental strain reject grafts from the hybrids:** a graft is permanently accepted only when essentially **all** its histocompatibility Ags are present in and therefore tolerated by the recipient.

Enhancement. Paradoxically, the survival of certain allografts may be prolonged in adult recipients by previous intensive immunization, either active (with the corresponding allogeneic cells) or passive (with Abs to the histocompatibility Ags of these cells). The mechanism for this graft "enhancement" is still not completely understood; it appears, however, that if Abs bound to cell surface histocompatibility Ags are not cytotoxic they can sometimes specifically protect the target cells against destruction by the "killer" lymphocytes responsible for cell-mediated immunity (Ch. 20, see "efferent enhancement" in discussion of Suppression of cell-mediated immunity by Abs). It is also possible that these Abs block immunogenicity of the graft's histocompatibility Ags, preventing induction of cell-mediated immunity (Ch. 20, "afferent" enhancement). Enhancement by serum Abs is less readily demonstrated with normal tissue allografts than with certain solid tumor allografts (Sarcomas and carcinomas, below).

Enhancement might be responsible for the long-lasting chimerism established in neonatal animals with allogeneic cells (Induction of immunological tolerance, above): the host, rather than being truly tolerant, might make Abs to the allogenic histocompatibility Ags, causing prolonged survival of the donor's cells. Thus, spleen cells from these chimeras appear, in in vitro cytotoxicity tests, to destroy donor cells, and the effect appears to be blocked specifically by the chimera's serum. (Other assays suggest, in contrast, that the chimera is truly tolerant; for example, his lymphocytes seem to be incapable of effecting a graft-vs.-host reaction in an appropriate host: see below.)

GRAFT-VS.-HOST REACTION

In establishing tolerance by injecting a newborn animal with viable allogeneic cells the inoculum is usually prepared as a suspension of spleen cells: when derived from an immunologically mature (adult) animal some T cells in the suspension can react with the alloantigens of the neonatal host.

Evidence of such a reaction was only occasionally observed with the particular donor-recipient strains used in the initial demonstration; but it has since been seen consistently with many other pairs of strains. In these graft-vs.-host reactions the inoculated newborn animal fails to gain weight normally, develops skin lesions and diarrhea, and dies after a few weeks **("runting syndrome").** This symptom complex has also been seen when immunologically competent cells from allogeneic donors are injected into an adult that cannot reject the cells, e.g., one depleted of lymphocytes by X-irradiation or cytotoxic drugs or an adult hybrid (F_1), who is tolerant because one of its parents is syngeneic with the donor (i.e., AA donor cells make a graft-vs.-host reaction against the B alloantigens in an AB recipient). For more on these reactions, see Ch. 20.

HISTOCOMPATIBILITY OR TRANSPLANTATION ANTIGENS

Partially purified histocompatibility Ags (obtained by limited proteolysis of mouse spleen cells) are glycoproteins (10% carbohydrate, MW ca. 35,000 to 50,000). The small amounts available so far have been able to induce allograft hypersensitivity (accel-erated rejection) and, in larger doses, to establish tolerance with respect to Ab formation. However, the purified Ags have not yet established tolerance of allografts, suggesting that they may have some defective (or missing) antigenic determinants.

The specificity of histocompatibility Ags seems to reside in the protein moiety (removal of most of the carbohydrate leaves the antigenic activity intact). Moreover, the allelic alloantigens of hybrid mice (one inherited from each parent are isolable as separate molecules; and in immunofluorescence with intact cells they appear to form separate aggregates ("patches") with the respective fluorescent Abs, labeled with a red (rhodamine) chromophore for one alloantigen and with a green one (fluorescein) for the other alloantigen (see Ch. 17, Fig. 17-10). These properties are in sharp contrast to the ABO blood group substances, whose alloantigenic determinants (A, B) are saccharides and where the final products of allelic genes (as well as some nonallelic ones) are joined covalently in a single heterosaccharide; moreover, the immediate products of the genes for blood group substances are enzymes that synthesize the antigenic determinants, whereas the immediate products of the genes that determine graft-host histocompatibility are almost certainly the histocompatibility Ags themselves (Histocompatibility genes, below).

HISTOCOMPATIBILITY GENES

Histocompatibility Ags are specified by histocompatibility or *H* genes.* Because a host immune response to any of a donor's transplantation Ags can lead to rejection of a graft, permanent acceptance (in the absence of chronic immunosuppressive therapy) requires that essentially all of the donor's histocompatibility alleles be present in the recipient. Hence the probability that an allograft will be accepted when donor and recipient are drawn at random from an outbred population, such as man, depends upon 1) the number of *H* genes or loci in the species, and 2)

---

* *H* is a convenient abbreviation but the reader must obviously not confuse it with the completely unrelated H (heterogenetic) antigen of blood group substances (earlier, this chapter).

the number of alleles at each locus and their frequencies in the population.

The *H* loci and their alleles have been characterized most extensively in the mouse, because its many inbred strains permit detailed genetic analysis with skin grafts. The *H* genes in this species seem to correspond closely to those in man, in whom methods of analysis are necessarily more limited.

HISTOCOMPATIBILITY GENES IN THE MOUSE

The number of independent *H* loci at which two inbred strains differ can be estimated by mating them (AA × BB), crossing the F_1 progeny (AB × AB), and using animals of the F_2 generation as recipients for skin grafts from the purebred parental strains. As is illustrated in Figure 21-6, the number, *n*, of *H* loci, is provided by the proportion (*x*) of F_2 animals that accept grafts from one of the purebred parental strains: $x = (3/4)^n$. This technic yields minimal values because some *H* genes are linked to one another and behave as single rather than as multiple genes, and some inbred strains have certain *H* alleles in common. In the mouse, where many pairs of strains have been subjected to this test, about 30 *H* loci have been detected.

These loci, and the number of alleles at each, have been characterized by more complex procedures that depend upon selected matings to produce **"congenic" lines*** that differ from a standard inbred strain by a small chromosomal segment containing a single locus (the one selected for; see Fig. 21-7). From the fate of grafts exchanged among various lines, and between these lines and standard inbred strains, it has been possible to establish pedigreed lines that differ only at single *H* loci and to enumerate the alleles at these loci (about 19 alleles at the *H-2* locus, 3 at *H-1*, etc.). Congenic lines are exceedingly valuable for analyzing the properties of various individual genes, not just those involved in transplantation, and a general method for their production is given in Figure 21-7.

H-2 Locus. The transplantation Ags specified by one locus, called *H-2,* are outstanding because of the intensity of the reactions they evoke: allografts exchanged between mice that differ only at this locus are usually rejected in about 11 days (first set), whereas those exchanged between mice that have the same *H-2* alleles but differ at any one of the

---

* Also called congenic "resistant" lines because of the assay originally used to detect alleles in the progeny of successive back-crosses of the type shown in Figure 21-7. A tumor arising in one purebred strain and carrying that strain's histocompatibility Ags was used as a graft: recipients that were **resistant** to the tumor (rejected it as an allograft) lacked one or more of the donor strain's histocompatibility Ags (and alleles).

Fig. 21-6. Estimate of the number of independent histocompatibility genes at which two inbred strains of mice differ. Shaded squares correspond to progeny in the F_2 generation that accept a graft from parent A. (Courtesy of Dr. Ralph J. Graff.)

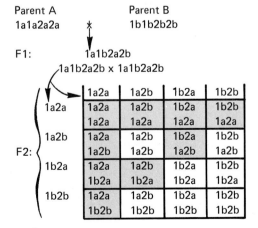

Parental Strains Differ by One H Gene

Parent A   Parent B
1a1a   x   1b1b

F1:   1a1b

1a1b x 1a1b

F2:
	1a	1b
1a	1a1a	1a1b
1b	1ab	1bb

$(\frac{3}{4})^1$ or 75% of F2 progeny accept grafts from parent A or parent B

Parental Strains Differ by Two Independent H Genes

Parent A   Parent B
1a1a2a2a   x   1b1b2b2b

F1:   1a1b2a2b

1a1b2a2b x 1a1b2a2b

F2:
	1a2a	1a2b	1b2a	1b2b
1a2a	1a2a 1a2a	1a2b 1a2a	1b2a 1a2a	1b2b 1a2a
1a2b	1a2a 1a2b	1a2b 1a2b	1b2a 1a2b	1b2b 1a2b
1b2a	1a2a 1b2a	1a2b 1b2a	1b2a 1b2a	1b2b 1b2a
1b2b	1a2a 1b2b	1a2b 1b2b	1b2a 1b2b	1b2b 1b2b

$(\frac{3}{4})^2$ or 56% of F2 progeny accept grafts from parent A or parent B

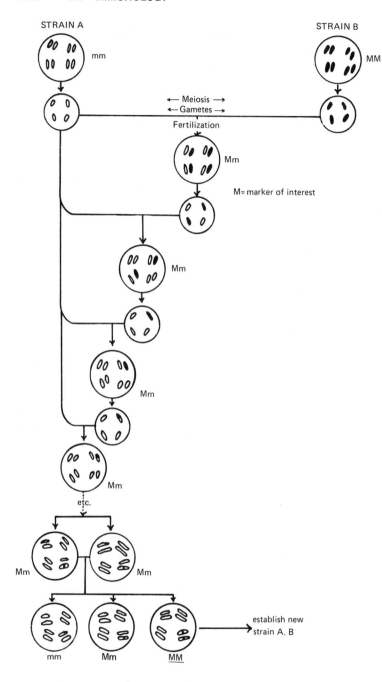

STRAIN A

STRAIN B

← Meiosis →
← Gametes →
Fertilization

M= marker of interest

etc.

establish new
strain A. B

Fig. 21-7. Production of congenic strain A.B. Following an initial cross between an inbred A mouse and an inbred B mouse and back-cross of the F₁ generation to strain A, a series of successive back-crosses to strain A is carried out with progeny that possess the B marker (M) of interest (e.g., their skin grafts are rejected by A-strain mice). Offspring of the tenth back-cross generation (N10) are intercrossed, and progeny that are homozygous for the B-strain marker (e.g., they reject skin grafts from A-strain donors) are then inbred by successive brother-sister matings to establish the new congenic A.B strain. This strain is essentially identical with inbred strain A except for a chromosomal segment (e.g., with a histocompatibility gene) of inbred strain B. The principle is a general one: a congenic strain can be established for any dominant gene. (Courtesy of Dr. Ralph J. Graff.)

other *H* loci have median survival times that range from 20 to upward of 200 days.

The H-2 alloantigens are also outstanding because they are present on red blood cells, which can be agglutinated by sera from animals that have been intensively immunized by appropriate skin grafts plus injections of allogeneic cells (especially lymphocytes). As

with many hyperimmune sera (Ch. 15), these sera also exhibit complicated cross-reactions: it appears that the Ag associated with each *H-2* allele has both a **unique ("private")** antigenic specificity and a variety of **broader ("public")** specificities, which it shares with certain other histocompatibility Ags, determined by other *H-2* alleles. Whether the shared specificities represent identical or similar structural elements in various H-2 Ags is uncertain and is not likely to be known until the detailed structure of these molecules is established.

With serological analysis to facilitate screening of many progeny from matings between inbred strains, it has been possible to detect rare crossovers within the *H-2* locus, which actually consists of two linked genes, called *H-2D* and *H-2K*. In between these genes there are several others (Fig. 21-8), including a number of so-called *Ir* genes,* which determine ability to make an immune response to various Ags (Ch. 17, Genetic control of Ab formation).

When surface macromolecules of intact

---

* About 1 in 200 progeny are recombinants between D and K. If the crossover frequency between two markers is proportional to the linear distance between them there is room between the D and K ends of the *H-2* locus for up to about 1000 genes.

cells are stained with differently colored fluorescent Abs of various specificities it is clear that the antigenic determinants specified by a *D* allele and those specified by the *K* allele of the same chromosome are located on separate molecules: i.e., anti-D and anti-K form separate aggregates in the same cell's membrane (Ch. 17, see Cap formation and Fig. 17-10). However the multiple determinants associated with any particular allele seem to be present in the same surface molecule. Thus *D* and *K* of a given chromosome (**haplotype;** see the human HL-A locus, below) specify different membrane molecules, each with multiple antigenic determinants (or specificities).

Non H-2 Loci. The other *H* loci determine Ags that are much less immunogenic in allogeneic mice. Not only are survival times much longer when grafts are exchanged between congenic lines that differ only at one *non H-2* locus, but many more inoculated cells are re-

Fig. 21-8. *H-2* locus in the mouse. Different *H-2* "alleles," designated by lower-case letters, correspond to different patterns of antigenic specificity (designated by numbers), which are found in the representative inbred mouse strains listed at the right. Each of the "alleles," representing a combination of linked alleles of two genes (*K* and *D*) in the locus, corresponds to a haplotype in the human *HL-A* locus. Genes *Ss* and *Slp* specify certain serum proteins; the *Ir* (immune response) region represents a cluster of genes that govern ability to make immune responses to about 20 different Ags (Ch. 17). Most of the numbered antigenic specificities shown are unique ("private") for a given allele. Some alleles (—) are associated with distinctive patterns of several specificities, each shared with various other alleles. [From Klein, J., and Schreffler, D. C. *Transplant Rev* 6:3 (1971).]

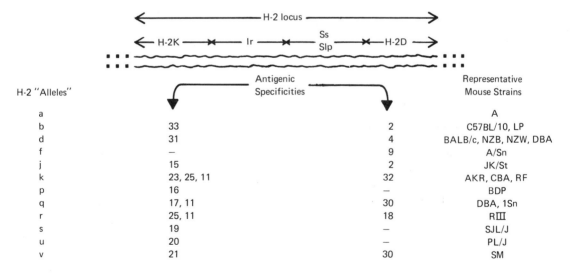

H-2 "Alleles"	Antigenic Specificities (H-2K)	Antigenic Specificities (H-2D)	Representative Mouse Strains
a			A
b	33	2	C57BL/10, LP
d	31	4	BALB/c, NZB, NZW, DBA
f	—	9	A/Sn
j	15	2	JK/St
k	23, 25, 11	32	AKR, CBA, RF
p	16	—	BDP
q	17, 11	30	DBA, 1Sn
r	25, 11	18	RIII
s	19	—	SJL/J
u	20	—	PL/J
v	21	30	SM

quired to induce transplantation immunity, and many fewer are needed to establish tolerance, with such strain combinations than with combinations that differ only at *H-2*. Nevertheless, the cumulative effect of many *non H-2* differences can approximate that of an *H-2* incompatibility and can lead to virtually as rapid allograft rejection.

Diverse *H* loci are associated with different genetic markers on various linkage groups (i.e., chromosomes): for example, the *H-1* locus is linked with albinism, and *H-2* with fused tail vertebrae. One of the *non H-2* loci appears to be associated with the Y sex chromosome. It is revealed by exchange of grafts (skin, spleen, thyroid, etc.) between males and females of a given inbred mouse strain: grafts from female to male are accepted permanently, but those from male to female are rejected (after long survival times). Male tolerance of female cells is due to the presence of X chromosomes in both sexes, but some product of the Y chromosome on cell surfaces of the male can apparently function as a weak histocompatibility Ag in otherwise isogenic females. Because this Ag is weak, tolerance of it is readily established; e.g., by transplanting an extra large piece of skin from male to female.

HISTOCOMPATIBILITY GENES IN MAN

When leukocytes from one mouse strain are injected into newborn mice of certain other strains the recipients became tolerant of grafts from the donor strain (Tolerance, above). Mouse histocompatibility Ags seem therefore to be fully expressed on these readily available cells. The analysis of human histocompatibility Ags has accordingly been largely based also on leukocytes.

Antisera to human leukocyte (HL) Ags are derived from three sources: 1) patients who have received multiple blood transfusions; 2) women who, through pregnancy, have been immunized against alien leukocyte alloantigens of their offspring, inherited from the father; 3) human volunteers immunized with leukocytes from selected donors.

These sera agglutinate appropriate leukocytes (leukagglutination) and, together with complement (Ch. 18), they also damage leukocyte membranes in a cytotoxic reaction that is revealed by "dye-exclusion" tests: ionic dyes, such as eosin and trypan blue, penetrate into and stain only those cells with damaged membranes (Ch. 17, Living vs.

dead cells). Monospecific sera, useful for typing, have been identified by screening many human sera against panels of leukocyte samples from many (100 or more) persons.

With standardized typing sera over 20 human leukocyte Ags have been identified. Their distribution in family pedigrees has established that they are determined by a single complex genetic locus that is remarkably like that of *H-2* in the mouse. Called **HL-A** (for human histocompatibility locus A), it consists of two closely linked loci (sometimes called the "first" and "second"), each with a large number of alleles (*HL-A1, HL-A2,* etc.). In a doubly heterozygous individual the cells carry four different HL-A antigens (called a "full house"). Because these Ags are produced by two closely linked genes (like *D* and *K* in the mouse *H-2* locus, see Fig. 21-8), they are associated in pairs or **"haplotypes"** (one pair inherited from each parent, Fig. 21-9).

Mixed Lymphocyte Cultures. Serological typing of HL-A Ags is still limited: monospecific sera for some of them are probably still not available and the results of cytotoxicity tests are not always unambiguous. More important, grafts are sometimes rejected when donor and recipient appear to have identical HL-A haplotypes, suggesting that incompatibility of other transplantation Ags can be significant. Other tests, resembling cross-matching in blood transfusions (above), are therefore used sometimes for further evaluation of HL-A matched pairs. In the mixed lymphocyte culture (MLC) test isolated blood

	Haplotype	Haplotype	
Father	1, 5	9, 12	
Mother	2, 7	10, 13	
Child No. 1	1, 5	2, 7	
2	1, 5	10, 13	HL-A
3	1, 5	10, 13	identical sibs
4	9, 12	2, 7	
5	9, 12	10, 13	

Fig. 21-9. A hypothetical family pedigree illustrating some features of the *HL-A* locus and its antigens. At gene 1 there are 9 alleles (*HL-A 1, 2, 3, 9, 10, 11, Ba, Li*); at gene 2 there are 14 alleles (*HL-A 5, 7, 8, 12, 13, 4C, BB, FJH, LND, AA, SL, Maki, 407*). Each haplotype consists of one allele (antigen) from gene *1* and one from gene *2*. Every child has one haplotype in common with each parent. With doubly heterozygous parents (as in the example) the probability that two sibs have identical HL-A antigens is 0.25.

lymphocytes from recipient and prospective donor are maintained together for several days in tissue culture. Under these conditions blast transformation occurs if allogeneic cells are present; i.e., the antigenically stimulated lymphocytes enlarge, become basophilic (owing to increase in content of ribosomes), and incorporate ³H-thymidine into DNA at an enhanced rate (Chs. 17 and 20). The test can be made unidirectional by treating one set of cells, say from the prospective donor, with mitomycin C before mixing with the prospective recipient's cells; DNA synthesis is blocked in the treated set and any increase in DNA synthesis in the mixed culture is due to the reaction of some of the recipient's lymphocytes against the treated cells, which must have surface Ags the recipient lacks.

Mixed lymphocyte cultures seem to be responsive primarily to HL-A Ags, for which they provide a sensitive measure of compatibility: e.g., the response is greater with cells from sibs that differ in two rather than in just one haplotype. However, a positive response has been obtained in rare instances with sibs that have two identical haplotypes; and among unrelated individuals with identical HL-A Ags a positive MLC response is seen more often. The lower frequency of discordant results among sibs suggests that other genes (the *MLC* locus), linked to HL-A, contribute to, or even determine, the MLC reaction: because of the linked relation, siblings having the same *HL-A* alleles usually have the same *MLC* locus, but unrelated persons with the same *HL-A* alleles differ more often at the *MLC* locus. These relations might account for the greater success with HL-A identical kidney grafts when donor-recipient pairs are siblings than when they are unrelated (Fig. 21-10).

The rare acceptance of an allograft when related donor-recipient pairs (e.g., uncle-nephew) differ in all HL-A Ags suggests that the Ag specified by the MLC locus might be the primary determinant of allograft immunity.

A positive MLC response has also been obtained with lymphocytes from congenic mouse strains that have identical *H-2D* and *H-2K* loci and differ only in the *Ir-1* locus. The human *MLC* locus might thus correspond to *Ir-1* of mice which, it may be recalled, occupies a position near the center of the *H-2* locus and determines the ability of mice to make immune responses to particular Ags (Ch. 17), perhaps because it codes for surface macromolecules that serve as Ag-binding receptors on T lymphocytes (Ch. 17).

ABO Blood Group Substances and Transplantation Immunity. ABO blood group substances are present on the surface membranes of many types of cells, in addition to erythrocytes, and these substances can also function as transplantation Ags: kidney grafts seem to be subject to especially rapid and violent rejection when donor and recipient belong to different ABO groups. Group O human volunteers injected with AB red cells (or with purified A and B substances; above) reject subsequent skin grafts from any AB donor in an accelerated manner (second set), but grafts from an O donor are rejected as a "first set." It is not clear if accelerated rejection of AB-incompatible grafts is due to conventional anti-A and anti-B alloantibodies (above) or to cell-mediated reactions.

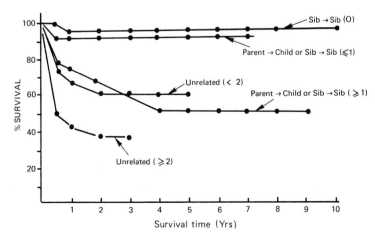

Fig. 21-10. Correlation between survival of human kidney grafts and HL-A compatibility. Number of incompatibilities based on leukocyte typing is given in parentheses. Since these are two linked genes (haplotypes) in the HL-A locus, every parent-child combination and half the sib-sib combinations will have at least one haplotype in common, or a maximum incompatibility of two. Uncertainties arise when fewer than four HL-A antigens are typed in donor and recipient. [From Dausset, J., and Hors, J. *Transplant Proc 3*:1004 (1971).]

If donor and recipient belong to the same ABO group, injected red cells from one donor do not induce accelerated rejection (second set) of a subsequent graft from the same donor: hence red cells lack HL-A Ags, at least in immunogenic form (or amount).

IMMUNITY AGAINST TUMORS

Tumor-specific Antigens. Immune reactions of experimental animals to tumor grafts, and of human subjects to their cancers, depend on **tumor-specific antigens (TSAs)** that are lacking or masked in normal cells. Because TSAs are usually present in the tumor cell's surface membrane, the host can react against his tumor as though it were an allograft. However, an intense host reaction can **select for tumor cell variants** with modified TSAs; this could account for the general finding that TSAs of most well-established tumors have little immunogenic potency in the **autochthonous host** (i.e., the individual in whom the tumor arose).

Tumor Transplantation. The fate of transplanted tumors depends upon the recipient's relation to the autochthonous host. When the latter and the recipient are **syngeneic** the outcome varies with the number of transplanted cells: with more than a critical number the tumor quickly becomes too massive to be destroyed by any first-set immune response that might be made against its TSAs.* However, an effective subthreshold number of cells can elicit a sufficient response to block the graft's growth; and the resistant host will then usually reject a much larger transplant of the same tumor (compare dose-response curves in immunized and unimmunized syngeneic recipients, Ch. 20, Tumor immunity, Fig. 20-7).

Recipients can also become specifically resistant to a tumor after injections of X-irradiated tumor cells (which are incapable of proliferating but have intact Ags) or after total excision of a tumor graft that has grown for 1 to 2 weeks in situ. Whichever method is used in syngeneic animals, the resistance is specific for the particular tumor used as immunogen or, in some instances, other tumors induced by the same oncogenic virus (see below). When the autochthonous host and the recipient are **allogeneic,** transplanted tumor cells are rejected, even in massive numbers, by the recipient's first-set response to the tumor's normal histocompatibility Ags (for rare exceptions see Loss of normal transplantation Ags, below).

Many tumors are weakly immunogenic in the autochthonous host. As noted before (Ch. 20), a mouse immunized with X-irradiated sarcoma cells, derived from its own totally excised tumor, can reject a subsequent graft of that tumor (maintained during the immunization procedure by successive transplants in syngeneic recipients), without becoming resistant to other sarcomas. (For other evidence, see Enhancement, below, and Tumor immunity, Ch. 20.)

Cell-mediated vs. Humoral Immunity. The rejection of solid tumor grafts in syngeneic or allogeneic hosts seems usually (like that of normal tissue allografts) to be due to cell-mediated immunity: resistance can usually be transferred adoptively with viable lymphocytes but not with antisera. In conjunction with C, however, serum alloantibodies against TSAs can destroy neoplastic lymphocytes (from leukemias and lymphosarcomas), just as other humoral Abs (plus C) can destroy allogeneic normal lymphocytes. With most other kinds of tumors, however, Abs to their TSAs are not destructive and some may even protect the tumor against cell-mediated immune reactions (Enhancement, below).

Enhancement. Many grafts of malignant epithelial or connective tissue cells (carcinomas or sarcomas, respectively) grow more rapidly and in a higher proportion of recipients if the recipients are first subjected to prolonged immunization or given antisera from syngeneic animals that were intensively im-

---

* The tumor is then lethal for the recipient. Experimental tumors are maintained routinely by serial transplantation of relatively large numbers of cells into animals that are syngeneic with the autochthonous host.

munized against the tumor. Evidently, TSAs on the tumor cell surface become covered by noncytotoxic Abs, blocking induction of immunity or recognition and attack by specifically reactive killer lymphocytes (Ch. 20, see afferent and efferent enhancement).

It is not clear why Abs to TSAs destroy leukemic lymphocytes but seem harmless or even protective for many carcinomas and sarcomas; possibly the target cells differ in susceptibility of the surface membrane to lytic attack by activated C or in the distribution of their surface TSAs: with widely dispersed TSAs, Abs might be less likely to activate C than if the TSAs were closely packed (Ch. 18). Even with the ordinarily susceptible neoplastic lymphocytes of leukemia some Abs to TSAs actually protect the cells against other, cytotoxic Abs: the difference could arise from differences in ability to activate the C cascade (Ch. 18).

Though enhancement by noncytotoxic Abs seemed initially a laboratory curiosity, there is growing evidence for its clinical importance. For instance, enhancing activity is present in the sera of many individuals with progressive tumors, but lacking in those with regressing tumors (below). As was noted above, enhancing Abs seem also, under certain circumstances, to prolong the survival of normal tissue allografts.

Unique vs. Shared Tumor-specific Antigens. Injection of methylcholanthrene or other chemical carcinogens into isogenic mice raises tumors that are antigenically distinct from one another; little or no cross-immunity has been detected when animals immunized with one tumor are challenged by grafts of other tumors, induced with the same carcinogen. Diverse tumors raised by a given carcinogen in one animal are also antigenically distinguishable by cross-grafting; and there is even evidence for antigenic variation within individual, chemically induced tumors, which could either have a multicellular origin, with different clones growing together in one tumor mass, or a unicellular origin, with the development of antigenic variants at subsequent cell divisions. The antigenic individuality of these tumors suggests that chemical carcinogens activate different host genes in different clones of tumor cells.

In contrast, different tumors induced in mice by a given oncogenic virus have the same TSAs, which differ from the TSAs of tumors induced by other oncogenic viruses. For instance, the histologically diversified tumors produced with polyomavirus in mice (Ch. 63) all have a common TSA, which is even shared (cross-reacts) with tumors induced by this virus in hamsters. This Ag, which induces resistance to tumor grafts, is not part of the virion; whether it is coded for by the virus or by a host gene activated by the virus is not known. In addition to such shared TSAs, some virus-induced tumors also have TSAs that seem to be unique for different tumors raised by the same virus.

Loss of Normal Histocompatibility Antigens. Some tumor cells differ from their normal counterparts not only in having gained TSAs, but also in having lost some normal histocompatibility Ags: in exceedingly rare instances a mouse tumor becomes freely transplantable in diverse allogeneic mice, and some human cancer cells seem also to have less HL-A antigen than normal cells of the same histological type.

A more restricted type of antigenic loss is seen when tumors originating in hybrid strains of mice (AB) develop specific subline variants capable of growing in one or the other of the parent strains (AA or BB). Thus, an AB tumor may develop variants that can grow in the AA parent, indicating an apparent loss of the histocompatibility Ags contributed by the B half of the hybrid's genome. This loss has been postulated to be the result of chromosomal deletion or of recombination in somatic cells (Ch. 43, Parasexual cycle in fungi).

Antigenicity of Human Tumors. Clinical observations have long suggested that a patient's immune response might suppress growth of his cancer cells. Thus tumors with slowed growth are often found to be heavily infiltrated by lymphocytes and plasma cells; on rare occasions tumors even undergo "spontaneous" regression.

Direct evidence for TSAs on human cancer cells has been provided by immunofluorescent staining, and C-dependent cytotoxicity tests show that serum from a patient may contain Abs that react wtih his own tumors cells and sometimes with tumor cells of the same type from other individuals (e.g., malignant lymphocytes of Burkitt's lymphoma, neuroblastoma).

Fetal Antigens. When rabbit antisera prepared against extracts of gastrointestinal tract carcinomas are absorbed with extracts of normal intestinal mucosa, the residual Abs react with an Ag (a glycoprotein with ca. 50% carbohydrate; MW 1×10^5 to 2×10^5) that is present not only in gastrointestinal carcinomas but also in embryonic gastrointestinal mucosa and in liver and pancreas (which are endodermal derivatives of the gut). Hence this **carcinoembryonic antigen (CEA)** appears to be specified by a normal gene that is expressed transiently in endodermal cells during fetal development, and in adult life if these cells undergo malignant change.

Serum from nearly all patients with colon or rectal adenocarcinoma contains CEA, and many also contain Abs to CEA. Both disappear with successful surgical removal of the cancer, and reappearance of CEA can be the first diagnostic clue of the tumor's recurrence. With widespread metastases the CEA concentration rises and anti-CEA disappears (masked by Ag excess). With highly sensitive radioimmunoassays that can detect ca. 1 ng, CEA (or a substance that cross-reacts with it) has also been detected in sera of some persons with carcinoma of lung or breast.

Other fetal Ags are associated with certain other human cancers: α-**fetoprotein** is found in serum of patients with hepatomas or embryonal carcinomas; γ-**fetoprotein,** a serum protein of fetal blood, is found in subjects with various types of cancer. The detection in adult serum of fetal Ags, by sensitive and rapid serological tests, promises to provide screening assays for the early detection of human cancers.

Cell-Mediated Immunity and Enhancement of Human Tumors. As noted before (Ch. 20), the prevalence of cell-mediated immune responses by human hosts to their own cancers has been revealed by the Hellstroms, who showed that under standard tissue culture conditions a patient's tumor cells usually form fewer colonies if incubated with his own lymphocytes than if incubated with lymphocytes from other persons. With certain types of cancer (e.g., neuroblastoma) the inhibitory effects of one patient's lymphocytes are also exerted on tumor cells from other subjects, suggesting that these tumors share common TSAs and might have been induced by a particular oncogenic virus.

Many human cancer cells seem, however, to be protected against the host's killer lymphocytes by the concomitant presence of "enhancing activities" in the patient's serum, which can specifically block his lymphocytes' inhibition of colony formation by his cultured tumor cells. Preliminary findings indicate that the enhancing activity could be due to Abs that bind to TSAs on tumor cells, or to soluble TSAs that block receptors on specifically reactive lymphocytes, or to soluble Ab-TSA complexes that combine with either target cell or killer lymphocyte. A further indication that tumor growth depends upon the net outcome of multiple, antagonistic immune responses is the further suggestion of "deblocking" activities that appear in serum of some mice with regressing tumors: these activities block enhancing activity, and thus reinforce the inhibitory effects of killer lymphocytes.

Immunological Surveillance. Increasing evidence for TSAs on almost every variety of tumor, and for host immune responses to these Ags, has raised hopes that serological or allergic skin tests might be developed for early detection of most human cancers, and that immunization might become practical in the prevention or treatment of certain tumors. It seems quite possible that neoplastic cells arise at frequent intervals in normal individuals but rarely establish cancers because they are rapidly detected and destroyed by host immune responses against their surface membrane TSAs. Indeed, some believe that this monitoring system, called immunological surveillance, may have been more important than protection against infection in promoting the evolution of the immune system.

When the possibility of immunological surveillance was first suggested (by Lewis Thomas) it seemed far-fetched. However, its credibility has grown with evidence for an increased incidence of neoplasms in animals and in humans with diverse spontaneous and induced immunological defects. In one striking episode, for instance, accidental contamination of an animal room with polyomavirus led to the appearance of tumors in all mice with severely defective cell-mediated immune responses (due to thymectomy and antilymphocyte serum), whereas no tumors appeared in any of the normal isogenic mice that shared the same space. Moreover, about 10% of persons with various immunological deficiency diseases (Chs. 17 and 20) develop diverse malignant tumors. And approximately 1% of patients under chronic immunosuppression therapy for maintenance of renal allografts develop a variety of cancers; this incidence is about five-fold higher than in the population at large (of the same age and sex distribution). Reticulum cell sarcoma accounts for almost half of the reported tumors in these chronically immunosuppressed patients, in whom the incidence of this lymphoma is increased about 4000-fold, perhaps because the normal precursors of the neoplastic lymphoid cells are targets for antilymphocytic serum and other immunosuppressive agents (Chs. 17 and 20).

CODA

Many genes, with multiple alleles at each, specify the great variety of macromolecular alloantigens that cover cell surfaces. The antigenic uniqueness of each individual arises from the distinctive combinations of these alloantigens on his cells. Immune responses to these antigens are responsible for both reactions to transfused blood and for rejection of transplanted tissues and organs.

About 60 human red cell alloantigens ("blood group substances") have been identified, largely with the aid of natural antibodies in normal human sera or antibodies formed in response to blood transfusions or to pregnancies in which the fetus carries paternal alloantigens that are foreign to the mother. The immunological specificity of the best characterized substances (with A, B, H, Le^a, and Le^b activities) resides in groups of four or five sugars at the free ends of oligosaccharide chains that branch from a polypeptide or lipoidal backbone. In the biosynthesis of these complex heteropolymers the critical sugar residues are added sequentially to a "core" polymer by enzymes (glycosyltransferases) that are determined by the corresponding blood group alleles.

The alloantigens (histocompatibility or transplantation antigens) responsible for allograft rejection are specified by histocompatibility genes, of which there are about 30 in the mouse with approximately 20 alleles at the most intensively studied locus (*H-2*). Polymorphism is doubtless as great in man and in other vertebrates. The antigenic individuality of a person's red cells may turn out to be no less distinctive that that of his tissue cells, but in blood transfusions the red cells need survive only a few weeks for the procedure to be scored as a success; whereas success of an allograft requires enduring survival, and therefore virtually complete antigenic identity of graft and host. Nevertheless, many human kidney allografts survive for many years. This impressive, but still limited, level of success occurs because 1) only a few of the great number of histocompatibility antigens are potent immunogens, 2) tissue-typing methods have improved to where badly matched donor-recipient pairs can be avoided, and especially because 3) host immune responses can be chronically depressed by skillful administration of immunosuppressive drugs. Though immunosuppressive measures greatly prolong graft survival, they increase susceptibility to overwhelming infection by ubiquitous "opportunistic" bacteria, viruses, and fungi, and they increase the risk of developing cancer, especially malignant lymphomas.

Tumor cells behave as allografts because their surface membranes possess tumor-specific antigens (TSAs) that are lacking or masked in normal cells. Host immune responses to tumors probably select for tumor cell variants with altered TSAs, which could account for the low-grade immunogenicity (in the autochthonous host) of TSAs of well-established tumors. Diverse host immune responses to TSAs can have antagonistic effects: some antibodies to TSAs protect tumor cells from destruction by cell-mediated immune reactions. TSAs are specified by various genes (of oncogenic viruses or host cells) and some are "fetal": they are normally expressed transiently on certain fetal cells during embryonic development, and later in life only on some kinds of tumor cells.

Immunological surveillance by the host immune system probably eliminates many of the potentially neoplastic cells that arise during a normal lifetime; hence individuals with long-term impairment of immune mechanisms (especially of cell-mediated immunity) have an increased probability of developing cancer.

SELECTED REFERENCES

Red Cell Isoantigens

KABAT, E. A. *Blood Group Substances: Their Chemistry and Immunochemistry.* Academic Press, New York, 1956.

KABAT, E. A. In *Blood and Tissue Antigens.* (D. Aminott, ed.) Academic Press, New York, 1970.

KOBATA, A., and GINSBURG, V. Uridine diphosphate N-acetyl-D-galactosamine: D-galactose α-3-N-acetylgalactosaminyltransferase, a product of the gene that determines blood type A in man. *J Biol Chem 245*:1484 (1970).

MOLLISON, P. L. *Blood Transfusions in Clinical Medicine,* 3rd ed. Blackwell, Oxford, 1961.

MORENO, C., LUNDBLAD, A., and KABAT, E. A. A comparative study of the reaction of A_1 and A_2 blood group glycoproteins with human anti-A. *J Exp Med 134*:439 (1971).

MORGAN, W. T. Croonian lecture: A contribution to human biochemical genetics: The chemical basis of blood group specificity. *Proc R Soc Lond (Biol) 151*:308 (1960).

RACE, R. R., and SANGER, R. *Blood Groups in Man,* 5th ed. Thomas, Springfield, Ill., 1968.

WATKINS, W. M. Blood-group substances. *Science 152*:172 (1966).

Transplantation Immunity

BACH, F. T. Transplantation: Pairing of donor and recipient. *Science 168*:1170 (1970).

BILLINGHAM, R., and SILVERS, W. *The Immunobiology of Transplantation.* Prentice-Hall, Englewood Cliffs, N.J., 1970.

DAUSSET, J., and RAPAPORT, F. T. (eds.). *Human Transplantation.* Grune & Stratton, New York, 1968.

KLEIN, J., and SHREFFLER, D. C. The H-2 model for the major histocompatibility systems. *Transplant Rev 6*:3 (1971).

LAFFERTY, K. J., and JONES, M. A. S. Reactions of the graft-vs.-host type. *Aust J Exp Biol Med Sci 47*:17 (1969).

MEDAWAR, P. B. The immunology of transplantation. *Harvey Lect 52*:144 (1956–57).

MEDAWAR, P. B. *The Uniqueness of the Individual.* Basic Books, New York, 1958.

SNELL, G. D. The H-2 locus of the mouse: Comparative genetics and polymorphism. *Folia Biol (Praha) 14*:335 (1968).

Symposium on biological significance of histocompatibility antigens. *Fed Proc 31*:1087 (1972).

Symposium on human histocompatibility antigens. *Fed Proc 29*:2010 (1970).

Tumor Immunity

DYKES, P. W., and KING, J. Progress report: Carcinoembryonic antigen (CEA). *Gut 13*:1000 (1972).

GOLD, P., and FREEDMAN, S. D. Specific carcinoembryonic antigens of the human digestive system. *J Exp Med 122*:467 (1965).

HELLSTRÖM, K. E., and HELLSTRÖM, I. Immunological enhancement as studied by cell culture techniques. *Annu Rev Microbiol 24*:373 (1970).

KALISS, N. Immunological enhancement. *Int Rev Exp Pathol 8*:241 (1969).

KLEIN, G. Tumor immunology in *Clinical Immunobiology.* (Bach, F. H. and Good, R. A., eds.) vol. 1, p. 219, Academic Press, New York, 1972.

KLEIN, E., and COCHRAN, A. J. Immunology and malignant disease. *Haematologica 5*:179 (1971).

OLD, L. J., and BOYSE, E. A. Current enigmas in cancer research. *Harvey Lect 67*:273 (1973).

SJÖGREN, H. O. Transplantation methods as a tool for detection of tumor-specific antigens. *Progr Exp Tumor Res 6*:289 (1965).

INDEX

Page numbers in *italics* indicate illustrations. Page numbers followed by the letter "t" indicate tabular material. Page numbers followed by the letter "n" indicate information in footnote.

A

ABO blood group system. See under *Blood group*.
ABO compatibility, kidney grafts and, 619
Actinomycin(s), immunosuppression by, 501
Addison's disease, 587
Adjuvants, 481, *481*
Adrenal steroid. See *Corticosteroid*.
Affinity-labeling, 443
Agammaglobulinemia
electrophoretic results in, *426*
infantile X-linked, 507–508
Agar. See *Gel*.
Age factors, in autoimmune disease, 588, *588*
Agglutination
as serologic reaction, history, 353
mechanisms, 391
of bacteria, 391
of erythrocytes, 391
by sera, human blood groups based on, 599t
passive, 393
sensitivity of, 394
Agglutination-inhibition assay, for human allotypes, *420*
Agglutination reaction, 391–394
in measuring bacterial adsorption of antibody, 391
prozone in, 392
sensitivity of, 393–394
serum titration by, 391–392
with surface versus internal antigens of cells, 392

Agglutinator(s)
rheumatoid serum (Ragg), 419
serum normal (SNagg), 419
Agglutinin(s), 392
Agglutinogen(s), 392
Albumin, bovine serum, proteolytic cleavage of, 376
Aleutian mink disease, 553
Alexin. See *Complement*.
Alkylating agents, immunosuppression by, 501
Allele(s). See also *Gene*.
codominant, 420n
for Gm allotypes, 420
Allergen(s), 530. See also *Antigen*.
Allergic reaction(s). 581–593. See also specific allergic reactions, e.g., *Hay fever*.
antibody-mediated, 529, 529t
at foci of bacterial infection, 594
cell-mediated, 11-oxycorticosteroid inhibition of, 580
cell-mediated versus humoral, 559t
due to IgE, 418
infectious diseases with, 593
serum sickness and, 550
to allotypes, 419n
to drugs. See under *Drug*.
to microbial antigens, 593, 594
with exotoxins, 593
Allergy(ies). See also *Hypersensitivity*.

Allergy(ies) (*continued*)
atopic. See *Atopy*.
bacterial. See *Hypersensitivity, delayed-type*.
definition, 528
history, 528
infectious. See *Hypersensitivity, delayed-type*.
inflammation in, corticosteroid therapy in, 501
SRS-A in, 543
to drugs. See under *Drug*.
to food, 481
to mycobacterial proteins, 594
to penicillin. See under *Penicillin*.
to quinidine, 585
to Sedormid, 585
Alloantibody(ies)
AB, 603–604
definition, 599
to leukocytic alloantigens, after transfusions and pregnancies, 609n
Alloantigen(s)
blood, transfusion reactions due to, 607
blood cell. See *Blood cell alloantigen*.
definition, 419, 454, 598
leukocytic, alloantibodies to, after transfusions and pregnancies, 609n
Ly A,B,C, 460
on cell surfaces, 597–624
on T lymphocyte surface, 460
Rh, notations for, 607t
theta, 460
T L, 460
Alloantiserum(a), 406, 460

74 75 76 77 78   9 8 7 6 5 4 3 2